Clinical Methods in ORTHOPEDICS

A Concise Guide

Clinical Methods in ORTHOPEDICS

A Concise Guide

Upendra Kumar
D Ortho (PMCH) DNB Ortho (DDUH)
Government Medical College
Bettiah, Bihar, India

Forewords

DK Taneja
NK Magu
VK Sinha

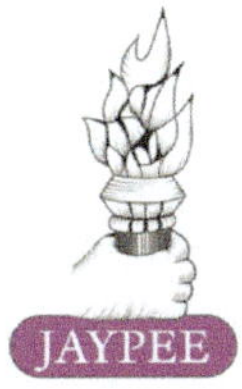

JAYPEE BROTHERS MEDICAL PUBLISHERS
The Health Sciences Publisher
New Delhi | London

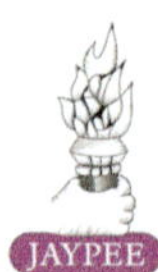

Jaypee Brothers Medical Publishers (P) Ltd

Headquarters
EMCA House
23/23-B, Ansari Road, Daryaganj
New Delhi 110 002, India
Landline: +91-11-23272143, +91-11-23272703
+91-11-23282021, +91-11-23245672
E-mail: jaypee@jaypeebrothers.com

Overseas Office
J.P. Medical Ltd
83 Victoria Street, London
SW1H 0HW (UK)
Phone: +44 20 3170 8910
E-mail: info@jpmedpub.com

Corporate Office
4838/24, Ansari Road, Daryaganj
New Delhi 110 002, India
Phone: +91-11-43574357
Fax: +91-11-43574314
E-mail: jaypee@jaypeebrothers.com

EU GPSR Authorised Representative
Logos Europe, 9 rue Nicolas Poussin
17000, La Rochelle, France
Phone: +33 (0) 6 67 93 73 78
E-mail: contact@logoseurope.eu

Website: www.jaypeebrothers.com
Website: www.jaypeedigital.com

Clinical Methods in Orthopedics: A Concise Guide

First Edition: 2020

Reprint: 2026

ISBN: 978-93-89587-51-7

Printed in india

Dedicated to

Indian Orthopaedic Association (IOA)
and its Bihar Chapter (BOA)

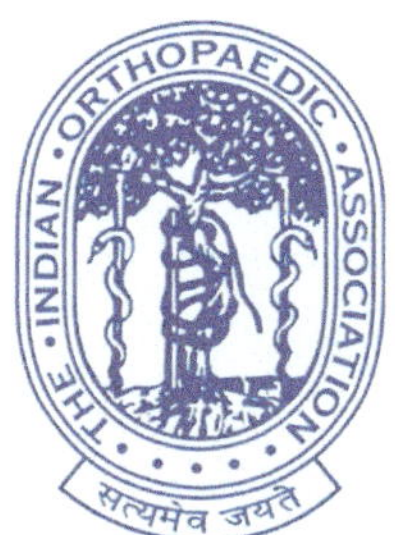

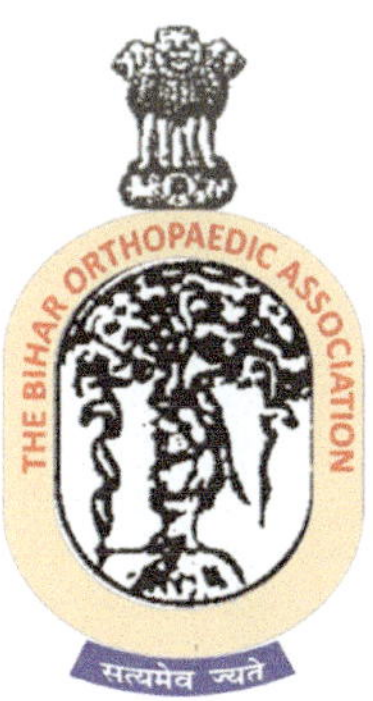

Special thanks to those who always beared with me

My Parents
Wife Dr Jyoti Bala and
Son Ishaan

Contributors

Ajay Rajput (DNB Ortho)
Lecturer Orthopedics
Uttar Pradesh University
of Medical Sciences
Etawah
Uttar Pradesh, India

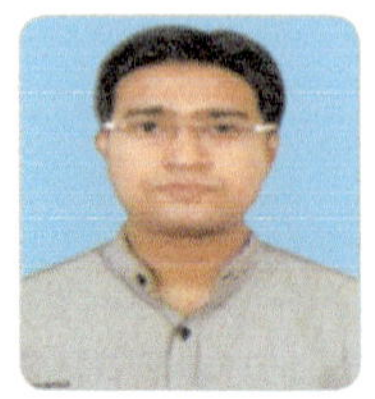

Anand Shankar (MS Ortho)
Consultant Orthopedic
Surgeon
Patna, Bihar, India

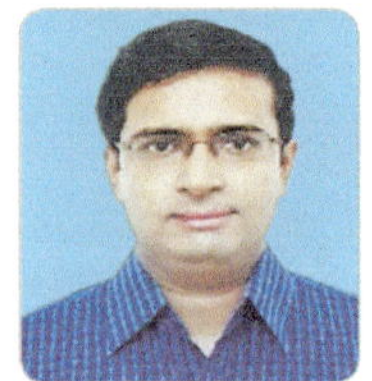

Anurag Sharma (DNB Ortho)
Consultant Orthopedic
Surgeon
Jalandhar, Punjab, India

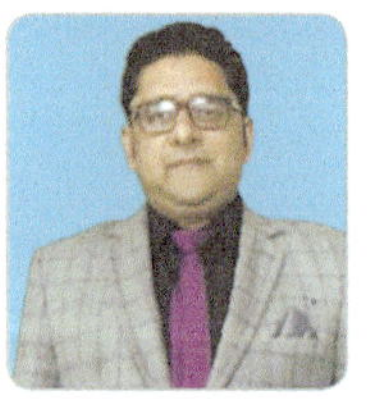

Arnab Sinha (DNB Ortho)
Consultant Orthopedic
Surgeon
Patna, Bihar, India

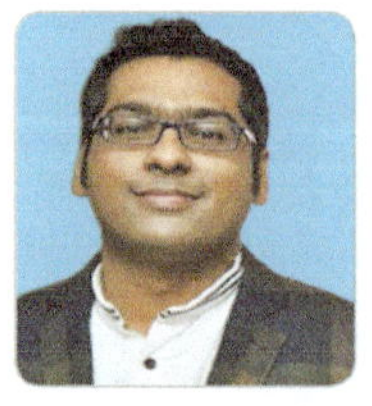

Chandan Sekhar
(DNB Ortho D Ortho)
Consultant Orthopedic
Surgeon
Patna, Bihar, India

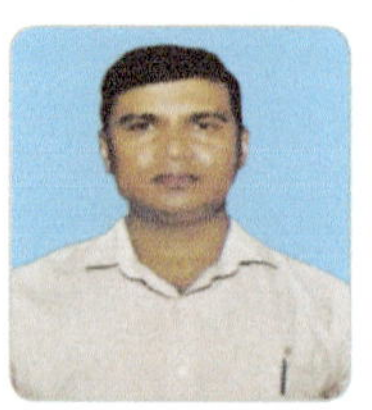

Deepak Kumar (MS Ortho)
Assistant Professor
Jannayak Karpuri Thakur
Medical College
Madhepura, Bihar, India

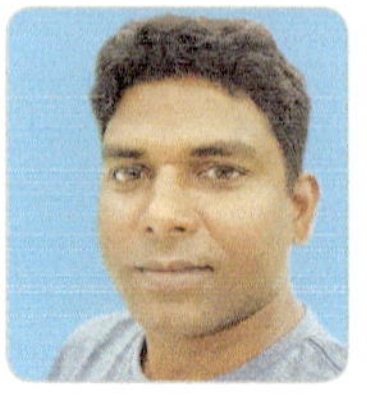

Deven Taneja
(D Ortho MS Ortho FAMS)
Medical Director and
Senior Consultant
Arihant Hospital and
Research Center
Indore, Madhya Pradesh
India

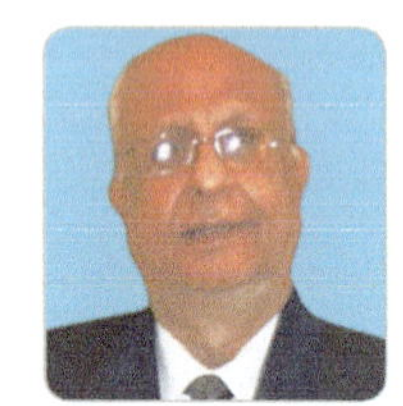

Gitika Khanna (MD Patho)
Incharge, CIO Laboratory
Safdarjung Hospital
New Delhi, India

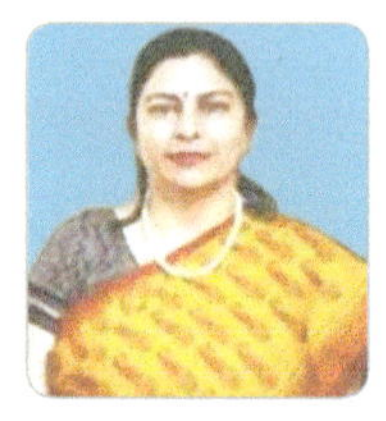

Govind Ballav Joshi
(DNB Ortho D Ortho)
Consultant Orthopedic
Surgeon
Sri Balaji Action Medical
Institute
Delhi, India

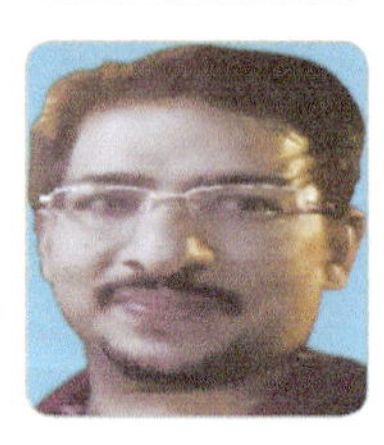

John Mukhopadhyay
(MCh Ortho, Liverpool)
Director Orthopedics and
Joint Replacement Paras
HMRI Hospital Patna,
Bihar, India

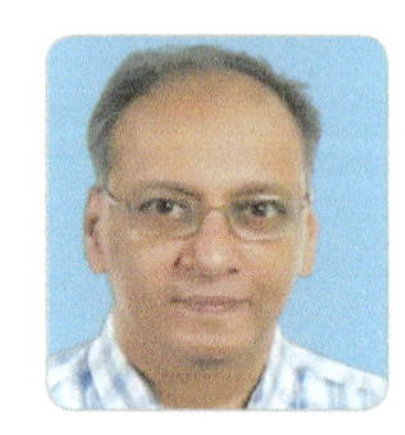

Khuswant Rathore
(DNB Ortho)
Consultant NIMS
University Hospital
Jaipur, Rajasthan, India

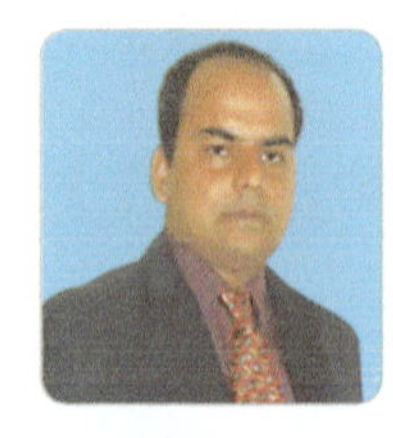

Kirti Gehlot
(DNB Radiodiagnosis)
Consultant Radiologist
Jalandhar, Punjab, India

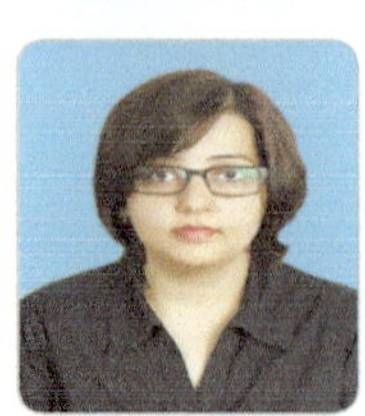

Kumar Kaushik (MS Ortho)
Senior Resident
Shrikrishna Medical College and Hospital
Muzaffarpur, Bihar, India

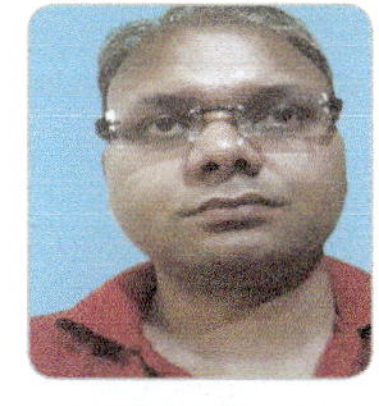

NA Khan (MS Ortho)
Consultant Orthopedic Surgeon
Bettiah, Bihar, India

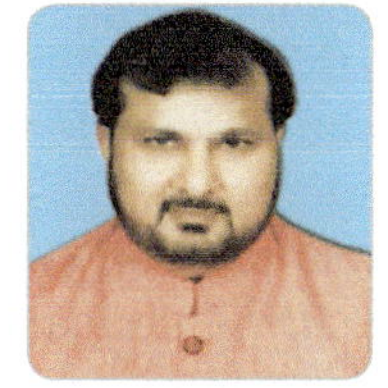

Naman Wahal (MS Ortho)
Ex-Senior Resident
All India Institute of Medical Sciences
New Delhi, India

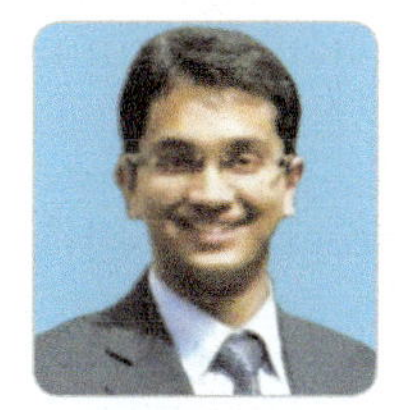

Naresh Chandra (MS Ortho)
Head
Department of Orthopedics
Guru Gobind Singh Government Hospital
New Delhi, India

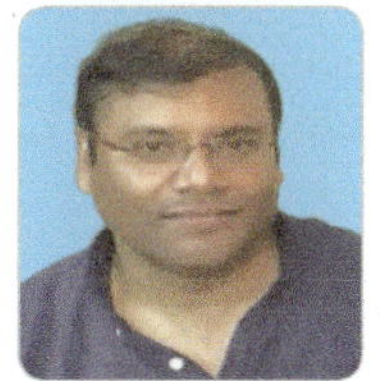

Nitesh Rustagi (MS Ortho)
Consultant Orthopedic Surgeon
New Delhi, India

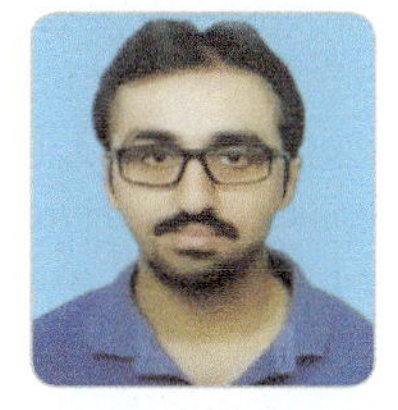

Oswald Anand (DNB Ortho)
Consultant Orthopedic Surgeon
Bettiah, Bihar, India

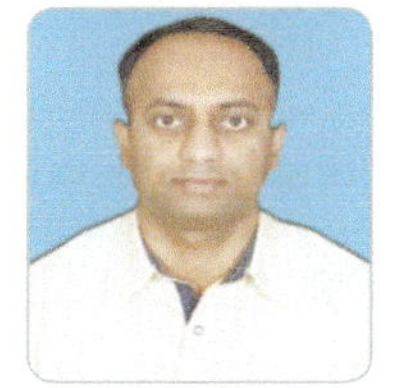

Piyush Kumar Singh
(DNB Ortho D Ortho)
Consultant Orthopedic Surgeon
Noida, Uttar Pradesh
India

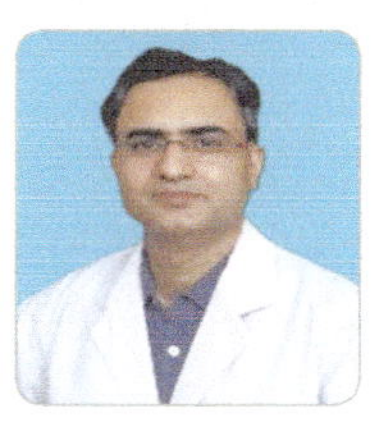

Preeti Goyal Varshney
(MD DNB Anesthesia)
Assistant Professor
Department of Anesthesia
Lady Hardinge Medical College
New Delhi, India

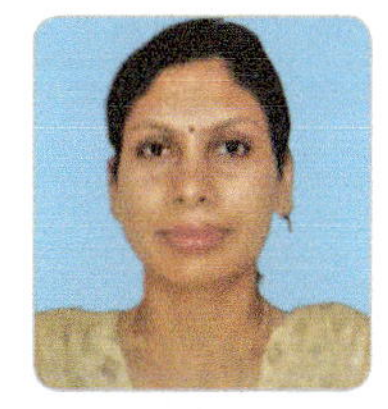

Sanjay Keshkar (MS Ortho)
Head
Department of Orthopedics
PGIMSR and ESI Hospital
Kolkata, West Bengal, India

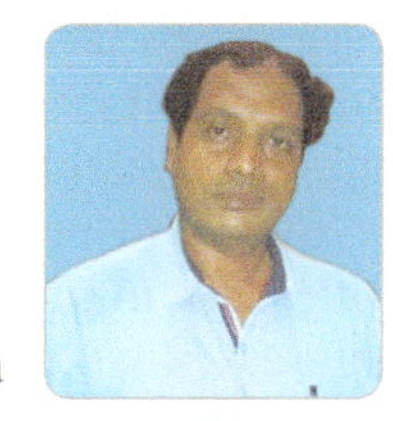

Sant Prakash Gautam
(BPO, MPO)
Prosthetist, Rishikesh
Uttarakhand, India

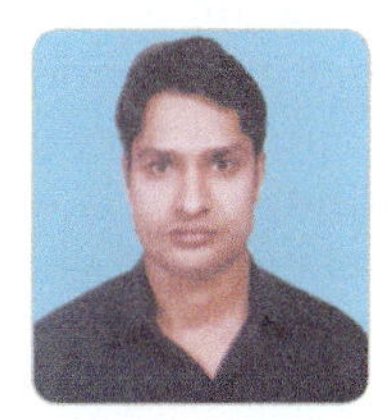

Shailendra Gupta
(MS Ortho)
Head
Department of Orthopedics
ESI Hospital, Rohini
New Delhi, India

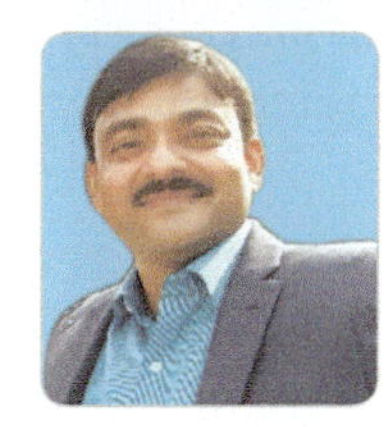

Shailendra Khare
(MS Ortho)
Consultant Orthopedic Surgeon
Safdarjung Hospital
New Delhi, India

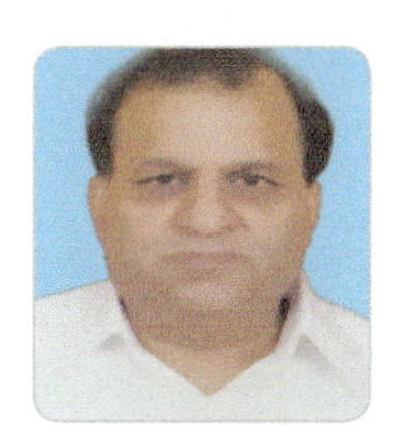

Surjit Kumar (BPO)
Prosthetist
Patna, Bihar, India

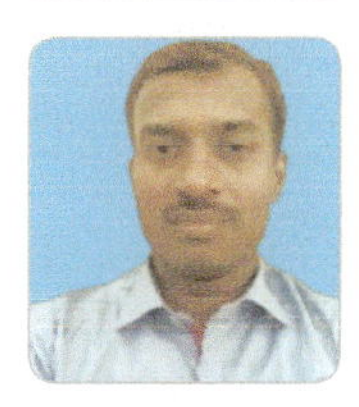

Tarun Solanki (MS Ortho)
Consultant Orthopedic Surgeon
Kashipur, Uttarakhand
India

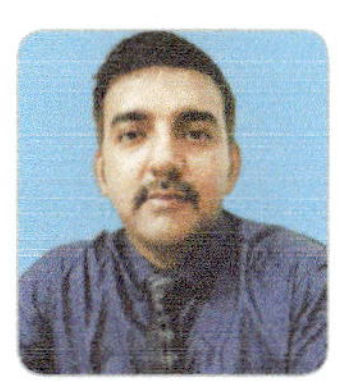

Foreword

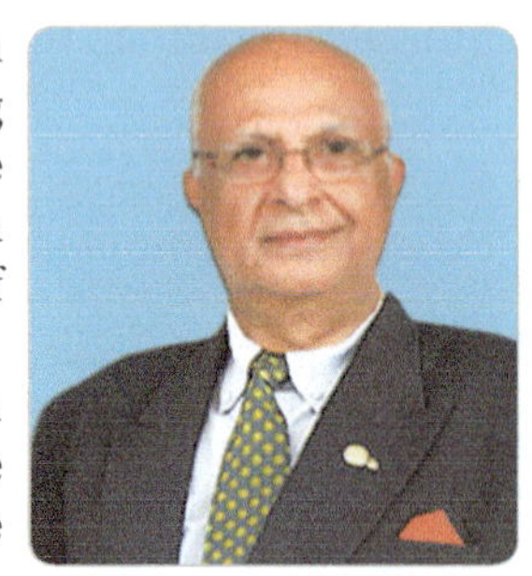

The practical examination is a clinical examination starting from bedside manners to history taking, eliciting clinical signs and making a clinical differential diagnosis. Unfortunately, all these aspects are very much lacking in the present set-up of training especially in undergraduate courses. In spite of the good theoretical knowledge of subject, students lack the clinical aspects of orthopedics.

In order to bridge this gap, endeavor of Dr Upendra will prove a milestone in undergraduate training. Side by side it will increase the interest of students towards orthopedics to opt for its postgraduate program. Dr Upendra has regularly attended Arihant PG courses in Indore and now he visits here as faculty too.

It is a very good effort by a young orthopedic surgeon which is commendable indeed. Undergraduate students will learn about common orthopedic cases with small history and related viva-voce questions and answers, side by side common orthopedic appliances and orthopedic radiographs, some instruments and implants along with bones are also covered in good details. After going through the book, I felt that it would prove to be very handy and useful for the undergraduate students as it covers all aspects of the examination and will help students to clear their practical examination in a single attempt.

DK Taneja
D (Ortho) MS (Ortho) FAMS
Medical Director and Senior Consultant
Arihant Hospital and Research Centre, Indore
Ex-Dean and CEO, MGM Medical College, Indore
Ex-Professor and Head, Department of Orthopedics
Mahatma Gandhi Memorial Medical College
Indore, Madhya Pradesh, India
Past President, Indian Orthopaedic Association
Past Secretary General, Orthopaedic Association of SAARC Nations
Secretary, Orthopaedic Research and Education Foundation, India
Secretary General, World Orthopaedic Concern

Foreword

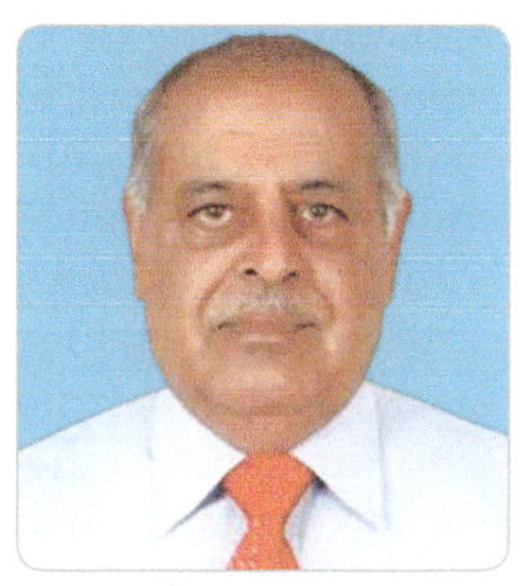

I am extremely happy to write the foreword for *Clinical Methods in Orthopedics: A Concise Guide*. Dear students, the book in the question is the commendable work of Dr Upendra who considers me as his teacher. Of course, I taught him in various postgraduate courses, hands on workshop and symposia organized in various conferences throughtout the India.

There is a big void in learning the art of clinical examination of patients. I take it seriously because learning of this art starts very early from undergraduates days. This book is a good effort to fill this gap and it will arouse interest among young buds to learn the art of clinical examination.

The book includes commonly seen orthopedic cases in viva voce pattern. Descriptions of radiographs, orthopedic appliances, instruments and implants including brief descriptions of bones make it a good clinical handbook.

I wish for its grand success and hope that it will solve the purpose for which it is treatised.

NK Magu
MS FAMS
Former Professor and Head
Department of Orthopedics
Postgraduate Institute of Medical Sciences
Rohtak, Haryana, India
Senior Consultant Orthopedic Surgeon
Max Smart Super Speciality Hospital
Saket, Delhi, India

Foreword

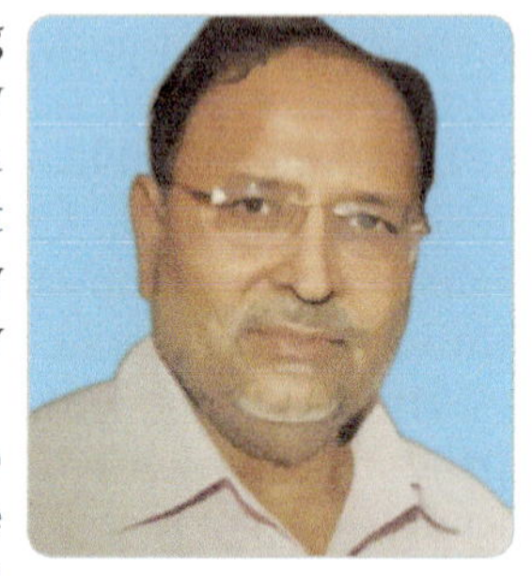

With this book Dr Upendra has given me an another thrilling experience. When I review and look back, it is surprising that how a student copes with such a vast courses of different subjects in undergraduate study. Side by side clinical examination of the subject is another nightmare for these students because it includes not only cases but many tables and viva-voce, and I don't think there is any special treatise to carry all these topics under one cover.

In this context the effort of Dr Upendra is commendable who was my student also in his PMCH days. The book is divided into five sections containing orthopedic cases in viva-voce manner, common orthopedic appliances, common radiographs, some instruments and implants along with bones. Being a teacher and examiner in orthopedics for many years I think this book will fill the lacunae of orthopedics in clinical study. I want to advise all undergraduates to increase one more true friend in the shelf in the form of this book. It will be helpful for all the undergraduate students during examinations.

VK Sinha
D Ortho MS Ortho PhD Ortho
Professor and Former Head
Department of Orthopedics
Patna Medical College
Patna, Bihar, India

Preface

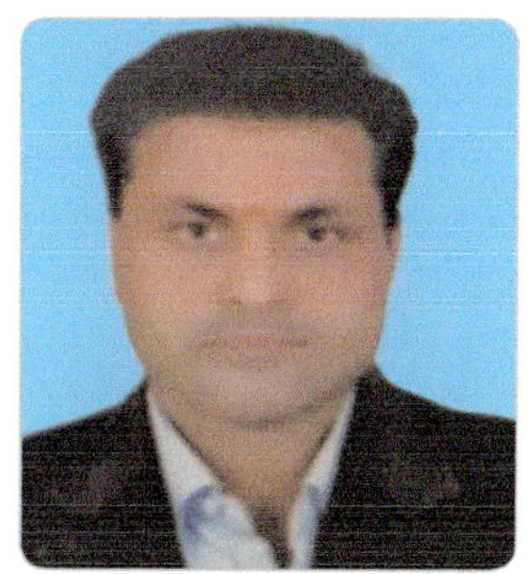

We all know necessity is the mother of invention. This story begins when I started my residency in Government Medical College Bettiah, Bihar, India. One day some undergraduate students asked me about some clinical orthopedic books for their practical orthopedic examination. And it was a kick for me to start thinking over it.

I discussed this issue with my teacher Dr VK Sinha, Professor, Department of Orthopedics, Patna Medical College, Patna. He told me that it was a very difficult task to concise the whole clinical orthopedic in few pages, if you can you should try. Then I started to think over it and discussed with my seniors, colleagues and juniors too. After a marathon debate we decided to construct this book and result is in front of you.

Section one contains common orthopedic cases along with related viva voce questions and answers. Section two is allotted for common orthopedic appliances like traction, plaster of Paris, etc. with brief and crispy descriptions. In section three instruments and implants pictorial presentation of these hardwares have been illustrated. In section four common radiographs are taken from fractures, tumors and metabolic and regional disorders. In the last section five bones are described with reasonable details.

The book stands up to the mark, which is informative, illustrative, comprehensive and with sufficient content. Although the facts included in the book are obtained from various sources, hence, we are thankful to all orthopedic personnel and publishers throughout the globe, who have given their direct or indirect contribution in this regard. Hence, please do not look this issue as copyright, but treat it as your contribution, if any.

Despite of meticulous corrections, there might be possibility of human error. Useful critics and suggestions are always invited from teachers, seniors, colleagues and juniors to make it more productive and fruitful. This is also a time to remember the living legends of orthopedics of India such as Dr Shailendra Bhattacharya (Kolkata), Dr Surendra Mohan Tuli (Delhi), Dr GS Kulkarni (Miraj), and Dr Hardash Singh Sandhu (Amritsar). Our generation is fortunate to have such great orthopedicians.

At the end I would like to thank Shri Jitendar P Vij (Group Chairman), Mr Ankit Vij (Managing Director), Mr MS Mani (Group President), Dr Madhu Choudhary (Publishing Head-Education), Ms Pooja Bhandari (Production Head), Ms Sunita Katla (Executive Assistant to Group Chairman and Publishing Manager), Dr Akanksha Singh (Development Editor), Ms Seema Dogra (Cover Visualizer), Mr Rajesh Sharma (Production Coordinator), Manoj Pahuja (Graphic Designar), Deep Kumar (DTP Operator), Narsingh Kumar (Proof Reader) of M/s Jaypee Brothers Medical Publishers (P) Ltd, New Delhi, India, for this opportunity. I can't forget my better half who supported a lot in the preparation of layout of this book. Finally, I offer this book to the young medi buds with a big salute to all my teachers throughout the country.

Share your views at: upenorthopmch@gmail.com

Upendra Kumar

Contents

SECTION 1: Orthopedic Cases and Viva Voce

SECTION 2: Some Orthopedic Appliances

SECTION 3: Some Orthopedic Instruments and Implants

SECTION 4: Some Common Orthopedic Radiographs

SECTION 5: Bones Catalogue

1

Section

Orthopedic Cases and Viva Voce

- Chronic Osteomyelitis
- Bony Swelling (Exostosis)
- Nonunion Fracture Long Bone
- Wrist Drop (Radial Palsy)
- Frozen Shoulder
- Cubitus Varus Deformity at Elbow (Malunited Supracondylar Fracture Humerus)
- Cubitus Valgus Deformity at Elbow (Nonunion Fracture Lateral Condyle Humerus)
- Malunited Colles' Fracture
- Congenital Clubfoot
- Genu Varus Deformity at Knee (Osteoarthritis Knee)
- Genu Valgus Deformity at Knee (Rickets)
- Nonunion Fracture Neck of Femur

Chapter

1

Chronic Osteomyelitis

CASE PRESENTATION

- **History**: My patient, a 12-year-old boy, presented with complaint of pain, swelling and discharge from his right lower thigh for last 4 months. He sustained an injury around his right knee during playing football. For this, he took treatment in the form of above knee slab along with analgesic. After 1 week of injury, he developed high fever with rigor, for that a symptomatic treatment was given. At the end of a month, he developed a discharging sinus at lower lateral area of thigh near the knee. For this occasional discharge, multiple dressings were done. There is no history of weight loss, appetite loss, night fever, perspiration or multiple joint pain.
- **Examination**: Patient is of poor built and of poor nutritional status. His general physical and systemic examination is within normal limit. Local examination showed a single purulent discharging sinus present on lower lateral part of thigh with wasting of its girth. The sinus is fixed with underlying bone and the skin around it was shiny and hyperpigmented. The underlying bone is thickened, irregular and tender. There is no abnormal mobility in the thigh. The range of motion at knee is decreased but normal at hip. There is no limb length discrepancy. Distal neurovascular examination was also normal.

VIVA VOCE FROM CASE

Q. What is your diagnosis?

Ans. This is a case of chronic osteomyelitis of femur (Fig. 1.1).

Q. Define chronic osteomyelitis.

Ans. Inflammation of bone and its marrow cavity is called osteomyelitis. Chronic osteomyelitis is said to be established when there is infected dead bone surrounded by a compromised covering of sclerotic, relatively avascular, thickened periosteum and scarred muscle.

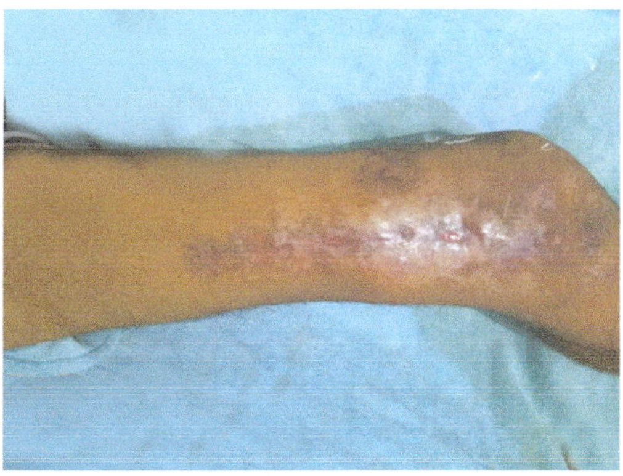

Fig. 1.1: A case of chronic osteomyelitis femur.

Etiological factors for chronic osteomyelitis.

- As a sequela of acute osteomyelitis
- Following compound fracture
- After surgical fracture fixation

Q. What are the points favoring your diagnosis?

Ans. The points favoring this diagnosis are as follows:
- History of trauma followed by pain and swelling
- History of fever with chill and rigor
- Gradual appearance of discharging sinus
- Sinus is adhered with underlying bone
- Thickening, irregularity and tenderness of underlying bone.

Q. Any other associative finding you like to search in this case.

Ans. These are as:
- Abnormal mobility due to pathological fracture
- Adjacent joint stiffness
- Limb length discrepancy
- Deformity at adjacent joint
- Any distal neurovascular deficit.

Q. What investigation you like to get in this case?

Ans. These are as:
- X-ray of the part anteroposterior (AP) and lateral view including adjacent joint (Fig. 1.2)
- Blood investigation
- Sinogram
- Culture sensitivity of discharging material.

Q. What is the interpretation of this investigation?

Ans. These are as:
- X-ray shows irregular thickening of bone, irregular bone destruction, loss of corticomedullary differentiation, sequestrum (free piece of bone) and involucrum (peripheral sclerosed bone).
- Blood investigation shows increased total count, increased erythrocyte sedimentation rate (ESR) and C-reactive protein.
- Sinogram shows the tract of the sinus.
- Culture and sensitivity of discharging material helps in selection of proper antibiotic.

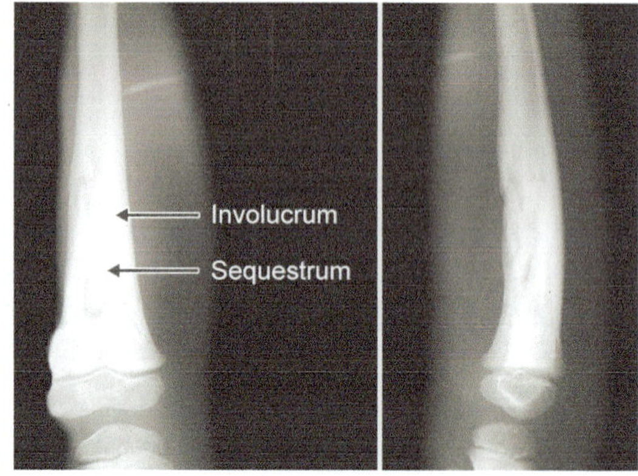

Fig. 1.2: X-ray of chronic osteomyelitis femur.

Q. What is sequestrum?

Ans. Sequestrum is a dead piece of bone present inside a living bone surrounded by an unhealthy granulation tissue (rough surface) and pus (smooth surface) around it (Fig. 1.3).

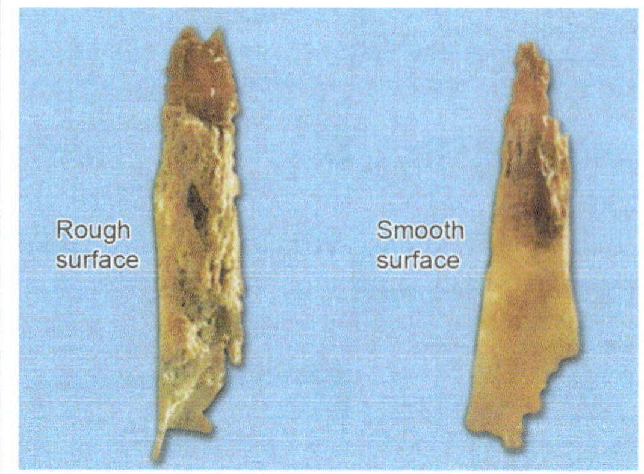

Fig. 1.3: Sequestrum.

Types of sequestrum.

- Pencil shaped—infants
- Cylindrical—infants
- Ring shaped—pin tract infection
- Coke like or sandy—tuberculosis
- Ivory—syphilis
- Black—calcaneal osteomyelitis

Q. What is involucrum?

Ans. It is a reactive new bone formation around sequestrum (weakened area of bone) to strengthen it.

Q. What is cloacae?

Ans. Cloacae is hole in involucrum that ejects out the small pieces of sequestrum gradually from parent bone.

Q. What treatment you like to offer to this case?

Ans. Sequestrectomy and saucerization along with proper antibiotic coverage as per culture and sensitivity of discharging material.

Q. What are the principles of treatment of chronic osteomyelitis?

Ans. These are as:

- Debridement of dead bone and soft tissue (e.g. sequestrectomy)
- Dealing with dead space: By bone grafting or antibiotic impregnated cement beads
- Overlying soft tissue coverage: By skin grafting or flaps if needed
- Eradication of infection: By proper and adequate antibiotic treatment (6–8 weeks)
- Dealing with complication as pathological fracture by some external fixator.

Q. What is sequestrectomy?

Ans. Removal of dead necrotic bone (sequestrum) from its native bone is called sequestrectomy. Sequestrectomy should be done till bleeding surface of underlying bone is achieved (**Paprika sign**).

Q. Is there any prerequisite for sequestrectomy?

Ans. Yes, for sequestrectomy at least 2/3rd circumference of parent bone must be surrounded by new protective involucrum.

Q. What may happen if you do not follow this guideline?

Ans. There are chances of pathological fracture during sequestrectomy.

Q. What is saucerization and what is its advantage?

Ans. After removal of sequestrum, the deroofing of osteomyelitis cavity is done in such a way that it shallows all around as a saucer plate (Fig. 1.4). It facilitates drainage of cavity and also increases the vascular bed that helps the approach of antibiotics in this area.

Q. How will you deal with the dead space created after debridement?

Ans. We obliterate this dead space by two means (1) with cancellous bone grafting and (2) by antibiotic impregnated bone cement beads which act as a local antibiotic delivery system (gentamicin or vancomycin) (Fig. 1.5).

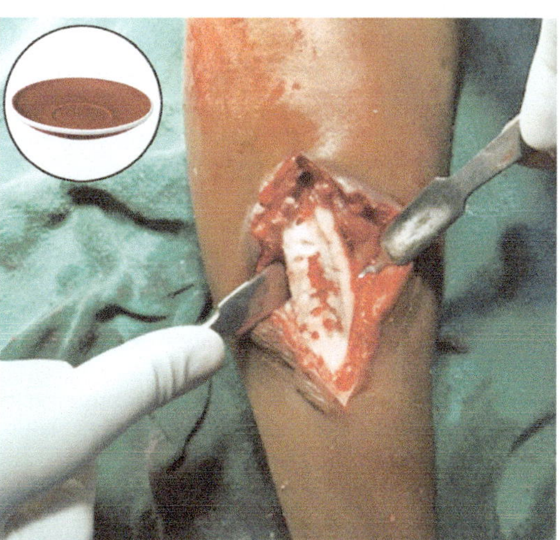

Fig. 1.4: Saucerization.

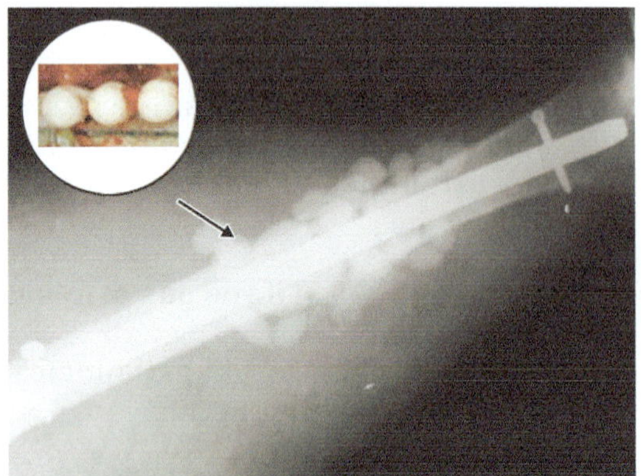

Fig. 1.5: X-ray showing antibiotic impregnated cement beads.

Q. How will you manage with soft tissue defect created after debridement?

Ans. The soft tissue defect over osteomyelitic area should be dealt with skin grafting or myocutaneous or fasciocutaneous or sometime free flaps.

Q. What is the protocol for your antibiotic treatment?

Ans. The protocol of antibiotic treatment is as follows:

- Initially broad-spectrum antibiotics covering gram-positive, gram-negative and anaerobic organism.
- Targeted antibiotic after culture and sensitivity report.
- Duration of antibiotic treatment is 8 weeks, 2 weeks intravenous and 6 weeks oral.

Other methods of treatment of chronic osteomyelitis.

- Instillation, i.e. continuous irrigation and suction of infected area with normal saline having some antibiotics.
- Ilizarov application.
- Osteotomy of infected area, e.g. fibular osteomyelitis.
- Papineau 3-stage procedure (1. Debridement with or without external fixation, 2. Cancellous bone grafting and 3. Skin coverage).

Q. What are the complications of chronic osteomyelitis?

Ans. These are as:

- Acute exacerbation
- Pathological fracture
- Septic arthritis if intra-articular metaphysis as upper femur, upper humerus, radius neck and lower fibula)
- Angular deformity around joint
- Limb length discrepancy (shortening due to physeal damage and lengthening due to physeal hyperemia)
- Metastatic abscess
- Amyloidosis
- Epidermoid or squamous cell carcinoma (after 15–20 years).

Q. What are the key features of tuberculous osteomyelitis?

Ans. These are as:

- Infecting organism is *Mycobacterium tuberculosis* or *Mycobacterium bovis.*
- Infection is always secondary, primaries exist in lung, lymph nodes and gastrointestinal area.
- Infection site is epiphysis and metaphysis both.
- Sequestrum is there but minimal periosteal reaction (due to low virulency).
- Constitutional symptoms may present along with local features.
- Multiple sinuses with serous discharge and adjacent blue-tinged area.
- Antituberculous therapy (ATT) is the mainstay of treatment along with debridement.

Q. What is spina ventosa?

Ans. Tuberculous dactylitis is called spins ventosa. It is common in small bones of hand and foot.

Q. What is subacute osteomyelitis?

Ans. It is insidious onset disease in high-immunity patient with low-virulent infection, e.g. Brodie's abscess and Garre's osteomyelitis (Table 1.1).

Table 1.1: Examples of subacute osteomyelitis.

	Brodie's abscess	Garre's osteomyelitis
Location	Metaphyseal	Diaphyseal
Suppuration	Cavity with sterile pus	Nonsuppurative lesion
Periosteal reaction	Some periosteal reaction	Sclerosed wall with obliterated marrow cavity
Treatment	Curettage and antibiotic	Multiple drilling and antibiotic

PYOGENIC OSTEOMYELITIS VERSUS SEPTIC ARTHRITIS (TABLE 1.2)

Table 1.2: Comparison between pyogenic osteomyelitis and septic arthritis.

	Pyogenic osteomyelitis	Septic arthritis
Etiological factors:	• *Staphylococcus aureus*—most common agent, also in postsurgical and open wound. *Salmonella* in sickle cell anemia, *Pseudomonas* in drug abusers, *Brucella* in spine • Most common site: Distal femur > upper tibia, in adult—spine is the most common site. Most common route of infection is hematogenous • Metaphyseal anatomy and physiology make it prone for infection: (1) Hairpin appearance of vessels. (2) Low macrophagic activity. (3) Rich-blood supply. (4) Repeated trauma producing microthrombi is good culture media for organism. (5) Batson plexuses of spine are comparable to hairpin arrangement of metaphyseal vessels	• *S. aureus*—most common agent • Most common site: Knee joint • Route of infection: (1) Hematogenous (2) as a complication of acute osteomyelitis • Septic arthritis of infant is also known as **Tom Smith arthritis**
Pathological staging:	• Stage of inflammation • Stage of suppuration or pus formation • Stage of necrosis or sequestrum formation • Stage of new bone (involucrum) formation	• Stage of synovitis and effusion • Stage arthritis • Stage ankylosis or instability
Clinical features:	• General features: Fever, chill, and rigor, shock and tachycardia • Local features: Pain, swelling, tenderness, fluctuation (abscess), erythema, limitation of movement	• General features: Fever, toxic look, shock and tachycardia, lymph node enlargement • Local features: Joint pain, swelling, warmth, tenderness, pseudoparalysis
Investigations:	Radiology: (1) First change in X-ray—loss of fat plane, after 24 hours (1st week). (2) First bony change—periosteal reaction at 7–10 days (2nd week). (3) Sequestrum is visible between 3–6 weeks. (4) MRI shows earliest changes as marrow edema within 6 hours. (5) Bone scan is 2nd best investigation Blood investigation: CBC, ESR and CRP Culture: (1) Bacterial culture from the lesion is gold standard. (2) bacterial blood culture is positive in 60% cases	• Radiology: (1) Soft tissue swelling. (2) Periarticular osteopenia. (3) Joint space alteration • Blood: CBC, ESR, CRP • Culture: Pus culture and sensitivity from joint aspirate and blood culture
Treatment:	• Medical treatment: (1) Intravenous antibiotics covering gram-positive, gram-negative and anaerobic infection. (2) Hydration with IV fluids. (3) Nutritional supplements. (4) Rest and splintage to the part • Surgical treatment is indicated in: (1) No improvement after 48 hours of intravenous antibiotics. (2) Fluctuant mass over affected limb. (3) Associated septic arthritis of adjacent joint	• Surgery is mainstay of treatment (arthrotomy) • Intravenous antibiotics • Hydration • Rest and splintage • Nutritional supplements

Contd...

Contd...

	Pyogenic osteomyelitis	Septic arthritis
	• Surgical methods are: (1) Aspiration of pus with wide bore needle. (2) Incision and drainage. (3) Multiple drilling of bone. (4) Making window at affected area (for thick pus)	
Differentials:	• Cellulitis • Pyomyositis • Trauma • Rheumatic fever • Scurvy • Syphilitic osteitis • Ewing sarcoma	• Transient synovitis • Juvenile rheumatoid arthritis • Trauma • Hemophilic arthritis • Gouty arthritis
Complication:	• Septicemia • Septic arthritis • Chronic osteomyelitis (most common) • Growth disturbance • Pathological fracture	• Septicemia • Arthritis • Subluxation or dislocation of joint • Ankylosis or joint fusion

Chapter

2

Bony Swelling (Exostosis)

CASE PRESENTATION

- **History**: My patient, a 13-year-old girl, presented with complaint of swelling in right lower thigh region from 3 years. She noticed that her swelling is painless and gradually increasing in size. She also felt some difficulty in sitting in cross-legged position and in squatting also. For this she took some physiotherapy but not relieved. There is no history of any trauma, fever or multiple joint pain.
- **Examination**: Patient is of average built and of average nutrition. Her general physical and systemic examination is also within normal limit. Local examination showed a single swelling in lower lateral aspect of thigh near knee joint. Swelling is globular, well defined, nontender, of bony consistency having smooth surface and continuous with femur. The range of motion at knee is slightly decreased. There is no limb length discrepancy. Distal neurovascular examination is also normal.

VIVA VOCE FROM CASE

Q. What is your case?

Ans. This is a case of exostosis of distal femur (Fig. 2.1).

Q. Is it a bone tumor?

Ans. It is a bony outgrowth also called osteochondroma, but not true bone tumor.

Q. What are the points favoring your diagnosis?

Ans. The cardinal features of exostosis are:

- Young growing age of patient (2nd decade)
- Single bony swelling
- Located in metaphyseal area (distal femur > upper tibia > proximal humerus)

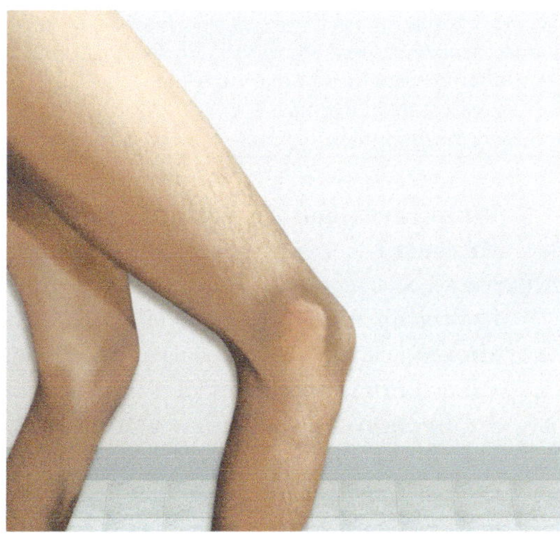

Fig. 2.1: A case of bony exostosis femur.

- Direction of growth is away from the joint (peripheral growth)
- Swelling is painless.

Swelling descriptions

- Number of swelling
- Location of swelling
- Shape and size of swelling
- Color and skin over swelling
- Surface of swelling
- Temperature (warmth) of swelling
- Tenderness of swelling
- Edge of swelling
- Consistency of swelling
- Fixity with overlying and underlying structure of swelling

Q. What else would you like to search in a case of exostosis?

Ans. These are as:
- Tenderness over swelling.
- Mechanical block of adjacent joint (decreases range of motion of joint).
- Neurovascular compression (in lower limb check dorsalis pedis or tibial pulsation, compression over common peroneal nerve near fibular neck may cause foot drop).
- Similar swelling in other body parts (**Hereditary multiple exostosis**).

Painful exostosis

- Inflammatory bursitis over swelling
- Any fracture in the mass
- Any malignant transformation in mass

Q. What investigation you like to get in this case?

Ans. X-ray of the part AP and lateral view including adjacent joint (Fig. 2.2). It shows:
- Location is metaphyseal
- Direction of growth is away from joint
- Stalk is pedunculated (some time sessile also)
- Cortex and medulla of growth is continuous with cortex and medulla of parent bone.

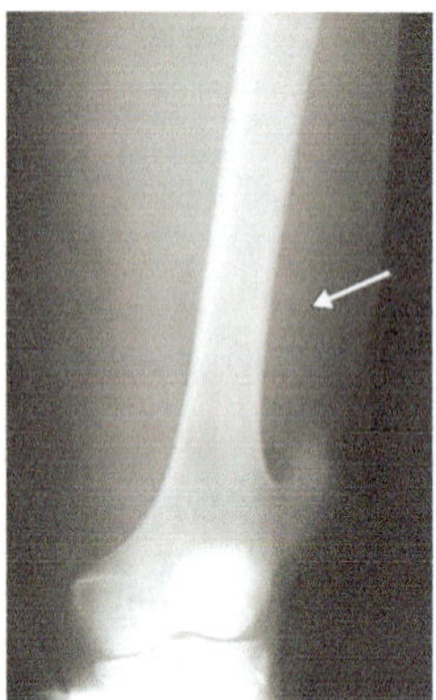

Fig. 2.2: X-ray of exostosis distal femur (arrows).
(*Courtesy*: Dr DK Taneja, Indore, Madhya Pradesh)

Q. Is there any difference in the clinical size and radiological size of swelling?

Ans. Yes, this swelling has two components, its proximal part is bony and distal part is cartilaginous. Hence, the size of the swelling in radiographs is smaller as its cartilaginous cap area is radiolucent.

Q. How will you confirm the diagnosis?

Ans. Tumor biopsy and its histopathological examination (hamartomatous lesion with outer mature cartilage resembling epiphysis and inner mature lamellar bone).

Q. What treatment you like to offer to this case?

Ans. As this swelling is producing mechanical blockade to knee joint its treatment is extraperiosteal resection of the mass (Fig. 2.3).

Q. What is meant by extraperiosteal resection and what is its advantage?

Ans. It means removal of whole tumor mass along with full covering of its periosteum. The removal of periosteum minimizes the recurrence of swelling.

Indications of surgical resection of exostosis.

- Mechanical blockade at joint
- Painful swelling
- Neurovascular compression
- Cosmetic (rarely)

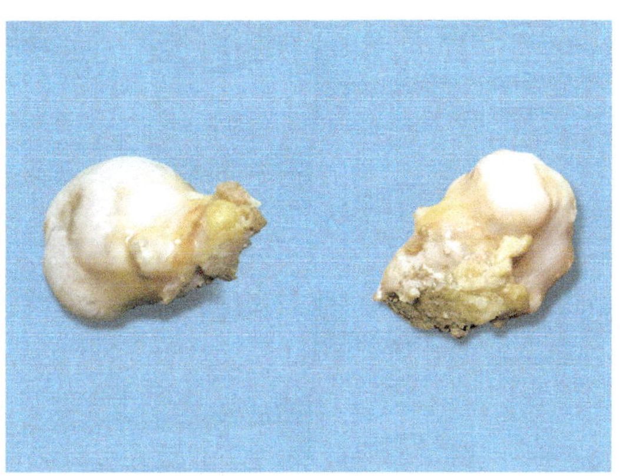

Fig. 2.3: Resected exostosis mass.

Q. What is the relation between age of patient and recurrence of swelling?

Ans. As the tumor grows up to skeletal maturity, hence there is great chance of recurrence if resection is done before maturity.

Q. What are the complications or risk of malignant transformation of osteochondroma?

Ans. Chondrosarcoma:
- Solitary exostosis: 1%
- Multiple exostosis: 5–6%.

Q. What are the signs of malignant transformation in exostosis?

Ans. These are as:
- Risk factor: Multiple exostosis and sessile growth
- Clinical: Sudden increase in size and painless swelling becomes painful
- X-ray: Irregular tumor margin and stippled calcification in cartilaginous cap
- CT/MRI: Increase in cartilaginous cap size (normally 2 cm in adult and few mm in children).

BENIGN VERSUS MALIGNANT BONY MASS (TABLE 2.1)

Table 2.1: Comparison between benign and malignant bony swelling.

	Benign bony swelling	Malignant bony swelling
Age group:	Mainly in younger age group	Common in middle age but also in younger age
General features: • Anemia • Cachexia • Loss of weight	 • Usually absent • Not common • Generally not seen	 • Usually present • Very common • Generally seen
Swelling descriptions: • Surface of swelling • Margin • Consistency • Skin over the swelling • Local adherence • Pressure effect	 • Smooth • Well defined • Firm • Normal • No • No	 • Irregular • Ill defined • Varrigated (soft to hard) • Shiny and venous prominence • May present • May present
Other features: • Secondary changes in tumor • Metastasis • Recurrence	 • Not seen • Not seen • Uncommon	 • May present • May present • Common
Histopathology:	Capsulated mass with cell differentiation and normal nuclei	Uncapsulated mass with no cell differentiation and nuclear atypia
Treatment:	Resection of mass	• Resection of bone with chemotherapy and radiotherapy

Chapter

3

Nonunion Fracture Long Bone

CASE PRESENTATION

- **History**: My patient, a 25-year young man, presented with complaint of inability to stand on right leg but is able to manage his walking with the help of walker. Nine months back he sustained an injury in his right leg in a road traffic accident. There was a fracture in his lower leg. For that he took treatment in form of above knee cast for 2.5 months. But even after removal of cast he could not be able to bear weight on his affected leg. There is no history of weight loss, appetite loss, night fever, perspiration or multiple joint pain.
- **Examination**: Patient is of average built and average nutrition. His general physical and systemic examination is within normal limit. In local examination, there is a painless abnormal mobility at the junction of middle third and lower third tibia (fracture site) in both anteroposterior and mediolateral direction. The affected leg is shortened by 3 cm and wasted in comparison to normal limb. The range of motion at ankle is decreased but normal at knee. Distal neurovascular examination is also normal.

VIVA VOCE FROM CASE

Q. What is your diagnosis?

Ans. This is a case of nonunion fracture tibia (Fig. 3.1).

Q. Define nonunion.

Ans. Nonunion is such a status of fracture where union is not possible without any surgical intervention. According to US Food and Drug Administration (FDA), nonunion is said to be exist if there is no

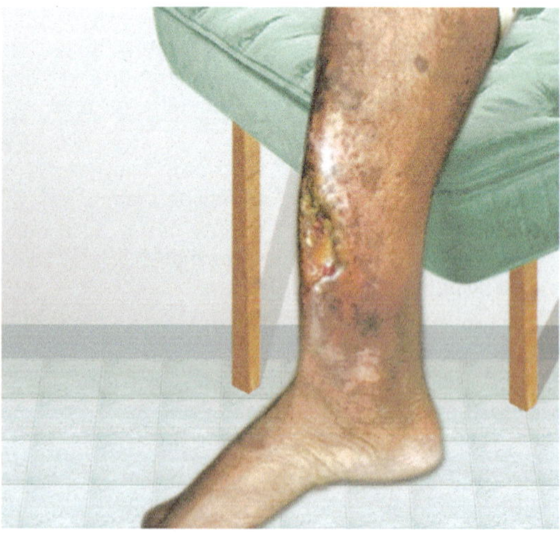

Fig. 3.1: A case of nonunion tibia.

Table 3.1: Causes of nonunion.

Fracture factor	Treatment factor	Patient factor
1. Compound fracture 2. Comminuted fracture 3. Segmental fracture 4. Infected fracture 5. Soft tissue interposition	1. Inadequate reduction 2. Improper immobilization 3. Improper fixation 4. Periosteal stripping 5. Hampered blood supply	1. Elderly and debilitated 2. Smoking and tobacco chewing 3. Steroid and anticoagulant therapy 4. Systemic illnesses 5. Alcohol intake

clinical, radiological or biological sign of progressive healing after giving adequate time (9 months) with failure of progression in 3 consecutive months. **Exception**—for fracture neck of femur and fracture lateral condyle of humerus, this time limit of only 3 months (Table 3.1).

Transmitted movement

In an intact bone when a movement is performed at its distal end, it passes over to the proximal end of bone. But in a broken bone this movement could not be transmitted from one end to another end and it is designated as absence of transmitted movement. Example: In an extended knee if a rotation is performed here which can be felt easily at greater trochanter level, which is not possible in a fractured femur (Fig. 3.2).

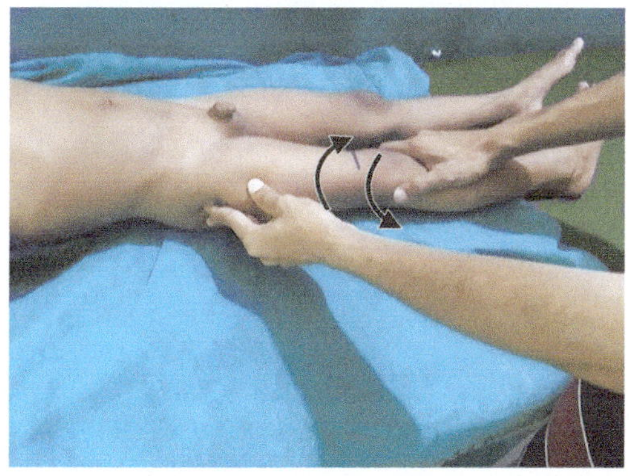

Fig. 3.2: Demonstration of transmitted movement.

Q. What are the points favoring your diagnosis?

Ans. The points favoring this diagnosis are as follows:
- History of trauma in past
- Treatment in form of above knee cast
- Painless abnormal movement at fracture site in both plane
- Shortening of affected leg.

Q. Any other associative finding you like to search in this case.

Ans. These are as:
- Any visible deformity at fracture site
- Any palpable gap
- Lack of transmitted movement.

Q. In what condition nonunion should be painful?

Ans. These are as:
- Infected nonunion
- Any live muscle or nerve impinging in between fracture ends.

Q. What are the features of infected nonunion?

Ans. These are as:
- Discharging sinus or wound at nonunion site
- Local tenderness present
- Local temperature raised
- Healing scar with adjacent puckering and tethering
- Thickening and irregularity of bone.

Q. What investigation you like to get in this case?

Ans. X-ray of the part anteroposterior (AP) and lateral view including adjacent joint (Fig. 3.3).
- Discontinuity in bone
- Obliteration of marrow cavity
- Sclerosis at the end of bones
- No visible calluses
- Inflammatory markers (CBC, ESR, CRP) for infected nonunion.

Q. Tell the classification of nonunion on the basis of radiology.

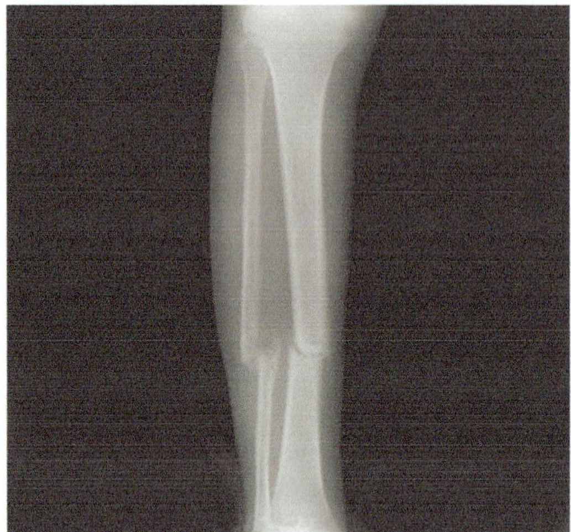

Fig. 3.3: X-ray nonunion tibia (N).

Ans. Two types:

- Atrophic nonunion: Here fracture ends have minimal or no callus formation due to poor vascularity hence no matter of fracture union even after good apposition at fracture ends.
- Hypertrophic nonunion: In this condition, exuberant callus formation due to poorly immobilized fracture hence fracture does not unite due to instability.

Q. What treatment you like to offer to this case?

Ans. Refreshening of sclerosed end of bone up to its bleeding, reduction and intramedullary nailing with cancellous bone grafting.

Q. What is the treatment principle of fracture nonunion?

Ans. These are as:

- Debridement of sclerosed end of bone and opening of medullary cavity
- Reduction of fracture
- Stable fixation
- Bone grafting
- Dealing with shortening with sole raising (up to 3 cm) or bone lengthening by Ilizarov.

Note: Ilizarov can deal infection, nonunion and shortening simultaneously (Fig. 3.4).

Q. Is the principle of treatment of infected nonunion is similar to above?

Ans. No, as the infected nonunion behaves like chronic osteomyelitis hence its treatment is similar to chronic osteomyelitis.

Q. How bone grafting works in nonunion?

Ans. It works in two manners:

1. Provides framework for bone growth between fracture ends (osteoconduction)
2. Increases the osteogenic potential at fracture site and enhances the progression of fracture union (osteoinduction) (Table 3.2).

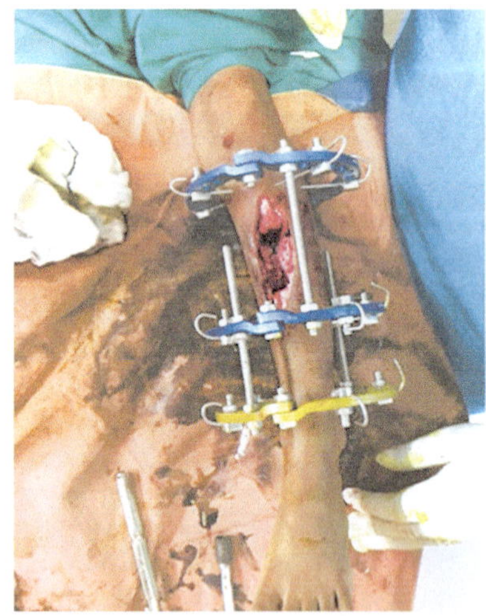

Fig. 3.4: Debridement of nonunion site and Ilizarov application.
(*Courtesy*: Dr NA Khan, Bettiah)

Table 3.2: Types of bone graft.

Cancellous bone graft	Cortical bone grafting
1. Harvested from iliac crest (Fig. 3.5) 2. Used at nonunion site or other bony defect	1. Harvested from fibula 2. To maintain continuity of bone in long defects

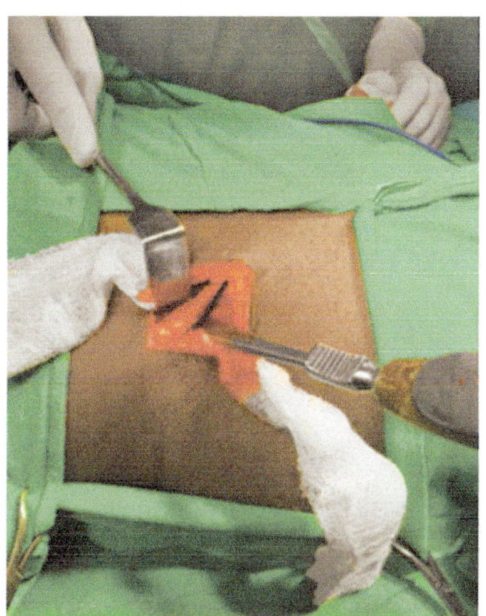

Fig. 3.5: Bone graft harvesting from iliac crest.
(*Courtesy*: Dr Oswald Anand, Bettiah)

Q. What are the common sites of nonunion and their possible causes?

Ans. These are as:

- Fracture neck of femur: (1) Precarious blood supply, (2) Absent cambium layer. (3) Washing of hematoma by synovial fluid. (4) Shearing forces at fracture site
- Fracture distal 1/3rd tibia: (1) Precarious blood supply. (2) Minimal muscular covering only tendinous
- Fracture talus neck: Precarious blood supply
- Fracture lateral condyle of humerus: Continuous traction of common extensor origin
- Fracture scaphoid: Precarious blood supply.

Q. What is delayed union?

Ans. When a fracture takes undue prolonged period than it is expected for union of a particular fracture, condition is called delayed union. Factors responsible for delayed union are similar to factors for nonunion but they are of lesser severity.

Q. What is the treatment of delayed nonunion?

Ans. These are as:

- Bone marrow injection or bone grafting
- Improve or strengthen immobilization
- Correct systemic factor like nutrition, patient general condition. etc.

Q. What are the stages of fracture healing?

Ans. These are as:

- Stage of hematoma formation and inflammation
- Stage of soft callus formation
- Stage of hard callus formation
- Stage of remodeling (Fig. 3.6).

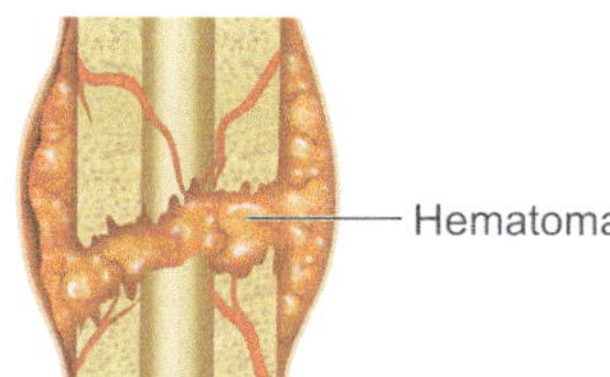

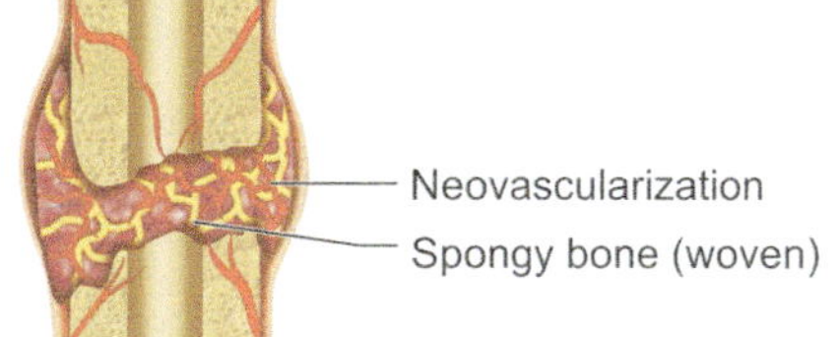

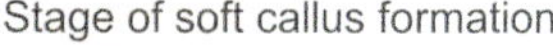

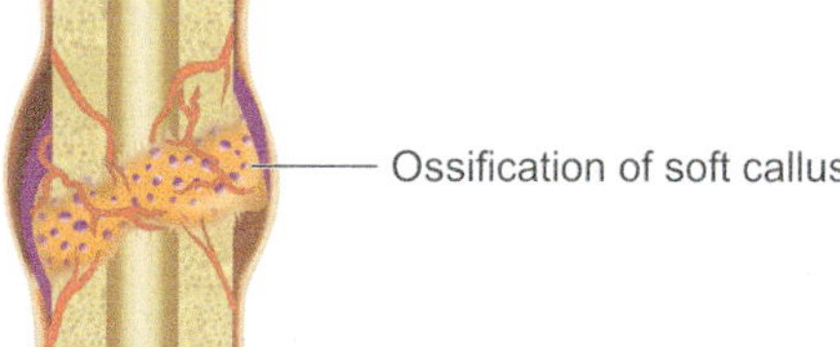

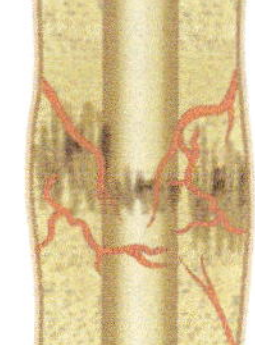

Fig. 3.6: Stages of fracture healing.

FRACTURE COMPLICATIONS (TABLE 3.3)

Table 3.3: Fracture complications.

Immediate complications (within hours)	Early complications (within days)	Late complications (within weeks or months)
• **Shock:** ➢ Decreased blood pressure, tachycardia and cold extremities are key features ➢ Blood and crystalloid perfusion are the mainstays of treatment	• **Fat embolism:** ➢ Common in fracture shaft femur and pelvis ➢ Appear after 24–72 hours ➢ Oxygenation and steroids are the mainstays of treatment	• **Nonunion or delayed union:** ➢ Causes may be fracture related, treatment related or patient related ➢ Painless abnormal mobility at fracture site is key feature ➢ Debridement of sclerosed bone, stable fixation and bone grafting are main steps of treatment
• **Neurological injury:** ➢ Common in limb injury ➢ Motor and sensory deficit in area of distribution is key feature ➢ Treatment is expectant or nerve repair	• **Deep vein thrombosis:** ➢ Occurs due to prolonged immobilization (lower limb or spine injury) ➢ Patient mobilization on bed and anticoagulant like heparin and warfarin are the mainstays of management	• **Reflex sympathetic dystrophy:** ➢ This is due to sympathetic overactivity in response to continuous painful stimuli at fracture site, e.g. Colles' fracture ➢ Disproportionate pain, swelling and stiffness are key features ➢ Physiotherapy, electrotherapy and sympathomimetic drugs are the mainstays of treatment
• **Head, chest and abdominal injury:** ➢ Life-threatening emergency ➢ Multidisciplinary approach is needed	• **Compartment syndrome:** ➢ Occurs due to increased pressure in osteofascial compartment in fracture, etc. ➢ Pain, pallor, paresthesia, paralysis and pulselessness are key features ➢ Decompression of compartment is the mainstay of treatment	• **Joint stiffness:** ➢ Commonly occurs in periarticular fracture or in prolonged cast immobilization ➢ Range of motion of joint is diminished ➢ Physiotherapy and sometime mobilization under general anesthesia are treatment tools
	• **Crush syndrome:** ➢ This syndrome develops due to rhabdomyolysis of crushed tissue of limb ➢ Serum electrolyte disturbances, acute renal failure, disseminated intravascular coagulation and cardiomyopathy are key features ➢ High urine output, crystalloid and forced alkaline diuresis are ways of treatment	

Contd...

Contd...

Immediate complications (within hours)	Early complications (within days)	Late complications (within weeks or months)
	• **Infection:** ➢ Common in compound fractures and causal agent is *Staphylococcus aureus* ➢ Debridement, external fixation and antibiotics are main treatment tools	
	• **Gas gangrene:** ➢ Causal agent is *Clostridium welchii* and common in compound fractures ➢ It is spreading myonecrosis of affected limb with foul smelling discharge ➢ Through debridement, antibiotics and antigas gangrene serum are the mainstays of treatment	

Chapter

4

Wrist Drop (Radial Palsy)

CASE PRESENTATION

- **History**: My patient, a 30-year-old male, presented with complaint of a mild pain in right arm and weakness in wrist and hand. One month back he was gone through a physical assault and sustained a fracture in his lower arm. For this he took treatment locally in form of U-slab. Next day he noticed that there is weakness in his wrist and hand. There is no history of fever, multiple joint pain, and any systemic illness or poisoning.
- **Examination**: Patient is of average built and average nutrition. His general physical and systemic examination is within normal limit. Local examination showed mild tenderness and irregularity at junction of middle third and lower third of affected arm. Forearm is slightly wasted. Neurological examination revealed grade 3 power in wrist extensors, grade 4 power in finger extensors, and hypoesthesia in dorsum of first web space of hand. Tinel sign and motor march is present. Examination of shoulder and elbow is normal. Distal pulsation palpable and comparable.

VIVA VOCE FROM CASE

Q. What is your diagnosis?

Ans. This is a case of wrist drop due to radial nerve palsy with fracture humerus under conservative treatment (Fig. 4.1).

Q. What is wrist drop?

Ans. When patient is unable to extend his wrist actively, situation is called wrist drop. If anyone is unable to extend his finger at metacarpophalangeal joint, condition is known as finger drop (Table 4.1).

Q. What are the points favoring your diagnosis?

Ans. The points favoring the diagnosis are as follows:

- History of trauma and fracture humerus in lower third zone.
- Unable to extend the wrist joint and metacarpophalangeal joint.
- Hypoesthesia in the dorsum of first web space of right hand.

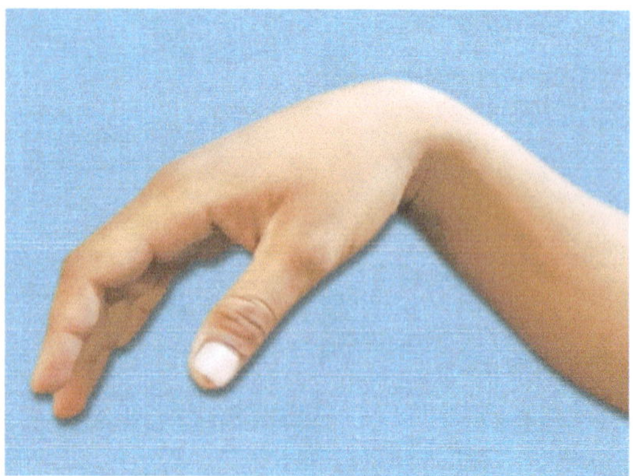

Fig. 4.1: A case of wrist drop.

Table 4.1: Types of radial palsy.

Very high type	High type	Low type
Injury above radial groove	Injury from radial groove to lateral condyle of humerus	Injury around elbow or below
For example—crutch palsy	Saturday night palsy, facture lower 1/3rd humerus with radial palsy	Posterior interosseous nerve (PIN) injury in Monteggia fracture dislocation or isolated nerve injury
One can not extend his elbow, wrist, and his finger	One can extend his elbow but unable to perform wrist and finger extension	One can extend his elbow and wrist but unable to do finger extension (finger drop)

Q. How you grade the power of a muscle?

Ans. The medical research council (MRC) London has graded the power of a muscle as follows:
- Grade 0: No power
- Grade 1: Flicker of contraction
- Grade 2: Contraction of muscle when gravity is eliminated
- Grade 3: Contraction of muscle against gravity
- Grade 4: Contraction against some resistance
- Grade 5: Normal muscle power.

Autonomous zone of a nerve for sensation.

- Axillary nerve: Upper arm (lower deltoid) regiment badge sign
- Radial nerve: Dorsum of first web space of hand
- Median nerve: Tip of index finger
- Ulnar nerve: Tip of small finger
- Deep peroneal nerve: Dorsum of first web space of foot

Q. Any other associative finding you like to search in this case?

Ans. These are as:
- Any history of fracture manipulation.
- Any scar on limb in course of the nerve (penetrating injury or glass cut).
- Any trophic changes (skin texture, soft tissue atrophy, nail changes, and hair changes).
- Sign of recovery (Tinel sign and motor march) (Table 4.2).

Q. What investigation you like to get in a nerve injury case?

Ans. I will go for X-ray of the limb (Fig. 4.2), it tells about:
- Fracture position
- Any evidence of foreign body (metal or glass piece).

Q. Is this a special fracture?

Ans. Yes sir, a oblique fracture present at the junction of middle third and lower third of humerus is called **Holstein-Lewis** fracture. This fracture is mostly associated with radial nerve injury, especially during reduction.

Q. Any other investigation relevant for a nerve injury case?

Ans. Yes sir, electrodiagnostic study of nerve.
- Nerve conduction velocity test: It is the study of propagation of nerve conduction

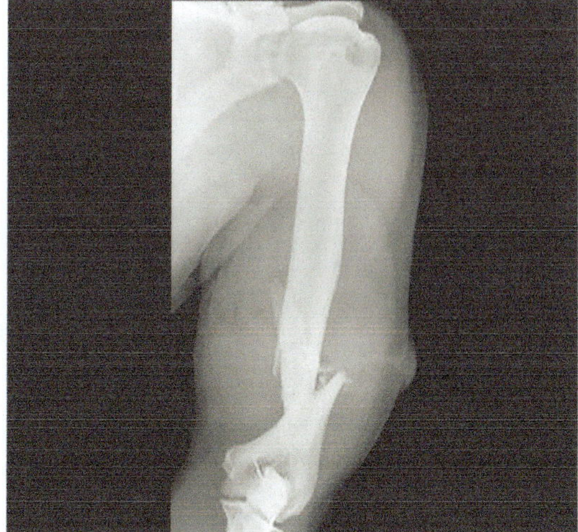

Fig. 4.2: X-ray of fracture distal one-third humerus (Holstein–Lewis fracture).

in response to electrical stimuli. It tells about the site of nerve injury.
- Electromyography: It is recording of electrical activity of muscle during rest and active phase. It tells about the type of nerve injury and recovery status.

Q. What treatment you like to offer to this case?

Ans. As patient is giving history of some recovery in sensation and power of affected limb, I will go for expectant treatment. If it fails then I will go for surgical intervention (Fig. 4.3).

Q. What do you meant by expectant treatment?

Ans. It is a conservative treatment method and its modalities are as:
- Splintage (dynamic cock-up splint)
- Physiotherapy
- Nerve stimulation.

Q. What is dynamic cock-up splint and how it works?

Ans. It is a functional wrist and hand orthosis where wrist joint is maintained in almost 45° of dorsiflexion and extension of the fingers are performed by recoiling activity of actively flexed fingers on rubber loop system (Fig. 4.4).

Q. What is your plan to follow this case?

Ans. I will go for clinical and electrodiagnostic evaluation at interval of 4 weeks:

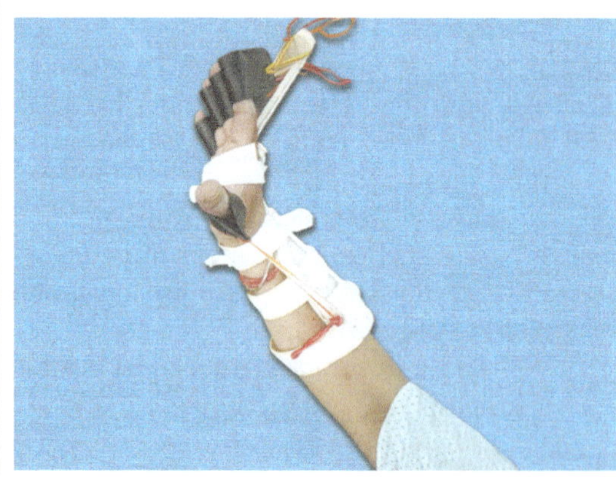

Fig. 4.4: Dynamic cock-up splint.

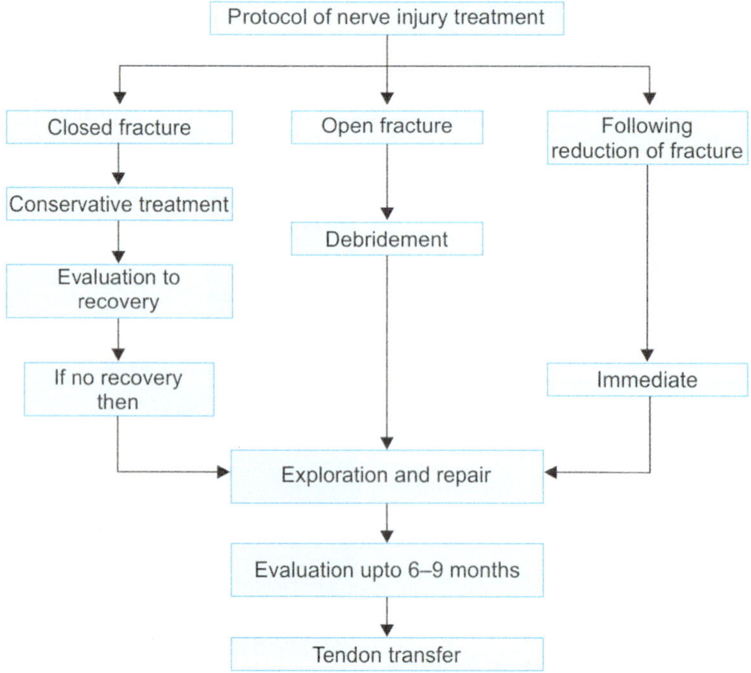

Fig. 4.3: Treatment protocol for nerve injury.

- Clinical examination: It includes sensory and motor examination along with Tinel sign. As the nerve grows at the rate of 1 mm per day; hence, advancing Tinel sign shows progressive recovery pattern but static Tinel sign indicates neuroma formation at nerve end.
- Electrodiagnostic test: It confirms the findings of our clinical examination.

Q. What are the definitive treatment methods?

Ans. This is surgical method and it includes neurolysis and neurorrhaphy.

- Neurolysis: Exploration of nerve by removing all adjacent fibrosis around it is called neurolysis. It relieves the nerve from compression.
- Neurorrhaphy: The repair procedure between two ends of the injured nerve is called neurorrhaphy.

Q. What will you do if your definitive treatment fails?

Ans. Sir, I will go for tendon transfer. Tendon transfer in wrist drop is as:

- For wrist extension: Pronator teres to extensor carpi radialis brevis.
- For finger extension: Flexor carpi radialis to extensor digitorum communis.
- For thumb abduction and extension: Rerouting of palmaris longus to extensor pollicis longus.

Principles of tendon transfer.

- Age of patient: More than 5 years otherwise difficulty in rehabilitation program
- Power of muscle: At least grade 4, because muscle looses its grade 1 power after its transfer
- Adjacent joint: Joint should be supple, i.e. without any contracture or deformity
- Tendon selection: Agonist should be preferred over antagonist
- Path of excursion: Transferred tendon should follow the similar path like original one
- Route: Subcutaneous route is preferred over intraosseous
- Tension of tendon: Newer tendon should insert in slightly greater tension

Q. What are different causes of nerve affection?

Ans. There are as:

- Traumatic fracture
- Infection: Leprosy and herpes
- Metabolic: Vitamin B12 deficiency and diabetic
- Collagen disorder: Amyloidosis
- Neoplastic: Neurofibroma
- Poisoning: Lead and arsenic
- Iatrogenic: Traction, manipulation, surgical, and esmarch bandaging.

Q. What are the prognostic factors for nerve injury?

Ans. These are as:

- Nerve type: Purely motor or sensory has better prognosis than mixed one, e.g. radial nerve.
- Type of nerve injury: Neuropraxia has always better prognosis than any other type.
- Location of nerve injury: Distal injury has better prognosis than nearer to proximal one.
- Age of patient: Younger patient had better prognosis.
- Nerve bed status: Healthy nerve bed has good prognosis than contaminated one.

Q. What do you meant by claw hand and how it happens?

Ans. Claw hand is defined as hyperextension at metacarpophalangeal (MCP) joint and flexion of interphalangeal (IP) joint.

- This deformity occurs due to affection of median nerve, ulnar nerve (partial) or both (complete).
- The hand muscle lumbrical is supplied my median nerve (lateral two) and ulnar nerve (medial two). The long flexor digitorum profundus is supplied by median nerve (lateral two sleeves) and ulnar nerve (medial two sleeves).
- Mechanism of clawing: As lumbricals are flexor of MCP joint and extensor of IP joint and supported by interossei in this movement too. Hence in

paralysis of either or both of these nerve, MCP joint attain the attitude of hyperextension and IP joint goes in position of hyperflexion and clawing ensues.

Q. What is ulnar paradox?

Ans. In lower ulnar nerve palsy (below elbow, i.e. around wrist) clawing is more prominent than higher lesion (around elbow) where deformity is less evident. This phenomenon is called ulnar paradox. The reason behind this is, escaping of flexor digitorum profundus (FDP) in lower lesion as it is innervated higher around elbow by ulnar nerve. Hence, unopposed action of FDP flexes the DIP joint and clawing becomes more evident.

Q. What are the clinical findings you like to get in median nerve palsy?

Ans. These are as:
- Thenar atrophy
- Loss of sensation in tip of index finger (autonomous zone)
- Pointing index or **Oschner clasp-knife** sign due to paralysis of lateral FDP
- Pen test shows palsy of abductor pollicis brevis
- Loss of thumb opposition due to palsy of opponens pollicis.

Q. What are the clinical evidences you like to get in ulnar nerve affection?

Ans. These are as:
- Hypothenar atrophy
- Loss of sensation in tip of small finger (autonomous zone)
- Book test or Froment sign shows palsy of adductor pollicis and overactivity of flexor pollicis longus
- Card test or finger adduction test shows palsy of palmar interossei
- **Egawa** test or finger abduction test shows palsy of dorsal interossei.

Q. Which splint you would like to use to correct the claw hand deformity?

Ans. Knuckle bender splint is used to correct the deformity of claw hand (Fig. 4.5). This splint maintains metacarpophalangeal (MCP) joints in flexion and interphalangeal (IP) joints in extension. This position is known as **James** position sometime also called functional position.

Q. What do you meant by foot drop and how it happens?

Ans. If anyone is unable to do active dorsiflexion at ankle, condition is called foot drop. This deformity is due to affection of common peroneal nerve around knee or sciatic nerve around hip and thigh (the outer boundary of sciatic nerve has fibers of common peroneal component).

Q. Which orthosis is used in this condition and why?

Ans. Ankle foot orthosis (AFO) also called foot drop splint is used in this condition

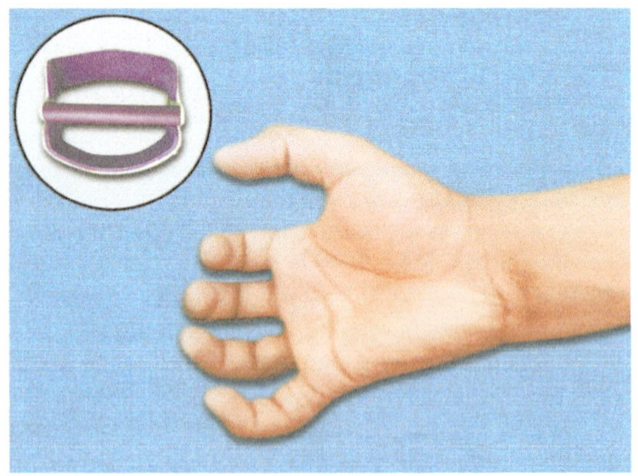

Fig. 4.5: Claw hand and knuckle bender splint.

(Fig. 4.6). In foot drop, foot remains in attitude of plantar flexion leading to equinus deformity if it is neglected for long period.

Q. What is Erb's palsy and how it happens?

Ans. This is due to paralysis of upper trunk of brachial plexus (C5 and C6). It occurs due to traction over shoulder during vaginal delivery (Fig. 4.7).

- The point affected is called Erb's point having following component: (1) root of C5, (2) root of C6, (3) suprascapular nerve, (4) nerve to subclavius, (5) ventral division of upper trunk (musculocutaneous nerve), and (6) dorsal division of upper trunk (axillary nerve).
- The affected limb get attitude of **porter tip or policeman tip** where shoulder is adducted and internally rotated, elbow extended and forearm pronated.
- Duration of antibiotic treatment is 8 weeks; 2 weeks intravenous and 6 weeks oral.

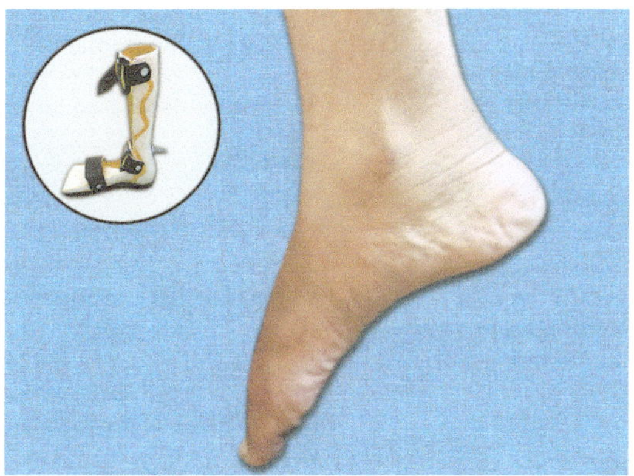

Fig. 4.6: Foot drop and foot drop splint.

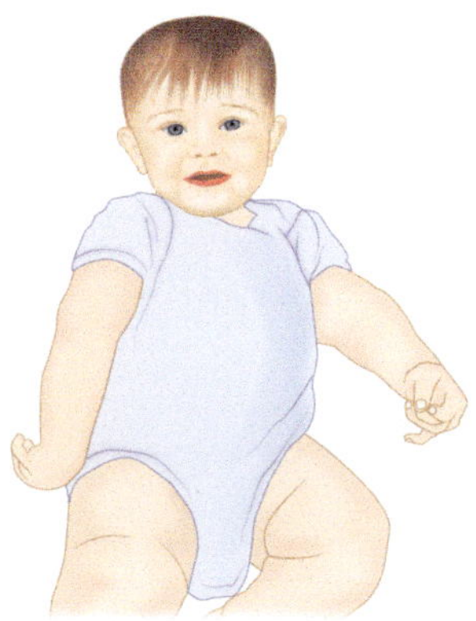

Fig. 4.7: A child of Erb's palsy.

Q. Which splint is used in this condition and why?

Ans. The aeroplane splint is used in this condition. It maintains shoulder in abduction and in externally rotated attitude. It also keeps elbow flexed and supinated.

NERVE INJURY PATTERN (SEDDON CLASSIFICATION) (TABLE 4.2)

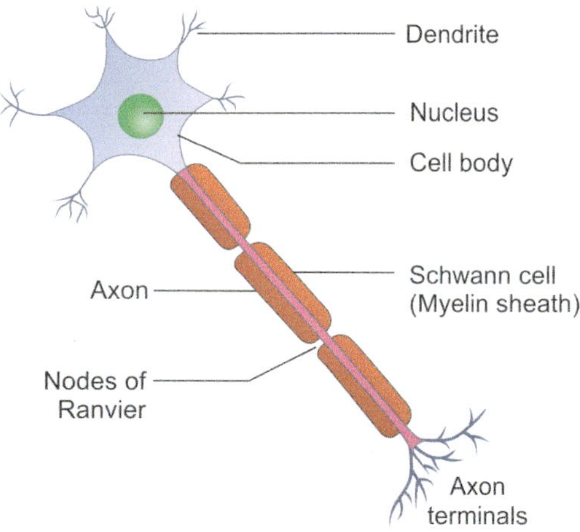

Fig. 4.8: An axon.

Table 4.2: Nerve injury pattern.

	Neuropraxia	Axonotmesis	Neurotmesis
Definition:	Physiological blockade of nerve conduction	Axonal disruption but nerve sheath intact	Complete anatomic dissection of the nerve
Status of myelination:	+/–	Myelin sheath disrupted	Myelin sheath disrupted
Status of axon	Intact	Axon cylinder disrupted	Axon cylinder disrupted
Wallerian degeneration: Degeneration of nerve from distal to proximal direction upto site of denervation.	No	Present	Present but forming neuroma at its end
Tinel sign: A current like spreading sensation from sprouting end of nerve to its distal most distribution, when nerve is tapped from distal to proximal direction.	Absent	Present	Present, but static due to neuroma formation
Motor March: Recovery of muscles takes place in order of their nerve supply from proximal to distal	Not seen	Present	Absent
Recovery:	Spontaneous recovery in one go (all and non phenomenon)	Recovery progressive	No recovery if not surgically repaired
Treatment:	Expectant	Expectant if failure then surgical intervention	Surgical intervention mandatory
Example:	Crutch palsy Saturday night palsy Tourniquet palsy	Closed fracture dislocation	Compound fracture dislocation

Chapter

5

Frozen Shoulder

CASE PRESENTATION

- **History**: My patient, a 41-year-old man, presented with complaint of pain and stiffness in his right shoulder from 7 months. Pain is of gradual onset, severe in nature, and increases in night and relieved with some analgesics. He has also a complaint of difficulty in combing hairs and other household activities. He is a known case of diabetes and taking pills for last 6 years. There is no history of previous trauma, any fever, and weight loss or any other multiple joint pain.
- **Examination**: Patient is of heavy built and good nutrition. Her general physical and systemic examination is within normal limit. Local examination showed some wasting around right shoulder so that underlying bones are prominent like acromion process. There is deep tenderness in anterior joint line. Shoulder range of motion is grossly restricted in all planes like abduction, flexion extension, and internal and external rotations. Opposite shoulder examination is normal. No distal neurovascular deficit.

VIVA VOCE FROM CASE

Q. What is your diagnosis?

Ans. This is a case of frozen shoulder (Fig. 5.1).

Q. What are the other names for this disease?

Ans. These are:

- Periarthritis shoulder
- Adhesive capsulitis (Table 5.1).

Q. What are the points favoring your diagnosis?

Ans. The points favoring this diagnosis are as follows:

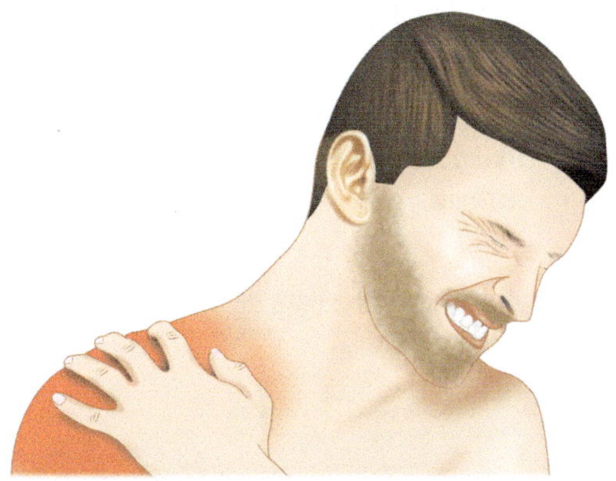

Fig. 5.1: A case of frozen shoulder.

Table 5.1: Risk factors for frozen shoulder.

Primary	Secondary
• Diabetes • Thyroid dysfunction • Hypercholesteremia • Hypertension	• Humeral head fracture • Infective arthritis • Inflammatory arthritis

- History of shoulder pain of gradual onset.
- Pain aggravates in night.
- Global restriction of shoulder range of motion (first rotation then abduction).

Q. Any other associative finding you like to search in this case?

Ans. These are as:
- Examination of opposite shoulder (in diabetics bilateral involvement is common)
- Cervical spondylosis is sometime preceder of frozen shoulder.

Q. What investigation you like to get in this case?

Ans. These are:
- X-ray of shoulder (Fig. 5.2)
- Blood investigation.

Q. What do you expect in X-ray of frozen shoulder?

Ans. Although X-ray of frozen shoulder is normal, but its gives some information like:
- Status of bone, if osteoporosis, mobilization under general anesthesia is contraindicated.
- Other findings for secondary causes like trauma, infection or inflammatory arthritis.

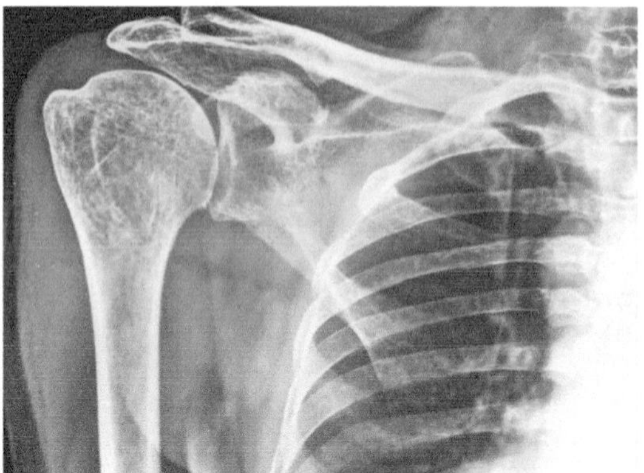

Fig. 5.2: X-ray of frozen shoulder.

- X-ray of cervical spine shows spondylosis changes as joint space reduction or osteophyte formation, etc.

Q. What you like to see in blood investigation?

Ans. It shows:
- Blood sugar (fasting and postprandial for diabetics)
- Serum T3, T4, TSH for thyroid dysfunction
- Lipid profile.

Q. What is your treatment plan for your case?

Ans. I will go for medication and physiotherapy first.
- Medical treatment: Analgesics (NSAIDs and opioids)
- Physiotherapy: Active or passive shoulder mobilization exercises and electrotherapy
- Intra-articular injection: Steroid methyl prednisolone is commonly used.

Q. What will you do if patient does not improve with this treatment?

Ans. Then I will go for active mobilization under general anesthesia after getting fitness from anesthetist.

Q. Is there any risk in this maneuver?

Ans. Yes, there is chance of fracture proximal humerus, especially in osteoporotic bones.

Q. Then what is next option for treatment in patient having osteoporosis?

Ans. Arthroscopic debridement of the joint.

Q. What is meant by adhesive capsulitis?

Ans. This term says about pathology of the disease as capsulitis means inflammation of capsule and adhesive means fibrosis of capsule. These two make a painful and stiff joint.

Q. What are the pathological staging of the frozen shoulder?

Ans. Although this is a self-limiting disease and it takes almost 18 months to complete its natural course. It has following three stages.

1. Stage of inflammation (4–6 month): Painful shoulder
2. Stage of stiffness (4–6 months): Decreased range of shoulder movement
3. Stage of thawing (4–6 month): Stage of recovery.

TWO DIFFERENTIALS FOR FROZEN SHOULDER (TABLE 5.2)

Table 5.2: Differentials for frozen shoulder.

	Shoulder impingement (painful arc syndrome)	Glenohumeral arthritis
Age group	Middle age	Elderly
Incidence	More common	Less common
Etiological factor	• Subacromial bursitis • Partial tear of supraspinatus • Calcific tendinitis of supraspinatus • Hooked acromion • Os acromiale • Acromioclavicular joint arthritis	Sedentary lifestyle Obesity
Pathology	Due to above mentioned etiological factor there is impingement of humeral head when it enters the subacromial space	Loss of proteoglycan in hyaline cartilage of joint leading to eburnation of this layer
Clinical presentation	• Painful arc: There is painful abduction between 60° and 120° of movement. Below 60° and above 120° movement is painless • Pain increases at night • Range of motion decreases gradually • Neer impingement test positive (Fig. 5.3): ➢ Position of patient: Standing ➢ Maneuver: Examiner steadizes the patient's scapula with one hand and fully flexes the shoulder with another hand and then produces a sudden jerk ➢ Inference: Patient feel pain, especially at the end of maneuver	• Painful shoulder joint • Crepitus may present • Range of motion decreased
Investigation	• X-ray shoulder for: ➢ AC joint arthritis: Arthritic changes in joint ➢ Calcific tendinitis: Radiopaque mass in supraspinatus tendon ➢ Os acromiale: A bony bump in under surface of acromion process ➢ Hooked acromion: Sharp and bent acromion process • USG/MRI: For tear in supraspinatus and bursitis	• X-ray shows (Fig. 5.4): ➢ Decreases joint space ➢ Osteophytes ➢ Subchondral sclerosis
Treatment	• Treatment of underlying disease is mainstay of treatment. Common modalities are: ➢ Analgesics (NSAIDs and opioids) ➢ Physiotherapy ➢ Intra-articular steroid injection ➢ Arthroscopic debridement	• Analgesics (NSAIDs and opioids) • Physiotherapy and habit change • Intra-articular injection of steroids • Arthroscopic debridement • Sometime total shoulder replacement

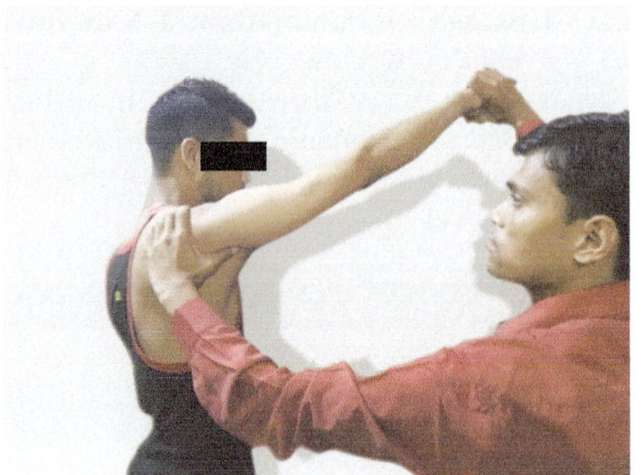

Fig. 5.3: Neer impingement test.

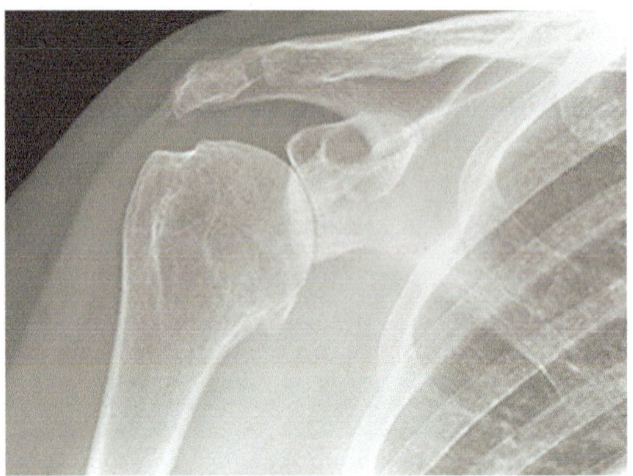

Fig. 5.4: X-ray of glenohumeral arthritis.

Chapter

6

Cubitus Varus Deformity at Elbow (Malunited Supracondylar Fracture Humerus)

CASE PRESENTATION

- **History**: My patient, a 12-year boy, presented with complaint of deformity at his right elbow for last 1 year. He fell down from a tree with outstretched hand and sustained an injury around his right elbow. He was carried to a local bonesetter who applied some bandaging with some wooden pieces and herbs in affected extremity. At the end of a month parents noticed a deformity and stiffness in his right elbow. For this he took physiotherapy and his elbow movement was improved completely, but deformity persisted. There is no history of any fever, weight loss, or multiple joint pain.
- **Examination**: Patient is of average built and of average nutrition. His general physical and systemic examination is within normal limit. Local examination revealed that there is an inward deviation of his forearm (cubitus varus) and a prominence over lateral aspect of elbow. Three bony point relationship is maintained. Both supracondylar ridges are thickened and irregular. The range of motion at elbow is near normal. There is no limb length discrepancy. Distal neurovascular examination is also normal.

VIVA VOCE FROM CASE

Q. What is your case?

Ans. This is a case of cubitus varus deformity of right elbow following supracondylar fracture of humerus (Fig. 6.1).

Q. What is the other name for cubitus varus deformity?

Ans. The other name for cubitus varus deformity is gunstock deformity as it looks like an old model long barrel guns.

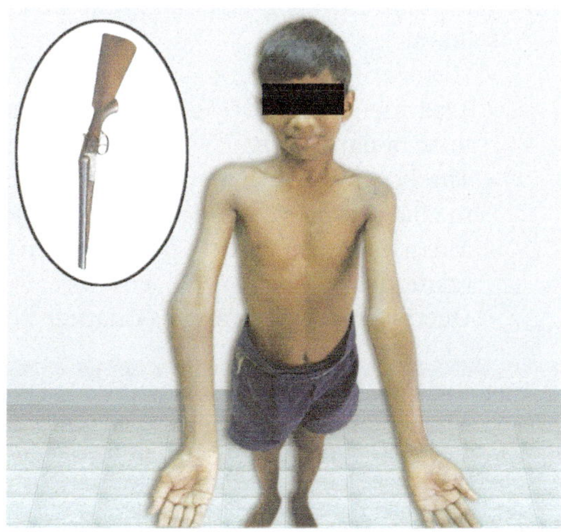

Fig. 6.1: A case of cubitus varus deformity.

Q. Define cubitus varus?

Ans. Cubitus varus deformity is defined as inward deviation of long axis of forearm in relation to arm when elbow is fully extended and supinated. *Do not use this term if elbow is not fully extended.*

Q. Is this progressive deformity?

Ans. No.

Q. Is it possible a progressive cubitus varus deformity after supracondylar fracture humerus?

Ans. Yes. Sometimes the progressive deformity is observed due to overgrowth of lateral condyle in supracondylar fracture but not common.

Different causes of cubitus varus deformity.

- Congenital cubitus varus
- Malunited supracondylar fracture humerus
- Malunited intercondylar fracture humerus
- Malunited medial condyle fracture humerus
- Malunited lateral condyle fracture humerus due to overgrowth

Q. Why you say that this deformity is due to malunited supracondylar fracture humerus?

Ans. The points favoring this statement are as follows:
- History of trauma in past.
- Treatment history by a bone setter in form of bandaging.
- Thickening and irregularity of both medial and lateral supracondylar ridges.
- Maintained three point bony relationship.
- Decreased carrying angle (Chapter 7).

Three point bony relationship at elbow (Fig. 6.2).

When elbow is flexed to 90°, its medial epicondyle (ME), lateral epicondyle (LE), and tip of olecranon process (OP) make a triangle which is identical to its opposite counter part. But in extended elbow these three points come into a straight line and triangular configuration is lost. This triangle and line is also called Hueter triangle and Hueter line. Implications of this three bony point relationship are as:

- Unaltered: Supracondylar fracture
- Altered: Intercondylar or condylar fracture
- Reversed: Posterior dislocation of elbow

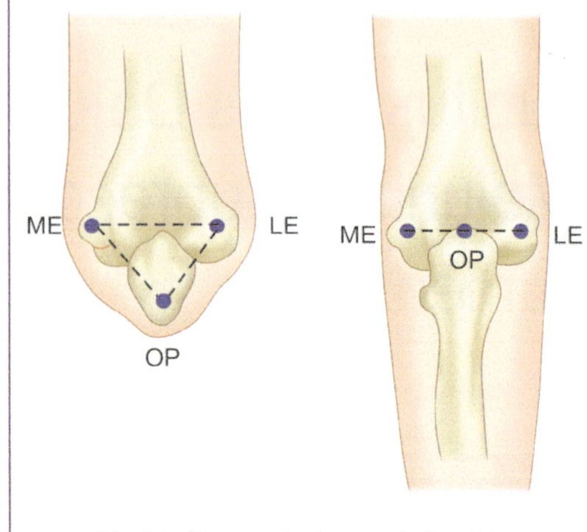

Fig 6.2: Three point bony relationship.

Q. Any other clinical finding you like to search in this case?

Ans. These are as:
- Associated deformity of cubitus varus like (1) internal rotation, (2) medial tilt, and (3) posterior tilt at elbow.
- Increased internal rotation and decreased external rotation of shoulder shows medial rotation deformity.
- Increased arm length (from angle of acromion to lateral epicondyle of humerus) shows medial tilt at deformity
- Increased extension and decreased flexion at elbow shows posterior tilt at deformity.

Q. What investigation you like to get in this case?

Ans. X-ray of the elbow AP and lateral view (Fig. 6.3)
- Cubitus varus deformity
- Healing supracondylar fracture with thickening of distal humerus.

Q. What is your treatment plan?

Ans. I will go for lateral closed wedge osteotomy. It is briefly explained as:

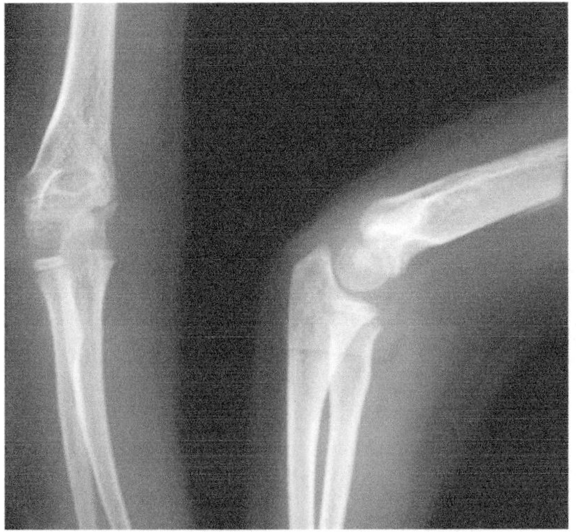

Fig. 6.3: X-ray of cubitus varus deformity.

- Making of adequate wedge at its lateral cortex.
- External rotation of distal fragment to correct the internal rotation deformity.
- Fixation of osteotomy site with K-wire, SS wire-screw assembly and sometimes low profile plate (Fig. 6.4).

Osteotomies for correction of cubitus varus deformity.

- Lateral closed wedge osteotomy (French osteotomy)
- Medial open wedge osteotomy
- Dome osteotomy
- Step cut osteotomy

Q. What is prerequisite for osteotomy?

Ans. There is a waiting period of at least 1 year between fracture and surgery so that adequate remodeling could take place at fracture site.

Q. Why supracondylar fractures are common in children?

Ans. The reasons behind this are as:

- Bone is thin anteroposteriorly in this area

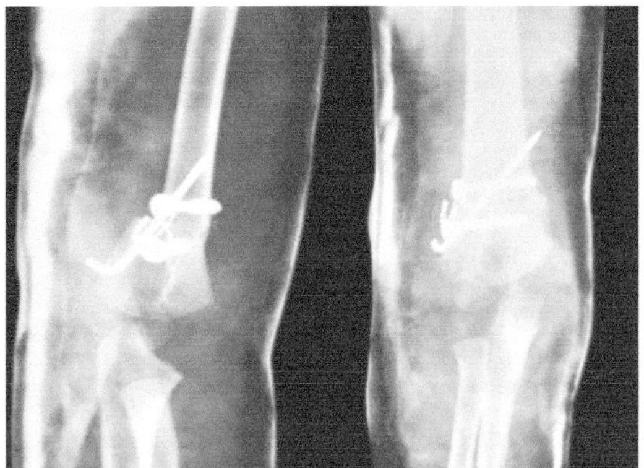

Fig. 6.4: French osteotomy and fixation.

- Bone is further weakened due to presence of fossae like olecranon, coronoid, and radial.
- Impinging leverage activity of olecranon process in olecranon fossa creating a stress point.
- Ligamentous laxity makes it prone for hyperextension.

Q. What is the puckering sign and what is its significance?

Ans. It appears in anterior aspect of elbow due to buttonholing effect of proximal fracture fragment (penetration) in brachialis muscle (Fig. 6.5). It makes fracture reduction difficult.

Q. What you expect in radiograph of supracondylar fracture?

Ans. These are as (Fig. 6.6):

- Medial shift (sometime lateral)
- Medial tilt (sometime lateral)
- Internal or medial rotation
- Posterior shift
- Posterior tilt
- Proximal migration.

Q. What is Baumann angle and what is its clinical implication?

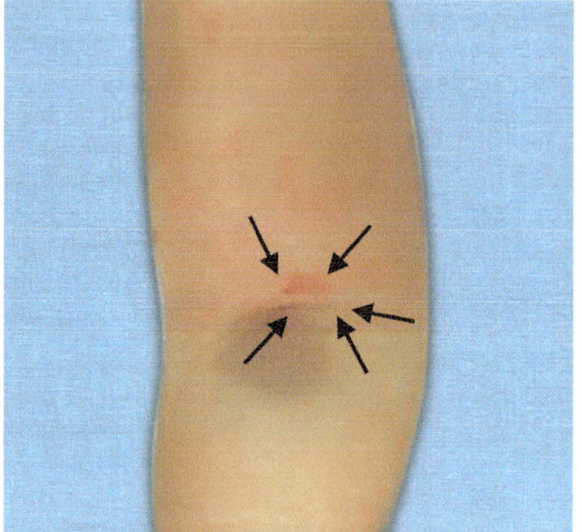

Fig. 6.5: Puckering sign.

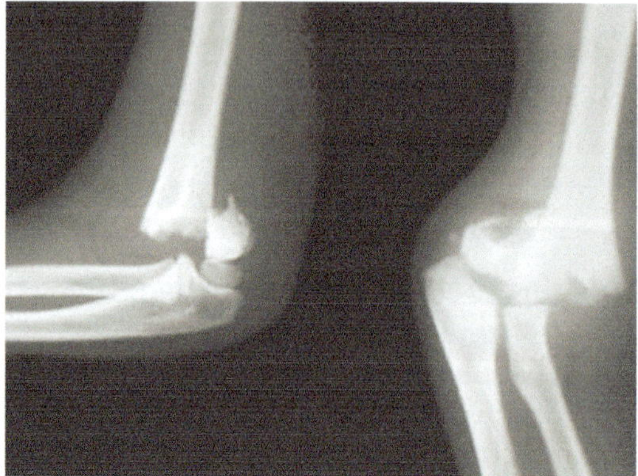

Fig. 6.6: Fracture displacement.

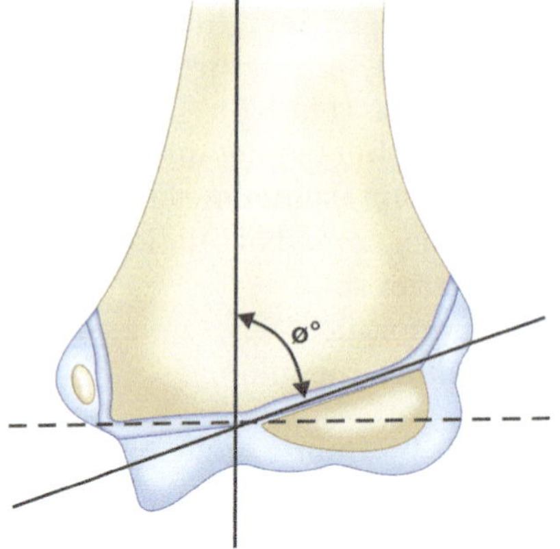

Fig. 6.7: Baumann angle.

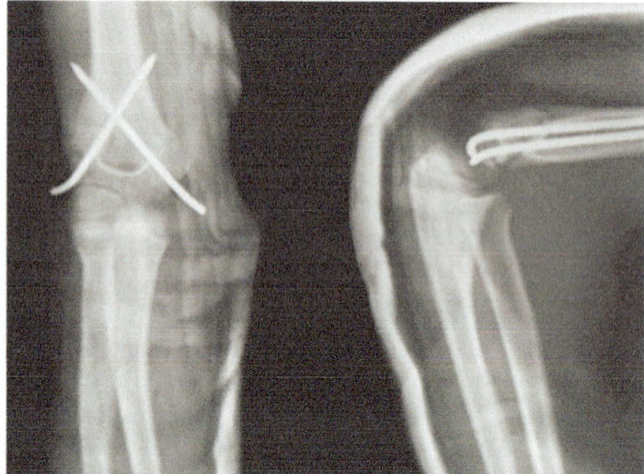

Fig. 6.8: Fracture reduction and K-wire fixation.

Ans. This is an angle subtended between following two lines: (1) long axis of humeral diaphysis and (2) tangent to lateral physis (Fig. 6.7). This angle measures between 64° and 81° (average 72°). It accesses the adequacy of reduction in coronal plane for axial deformity.

Q. What are the treatment methods for supracondylar fracture?

Ans. These are as:
- Conservative: Close reduction and above elbow slab for 4 weeks.
- Surgical: Close or open reduction and pinning (K-wire fixation) (Fig. 6.8).

Q. What are the complications of supracondylar fracture?

Ans. These are as:
- Early complication:
  - Compartment syndrome
  - Neurological injury
  - Vascular injury (brachial artery)
- Late complication:
  - Malunion (varus or valgus)
  - Volkmann ischemic contracture
  - Myositis ossificans (due to massage, brachialis is most commonly involved muscle)
  - Nerve entrapment in healed callus (Metev sign).

EXTENSION AND FLEXION TYPE OF SUPRACONDYLAR FRACTURE HUMERUS (TABLE 6.1)

Table 6.1: Comparison between extension and flexion type of supracondylar fracture humerus.

	Extension type (Fig. 6.9)	Flexion type (Fig. 6.10)
Mechanism of injury	Fall in outstretched hand with extended elbow and forearm in pronated attitude	Fall on olecranon
Incidence	97%	3%
Classification of fracture	Gartland classification • Type I: Undisplaced • Type II: Displaced with intact posterior cortex • Type III: Completely displaced	• Type I: Undisplaced • Type II: Displaced with intact anterior cortex • Type III: Completely displaced
Nerve involvement	• Posteromedial displacement: Radial nerve (commonest displacement but incidence of nerve involvement is less) • Posterolateral displacement: Anterior interosseous nerve > median nerve (more incidence)	• Ulnar nerve
Treatment	• Type I: Above elbow POP slab in 90° flexion and supinated forearm • Type II: Close reduction and above elbow POP slab in hyperflexion at elbow with pronated forearm (in posteromedial displacement) or supinated forearm (in posterolateral displacement) • Type III: Closed or open reduction with K-wire pinning **Note:** Hyperflexion at elbow provide internal splintage of triceps at fracture site	• Reduction either closed or open followed by pinning is mainstay of treatment. Sometimes closed reduction and above elbow slab in extension is also applicable.

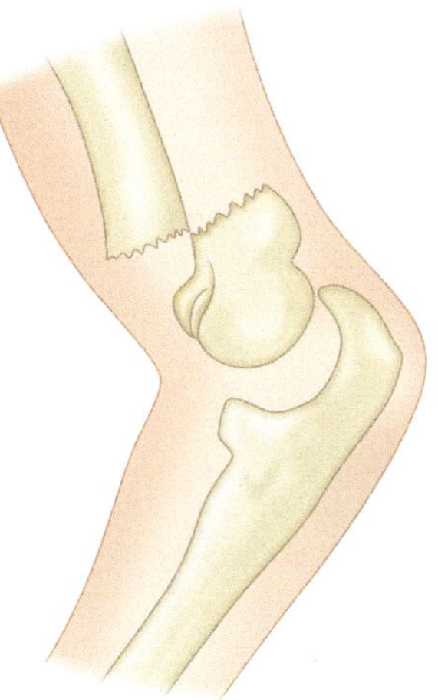

Fig. 6.9: Extension type.

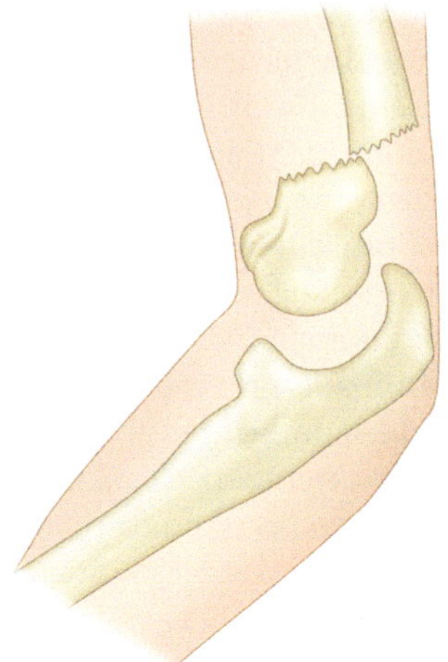

Fig. 6.10: Flexion type.

Chapter

7

Cubitus Valgus Deformity at Elbow (Nonunion Fracture Lateral Condyle Humerus)

CASE PRESENTATION

- **History**: My patient, a 18-year-old girl, presented with complaint of deformity at her left elbow for last 2 years. She fell down by the side of road and sustained injury in her left elbow. She took treatment locally with a bonesetter in the form of above elbow cast for 2 months. After removal of cast she noticed a deformity and some stiffness at her affected elbow. She further took some physiotherapy that cured her stiffness but deformity persisted. For last few months she noticed that her deformity is progressing and it became her concern for consultation. There is no history of any fever, weight loss, or multiple joint pain.
- **Examination**: Patient is of average built and of average nutrition. Her general physical and systemic examination is within normal limit. Local examination revealed that there is an outward deviation of her forearm (cubitus valgus) and a prominence over medial aspect of elbow. Three bony point relationship is altered. The lateral supracondylar ridge is thickened and irregular. There is palpable bony mass at the lower end of lateral supracondylar ridge which is showing some painless and free mobility. The range of motion at elbow is near normal. Carrying angle is also increased. There is no upper limb length discrepancy. Distal neurovascular examination is also normal.

VIVA VOCE FROM CASE

Q. What is your case?

Ans. This is a case of cubitus valgus deformity at elbow following nonunion fracture lateral condyle of humerus (Fig. 7.1).

Q. Define cubitus valgus?

Ans. It is defined as abnormal outward deviation of long axis of forearm in relation to arm when elbow is fully extended and supinated. *Do not use this term if elbow is not fully extended.*

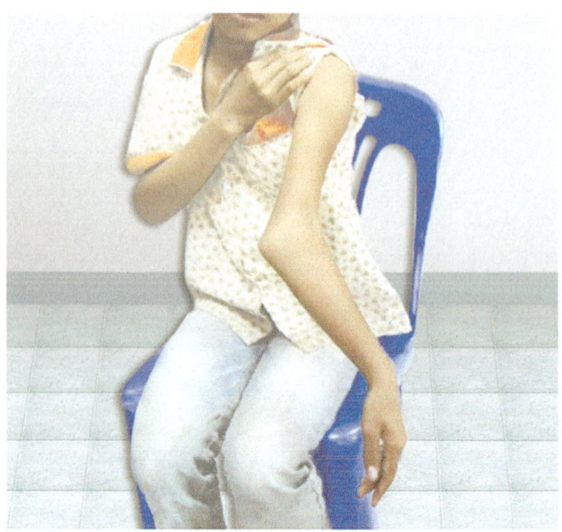

Fig. 7.1: A case of cubitus valgus deformity.

Q. Is this progressive deformity and why?

Ans. Yes. The damage of lateral physis and overgrowth of medial physis is responsible for its progression.

Different causes of cubitus valgus deformity.

- Congenital dislocation of radial head
- Nonunion fracture lateral condyle humerus
- Monteggia fracture dislocation
- Neglected pulled elbow
- Malunited radial neck fracture

Q. Why you say that this deformity is due to nonunion of fracture lateral condyle?

Ans. The points favoring this statement are as follows:
- History of trauma in past.
- Treatment given in form of above elbow cast.
- Thickening of lateral supracondylar ridge.
- Painless abnormal mobility with crepitus at lateral condyle (sometime painful).
- Three bony point relationship is disturbed.
- Increased carrying angle (Fig. 7.2).

Carrying angle at elbow

- There is an angle between long axis of arm and forearm when elbow is fully extended and supinated, this is called carrying angle. It disappears when elbow is pronated or flexed. It provides the pelvic clearance in female.
- Normal value:
  - Male: 5–10°
  - Female: 15–20°.
- Increased in carrying angle is called valgus.
- Decrease, neutralization or reversal of carrying angle is called varus.
- Sometimes neutralization of carrying angle is also called cubitus rectus.

Q. Any other clinical finding you like to search in this case?

Ans. I will look for tardy ulnar palsy (neurological examination).

Q. What investigation you like to get in this case?

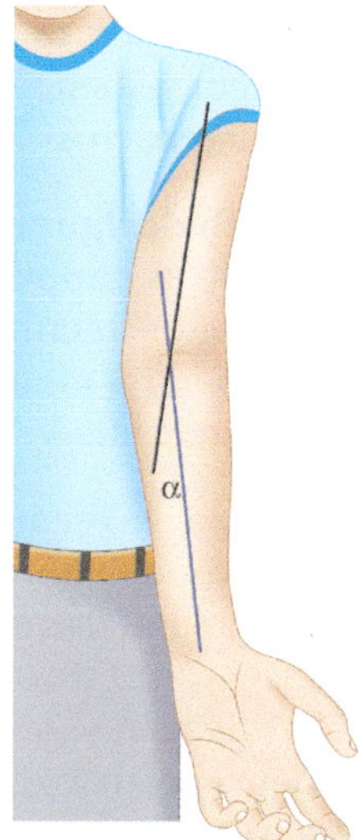

Fig. 7.2: Carrying angle.

Ans. X-ray of the elbow AP and lateral view (Fig. 7.3).
- Cubitus valgus deformity
- A displaced free fracture fragment of lateral condyle.

Q. What is your treatment plan?

Ans. I will go for in situ fixation of fracture fragment and bone grafting.

Q. What is meant by in situ fixation and what is its advantage?

Ans. Fixation of fracture fragment in displaced position without mobilizing it into a

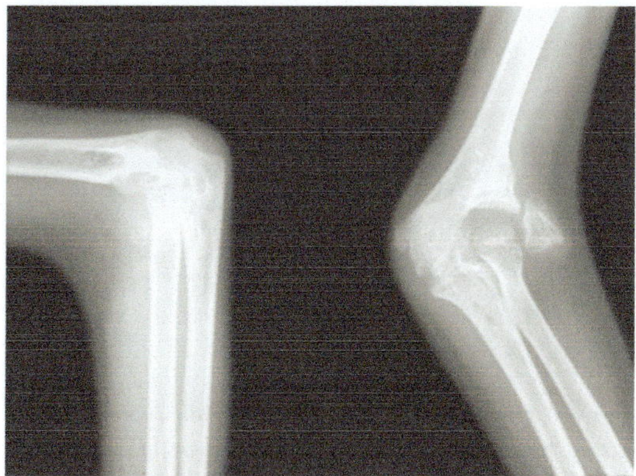

Fig. 7.3: X-ray of cubitus varus deformity.

reduced position is called in situ fixation (Fig. 7.4). It maintain the vascularity of displaced fragment hence minimizes the risk of avascular necrosis.

Q. When you will designate the fracture lateral condyle as nonunion?

Ans. If the duration of fracture has crossed the time period of 3 months, nonunion is said to be established.

Q. Why fracture lateral condyle of humerus is prone to nonunion?

Ans. The reasons behind this are as:
- Continuous traction of common extensor origin.
- Great chances of damage to vascularity of lateral condyle.
- Displacement and rotation of fracture fragment makes it unopposed to humeral fracture surface.

Q. Why valgus is of so much concern in nonunion lateral condyle fracture?

Ans. Because progressive valgus may lead to tardy ulnar palsy.

Q. What is tardy ulnar palsy?

Ans. As name suggest, tardy means late. Basically it is friction neuritis of ulnar nerve due progressive valgus at elbow.

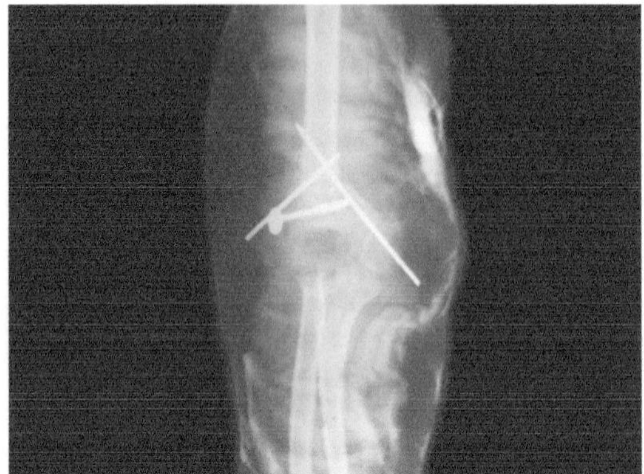

Fig. 7.4: In situ fixation of lateral condyle nonunion along with supracondylar osteotomy.

It is characterized by tingling and numbness in ulnar aspect of hand and fingers (small and ring). This might shows positive tests for ulnar nerve paresis.

Q. Why fracture fragment of lateral condyle appears smaller in radiograph than its original size?

Ans. As the most part of lateral condyle is articular and made up of hyaline cartilage; hence, it remains radiolucent in X-ray and appear smaller than its original size.

Q. What are the absolute indications of surgery in nonunion fracture lateral condyle?

Ans. These are as:
- Continuous pain
- Progressive valgus deformity
- Instability
- Tardy ulnar palsy.

Different treatment modalities in nonunion lateral condyle fracture.
- Open reduction and internal fixation with bone grafting
- In situ fixation and bone grafting
- Supracondylar valgus correcting osteotomy
- Anterior transposition of ulnar nerve

Q. Is there any indication of open reduction and fixation of fracture fragment in lateral condyle nonunion cases?

Ans. Yes, if there is minimal displacement (< 1 cm) of fracture fragment, open reduction, and internal fixation is advisable along with bone grafting.

Q. How fixation works in lateral condyle nonunion?

Ans. It acts in following ways:
- It makes elbow painless.
- It establishes lateral column hence stop the progression of valgus.
- It minimizes the chance of tardy ulnar palsy.

Q. What is indication of osteotomy in nonunion lateral condyle fracture?

Ans. When valgus deformity is more than 20°, a supracondylar osteotomy is indicated. It may be of following type: (1) lateral open-wedge osteotomy, (2) medial closed-wedge osteotomy, and (3) step-cut osteotomy.

Q. What is anterior transposition and when it is advisable?

Ans. Normally ulnar nerve runs in posterior aspect of medial epicondyle of humerus in an ulnar groove. After neurolysis nerve is placed anterior to medial epicondyle (subcutaneous or submuscular plane); procedure is called anterior transposition. This is mandatory if there is any sign of friction neuritis of ulnar nerve in case of lateral condyle nonunion. Most orthopedician have common consensus to do anterior transposition in all surgically treated cases due to fear of future tardy ulnar palsy under effect of progressive valgus deformity.

COMPARATIVE STUDY OF LATERAL AND MEDIAL CONDYLE OF FRACTURE HUMERUS (TABLE 7.1)

Table 7.1: Comparative study of lateral and medial condyle of fracture humerus.

	Lateral condyle fracture (Fig. 7.5)	Medial condyle fracture (Fig. 7.6)
Mechanism of injury	Fall in outstretched hand with varus stress on extended elbow	Fall in outstretched hand with valgus strain and direct trauma
Age group	More common in children	More common in adolescent
Fracture classification	• Milch Type I: Fracture line passes through capitotrochlear groove (Salter-Harris type IV) • Milch Type II: Fracture line extends into apex of trochlear groove. (Salter-Harris type II)	• Milch Type I: Fracture line passes through apex of trochlear groove (Salter-Harris type II) • Milch Type II: Fracture line passes through capitotrochlear groove (Salter-Harris type IV)
Displacement	More prone	Less prone
Treatment	• Conservative: For undisplaced fracture, above elbow cast for 6 weeks • Surgery: For displaced fracture, open reduction and internal fixation with K-wire or 4 mm cancellous screw	• Conservative: For undisplaced fracture, above elbow cast for 4 weeks • Surgery: For unstable displaced fracture, open reduction and internal fixation with K-wire or 4 mm cancellous screw
Complication	• Nonunion • Cubitus valgus due to growth arrest (tardy ulnar palsy) • Avascular necrosis and elbow osteoarthritis	• Delayed union • Cubitus varus • Ulnar nerve injury

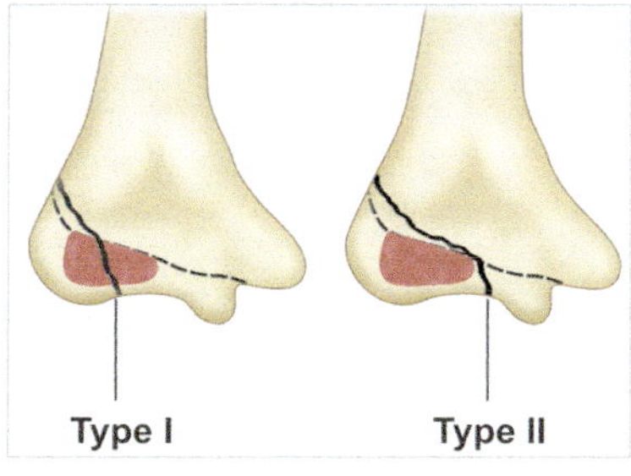

Fig. 7.5: Fracture pattern of lateral condyle.

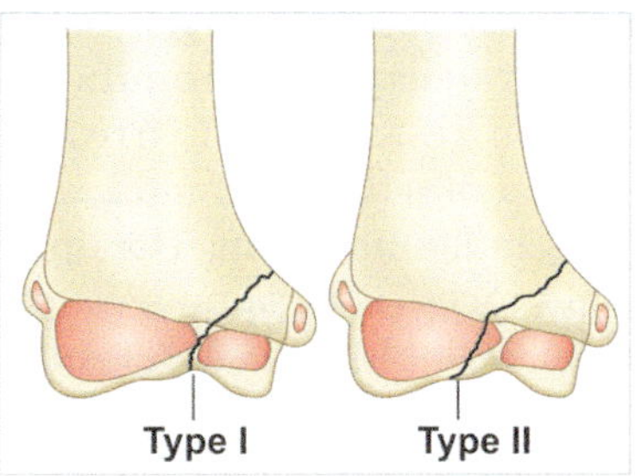

Fig. 7.6: Fracture pattern of medial condyle.

Chapter

8

Malunited Colles' Fracture

CASE PRESENTATION

- **History**: My patient, a 55-year-old lady presented with complaint of deformity at her right wrist for last 5 months. She fell down on a slippery surface with her outstretched hand. She sustained an injury in her left wrist that produces a peculiar attitude of her hand. She was carried to a local bonesetter who applied some bandaging for 4 weeks. After removal of bandaging patient noticed a deformity in her left hand which was associated with pain and stiffness. For this she took some physiotherapy and her stiffness was resolved partially but deformity and pain persisted. There is no history of any fever, weight loss, or multiple joint pain.
- **Examination**: Patient is of average built and of average nutrition. Her general physical and systemic examination is within normal limit. Local examination showed an outward deviation of hand (manus valgus) with prominent ulnar styloid process. There is irregularity at lower end of radius and mild tenderness at distal radioulnar joint. The tip of radial styloid process is at same level of the tip of ulnar styloid process. All movement, such as palmar flexion, dorsiflexion, supination, and pronation are restricted. There is no limb length discrepancy. Distal neurovascular examination is also normal.

VIVA VOCE FROM CASE

Q. What is your case?

Ans. This is a case of right-sided malunited Colles' fracture (Fig. 8.1).

Q. What deformity you are getting at wrist?

Ans. Manus valgus deformity.

Two deformity at wrist of attention.

- Madelung deformity
- Malunited Colles' fracture.

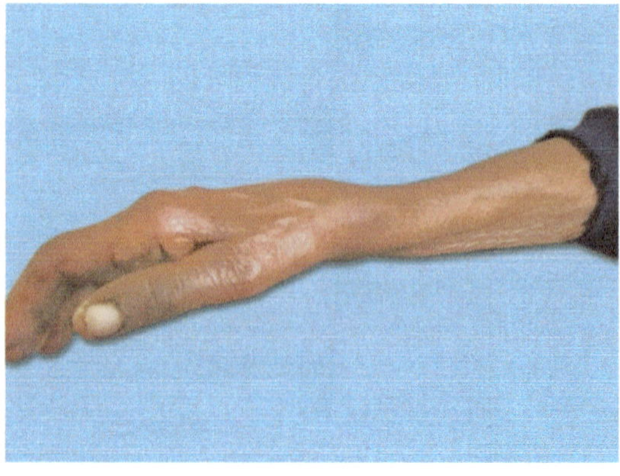

Fig. 8.1: A case of malunited Colles' fracture.

Q. Why you say that this deformity is due to malunited Colles' fracture?

Ans. The points favoring this statement are as follows:
- History of trauma in past.
- Treatment history by a bone setter in form of bandaging.
- Peculiar deformity at wrist (manus valgus).
- Irregularity at lower end of radius.
- Tenderness at distal radioulnar joint.
- Tip of radial styloid process is at same level of the tip of ulnar styloid process (Fig. 8.2).
- Range of motion at wrist is restricted.

Correlation between tip of radial styloid process and tip of ulnar styloid process.
- Normally the tip of radial styloid process lies approximately 1 cm (11–12 mm) distal to the tip of ulnar styloid process.
- This difference is also known as radial height.
- After Colles' fracture, both styloid processes come at same level or tip of radial styloid process goes higher due to proximal impaction of fracture fragment.

Q. Any other clinical finding you like to search in this case?

Ans. I will try to search any involvement of **distal radioulnar joint**. It could be identified by two ways:

1. Restricted and painful pronation and supination.
2. Instability at distal radioulnar joint (ballottment of ulnar head antero-posteriorly—piano-key sign).

Q. What investigation you like to get in this case?

Ans. X-ray of the wrist, AP and lateral view (Fig. 8.3).
- Manus valgus deformity
- Healed fracture (in healing fracture there is presence of varying amount of callus)
- Both radial and ulnar styloid processes tips are at same level.

Q. What is your treatment plan?

Ans. Here the main problem is pain and stiffness and there is no functional loss in wrist and hand, hence I will go for conservative treatment in form of:
- Analgesics
- Activity restriction like lifting heavy weight, etc.
- Physiotherapy and electrotherapy (ultrasound) for improvement of wrist movement and hand function.

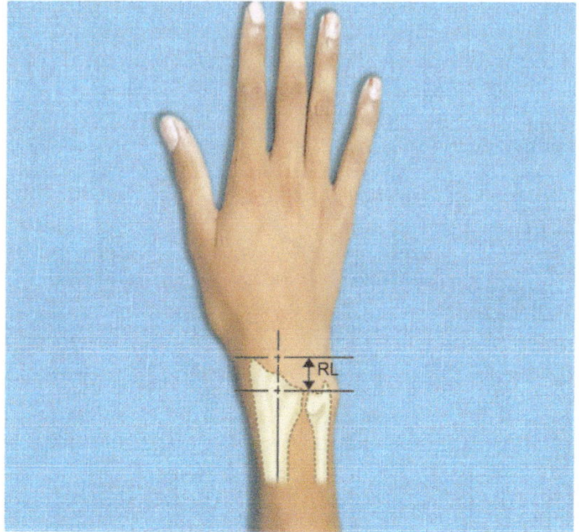

Fig. 8.2: Relationship between radial and ulnar styloid process.

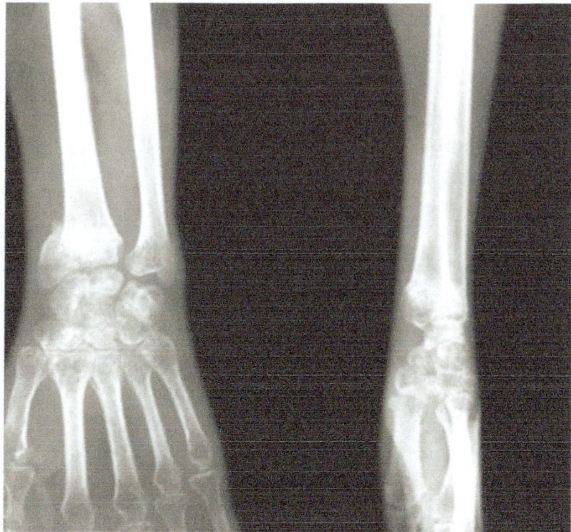

Fig. 8.3: X-ray of malunited Colles' fracture.

Q. About which function of hand you are talking about?

Ans. I am quoting about basic functions of hands; these are (Fig. 8.4):
- Grip
- Hook
- Pinch.

Q. What is Colles' fracture?

Ans. It is a fracture at distal end of radius within 2 cm of wrist joint. It is named in respect of sir Abraham Colles from Ireland.

Q. What is mechanism for Colles' fracture?

Ans. A fall in outstretched hand with wrist in slight dorsiflexion mode. Here a bending force acts at corticocancellous junction and fracture happen.

Q. Is there any relation between age and sex with this fracture?

Ans. Yes, it is common in elderly female with osteoporotic bone mainly after menopause.

Q. What special deformity you get at wrist after Colles' fracture?

Ans. It is known as dinner fork deformity (Fig. 8.5).

Q. What are different injuries associated with fracture distal radius?

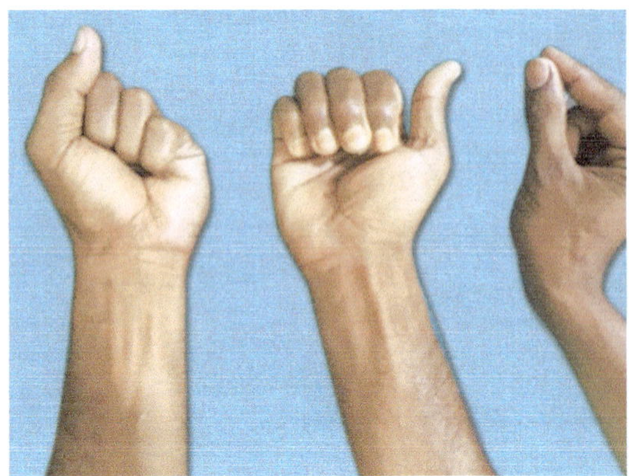

Fig. 8.4: Grip, hook, and pinch.

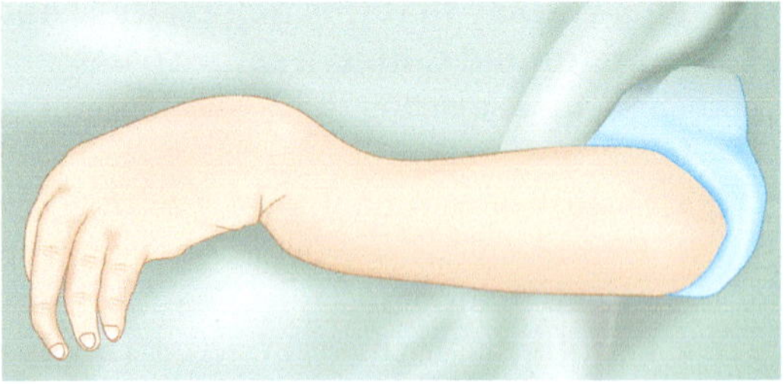

Fig. 8.5: Dinner fork deformity.

Ans. These are as:
- Fracture distal ulna
- Fracture ulnar styloid process
- Distal radioulnar joint injury.

Q. What are the classical displacements you get in radiographs of Colles' fracture?

Ans. These are as (Fig. 8.6):
- Lateral tilt
- Lateral shift
- Dorsal tilt
- Dorsal shift
- Proximal impaction
- Supination.

Q. How will you treat this fracture?

Ans. I will go for close reduction and Colles' cast application.

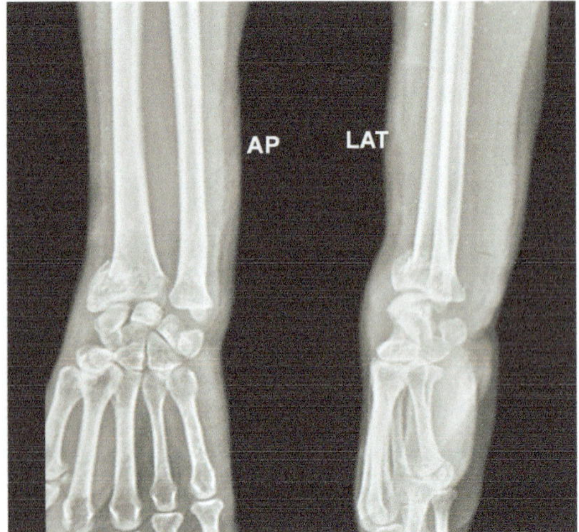

Fig. 8.6: Colles' fracture showing displacements in AP and lateral view.

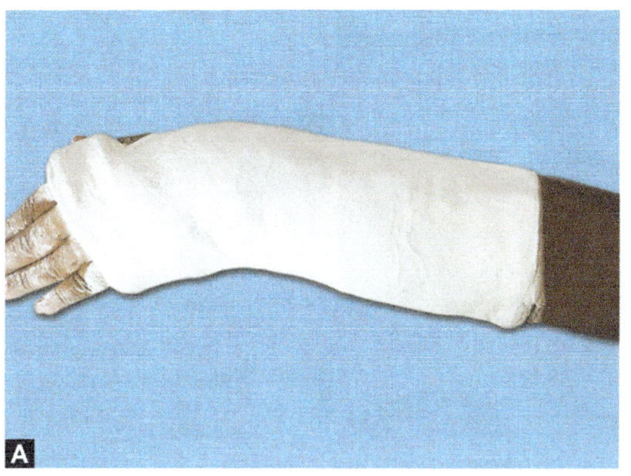

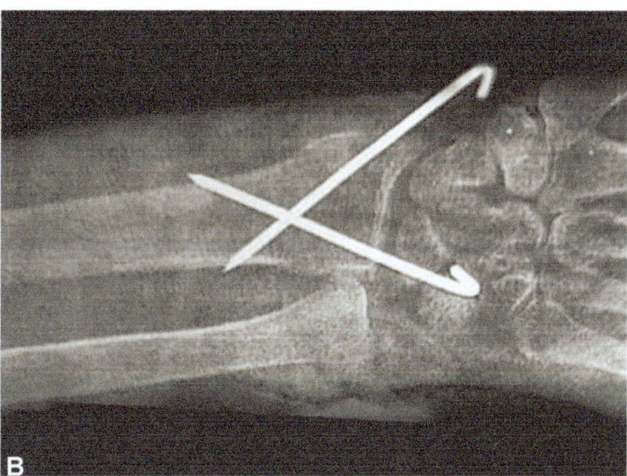

Figs. 8.7A and B: A. Colles' cast and; B. Colles' fracture fixed with K-wire.

Q. What is Colles' cast?

Ans. Colles' cast is a below elbow cast with a special position to counteract the displacements of Colles' fractures.

- Forearm position: Pronated
- Palmar flexion
- Ulnar deviation.

Note: Traction forces reduce the proximal impaction and maintain radial height.

Q. Is there any indication of surgical fixation in Colles' fracture?

Ans. Yes. If there is unacceptable or unstable reduction, fracture should be fixed with K-wire or distal radius plate (Figs. 8.7A and B).

Q. What are the complications of Colles' fracture?

Ans. These are as:

- Stiffness of wrist and hand
- Malunion (manus valgus)
- Carpal tunnel syndrome
- Reflex sympathetic dystrophy
- Distal radioulnar joint instability
- Rupture of extensor pollicis longus
- Shoulder hand syndrome (due to cast application).

OVERVIEW OF FRACTURE AROUND DISTAL RADIUS (FIGS. 8.8 TO 8.10)

Smith Fracture (Fig. 8.8)	Barton Fracture (Fig. 8.9)	Chauffeur Fracture (Fig. 8.10)
• Reverse of Colles' fracture is called smith fracture. • Mechanism: Fall on dorsum of wrist in palmar flexion attitude. • Displacement: Volar tilt and volar shift. • Deformity: Garden spade deformity. • Treatment: Close reduction and above elbow cast. In unstable reduction cases surgical fixation is done with K-wires or distal radius plate.	• Intra-articular vertical split fracture of distal radius in coronal plane extending from joint to dorsal cortex (dorsal Barton) or ventral cortex (volar Barton). • Mechanism: Fall on outstretched hand under effect of shearing forces. • Displacement: Displacement of entire carpals bones with dorsal fragment. • Treatment: Close reduction and below elbow cast with wrist palmar flexion and dorsiflexion. Unstable reduction cases are surgically fixed with distal radius plating.	• Intra-articular radial styloid fracture. • It occurs due to backfire of handle during genset starting. • Treated by a below elbow cast in Colles' position.

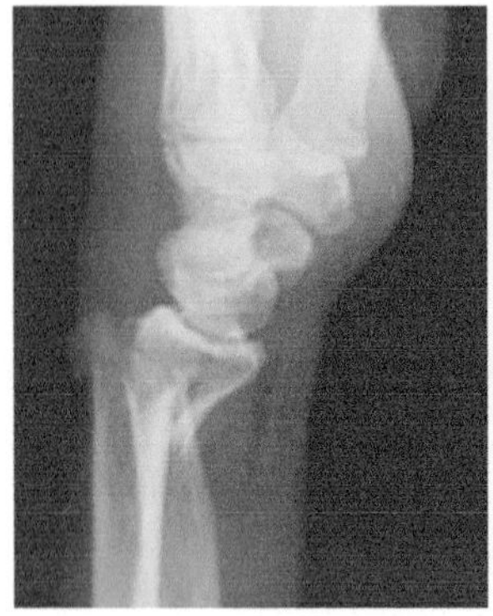

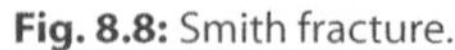

Fig. 8.8: Smith fracture.

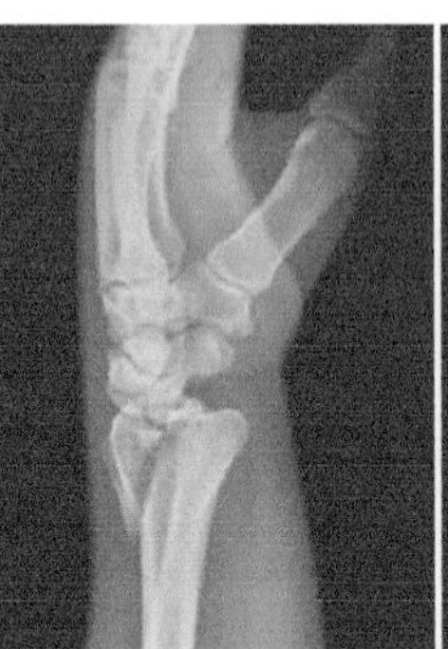

Fig. 8.9: Dorsal and volar Barton fracture.

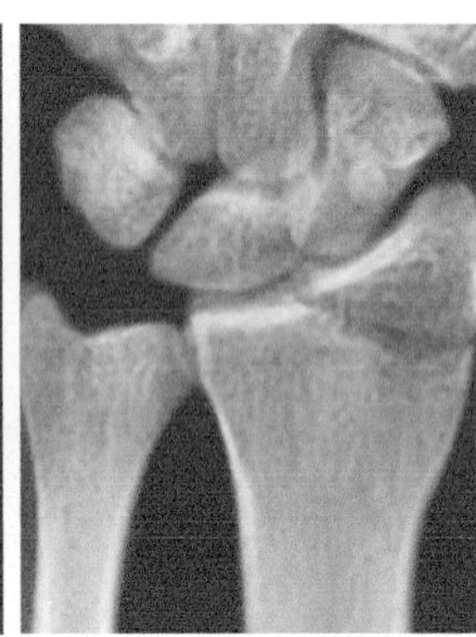

Fig. 8.10: Chauffeur fracture.

Chapter

9

Congenital Clubfoot

CASE PRESENTATION

- **History**: The parents of a 7-month-old child presented with complaint of a peculiar deformity in their kid's right foot. This deformity is present by birth, nonprogressive, painless, and not associated with any other congenital anomalies. His prenatal, perinatal, and postnatal history is uneventful. His developmental milestones are also normal. His vaccinations are also up-to-date. There is no history of any trauma, fever, and diarrhea.
- **Examination**: General health of child is good. Examination of foot revealed an equinovarus deformity in his foot. There equines in ankle, varus in heel, adduction in forefoot, and cavus in midfoot. Foot appears to be smaller in comparison to other side. Calf is atrophied with prominent creases over heel and medial border. Distal neurovascular examination is also normal. Examination of neck, spine, and hip is also normal.

VIVA VOCE FROM CASE

Q. What is your case?

Ans. This is a case of congenital idiopathic talipes equinovarus (CTEV) (Fig. 9.1).

Q. What is literal meaning of talipes and equinus?

Ans. Talipes is composed of two words; talus and pes (foot) it means walking on talus. Equinus means horse as their ankle appears to be in plantar flexion.

Q. Why you say that it is congenital and idiopathic?

Ans. Because deformity is present since birth hence congenital and no other cause was found responsible for deformity that is why idiopathic (Table 9.1).

Q. What are the deformities in CTEV?

Ans. These are as:

- Equinus at ankle (tibiotalar joint)
- Heel varus at subtalar joint (talocalcaneal)

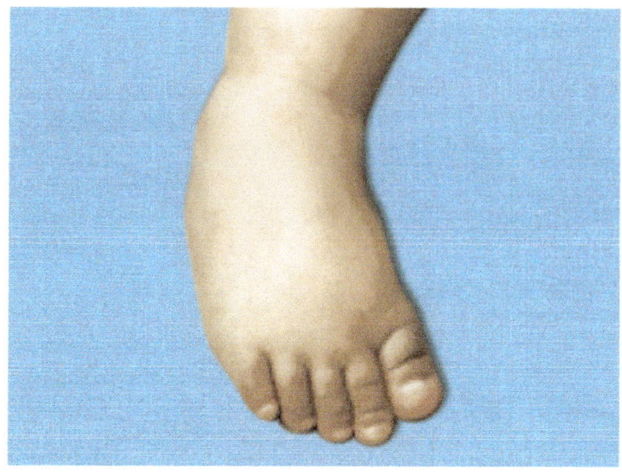

Fig. 9.1: A case of clubfoot.

Table 9.1: Causes of CTEV.

Congenital	Acquired
• Idiopathic • Spina bifida • Arthrogryposis multiplex congenita (multiple contractures in limb)	• Cerebral palsy • Postpolio palsy • Post-leprosy stigmata • Volkmann ischemic contractures • Postburn contractures

- Forefoot adduction at midtarsal joint (talonavicular and calcaneocuboid)
- Midfoot cavus (exaggeration of longitudinal arch due to forefoot pronation).

Q. What are the special features of a clubfoot?

Ans. These are as:
- A relatively small foot.
- Medial rotation of foot so that sole facing inward and downward.
- A small heel.
- Calf atrophy of varying degree.
- Prominent creases in medial side of foot, sole of foot, and above the heel.
- Lateral border of foot longer than medial border.
- Palpable talus head due to its lateral subluxation.
- Callosities over anterorlateral part of foot in walking child.

Q. Any other associative finding you like to search in this case?

Ans. I will search for other intrauterine packaging defects like:
- Torticollis in neck
- Developmental dysplasia in hip.

Q. How can you say that it is flexible or rigid clubfoot?

Ans. I can say this by a simple test. If all the deformities are correctible by passive manipulation it is flexible and if not correctible then that is of rigid variety.

Q. What is the role of radiologic investigation in clubfoot?

Ans. For all practical purposes idiopathic clubfoot need not any investigation for planning of their treatment.
- Plain radiographs are useful to see the maturity status of bone.
- MRI to explore the involvement of cord in spina bifida.

Q. How will you manage your case?

Ans. I will go for serial manipulation and CTEV casting.

Q. What is CTEV cast?

Ans. It is a special type of above knee casting where knee is maintained in flexed position (Fig. 9.2).

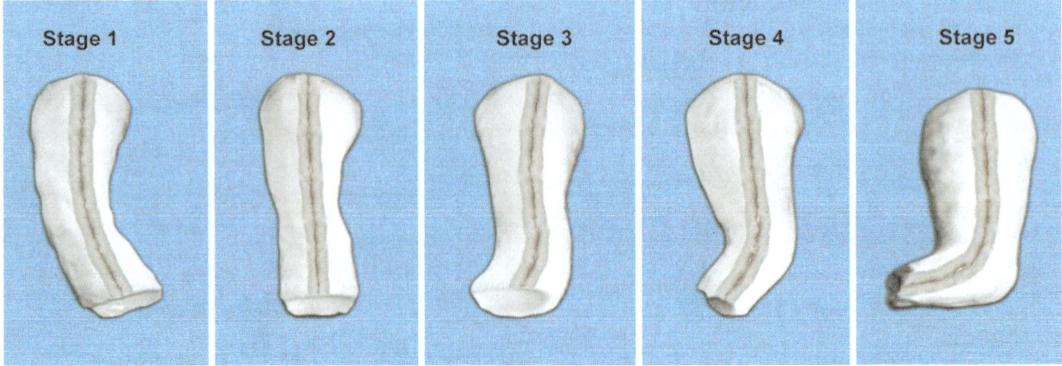

Fig. 9.2: CTEV casting.

Q. What is the order of deformity correction?

Ans. The order of correction is as: (1) **c**avus (2) forefoot **a**dduction and **v**arus, and (3) **e**quinus (CAVE).

Q. What will happen if you will not follow this order of correction?

Ans. The foot will converted into rocker bottom foot having a convex sole.

Q. What are the advantages of flexed knee position?

Ans. It acts as follows:
- Relaxes the gastrocnemius pull hence helpful in equinus correction.
- Prevent slippage of cast from child leg.
- Provide support to plaster bandages during correction of varus deformity.

Q. Which technique of casting is famous nowadays and why?

Ans. The **Ponseti** (Ignacio Ponseti) method of manipulation and casting is very famous and widely accepted nowadays. Its reasons are as:
- Easy method of correction.
- Rapid correction possible.
- Provide a constant correction (Table 9.2.)

Table 9.2: Difference between Ponseti method and Kite method.

	Ponseti method	Kite method
Fulcrum for correction	Talar head	Calcaneocuboid joint
Cavus correction	First to correct	No detailing
Tenotomy for equines correction	For residual equines	Not mentioned
Order of correction	One by one (CAVE)	All at a time
Rocker bottom foot	Less chances	More chances

Q. At what age one can start the correction of deformity?

Ans. We should start the treatment as early as possible. In neonates we can wait for 4–6 weeks for getting of some skin maturity.

Q. Will you advise anything to mother for these waiting period?

Ans. Yes, I will explain her, how to correct these deformity passively especially when the child is on feed. This is called mother manipulation.

Q. What are the protocols of Ponseti technique of casting?

Ans. These are as:
- Place: Outpatient procedure
- Manipulation time: 2 or 3 minutes manipulation before casting
- Total number of cast: 5–7, sometimes needed more
- Duration between two cast: 5–7 days
- First 2 or 3 cast: For correction of cavus (pronated forefoot is supinated by elevating the first ray)
- Successive cast: For correction of forefoot adduction, heel varus, and equinus.

Q. What are the instructions to mother before leaving the plaster room?

Ans. These are as:
- Aware about any skin discoloration, it must be always pink.
- Keep baby casted foot away from water or other liquid.

Q. Is there any place of surgery in Ponseti method?

Ans. Yes, residual or uncorrected equines is corrected by percutaneous tenotomy of tendoachilles (Fig. 9.3).

Q. When you decide to end the manipulation and casting?

Ans. We look for two things:
- Ankle dorsiflexion: 10–15°
- Foot abduction: 60–70°

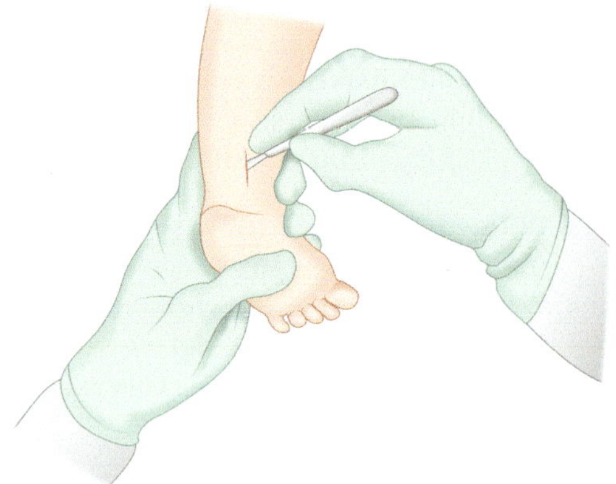

Fig. 9.3: Percutaneous tenotomy of tendoachilles.

Q. What you do next once you get the correction of deformed foot and why?

Ans. After correction of deformity, I will maintain the correction in foot splints. Otherwise there will be great chances of recurrence of deformities.

Q. What splint you prefer before walking period (1 year) of child?

Ans. **Dennis Brown** (DB) splint (Fig. 9.4) or Steinbeck abduction brace.

Q. What are the special features of DB splint?

Ans. It is a dynamic splint as child kicks off its one side of splint, another foot is dorsiflexed and everted. It has following components.

- A bar equal to the width of shoulder of child.
- A pair of CTEV shoes attached at the ends of bar.
- Winged nuts to allow abduction of each foot.

Q. What is the wearing schedule of DB splint?

Ans. These are:

- Apply splint immediately after removal of last cast.
- Wear it for 23 hours in day and rest 1 hour is left for foot caring and mother manipulation.

Q. What splint you recommend for walking child?

Ans. I will recommend CTEV shoes (Fig. 9.5).

Q. What are the features of a CTEV shoe?

Ans. These are as:

- No heel
- Straight medial border
- Raised lateral border.

Q. Up to what age you will follow such child?

Ans. The child should be followed up to 4 years of age.

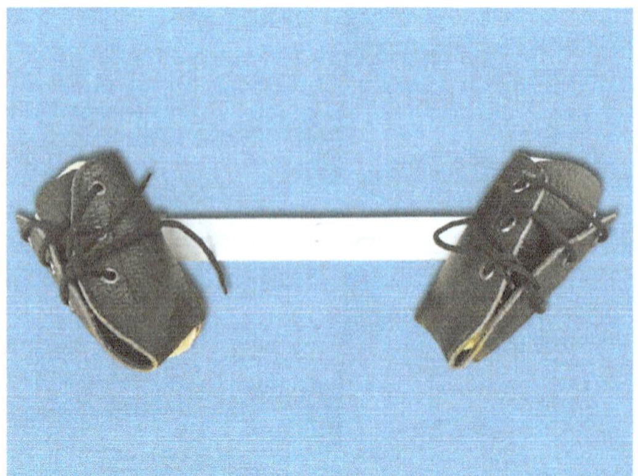

Fig. 9.4: Dennis Brown splint.

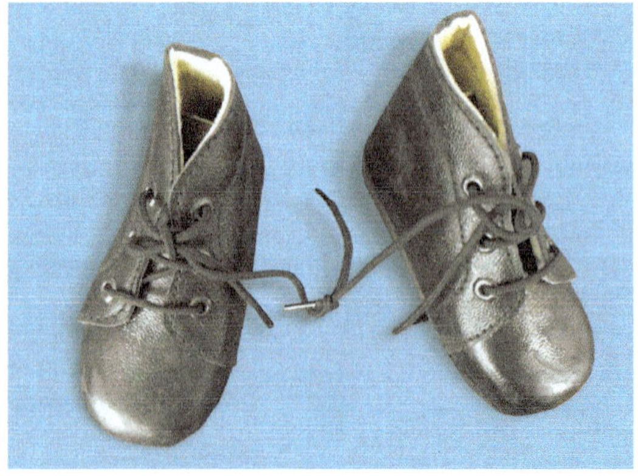

Fig. 9.5: CTEV shoes.

Different terminologies regarding treatment of clubfoot.

- Complete treatment means full correction of all deformities by serial casting along with completeness of splint wearing schedule.
- Fresh cases/untreated: Child visited to clinician before walking age (1 year) without any treatment.
- Neglected: Child visited to clinician after walking age (1 year) without any treatment.
- Recurrence: Reappearance of any deformity during treatment.
- Relapsed: Reappearance of a deformity after completion of treatment schedule.
- Resistant: Not possible to correct the deformity by any means. It happens mainly due to inappropriate technique.

Q. Which deformity commonly recurs?

Ans. Equinus.

Q. In what sense neuroparalytic clubfoot are different from idiopathic clubfoot?

Ans. These are as:

- Etiological conditions are spina bifida, cerebral palsy, postpolio residual paralysis, etc.
- Muscle imbalance is cause of deformity.
- Serial manipulation and casting is not sufficient.
- Soft tissue procedure (release of contracture and tendon transfer) and bony procedure (osteotomy and arthrodesis) are used in combination.

IDIOPATHIC CLUBFOOT AT A GLANCE (TABLE 9.3)

Table 9.3: Idiopathic clubfoot.

Incidence	1 per 1,000 birth			
Sex preponderance	Male: female—2:1			
Genetics	Multifactorial inheritance			
Laterality	Bilateral in 50% cases, R > L			
Etiological factors	1. Fetal theory: Intrauterine packaging defect 2. Germ plasm theory: Defect in talar germ plasm 3. Myogenic theory: Myoblast contraction leading to fibrosis 4. Neurogenic theory: Increased ratio of type 1 fibers in calf muscle 5. Vascular theory: Hypotrophied anterior tibial vasculature			
Pathoanatomy	1. Navicular subluxation medially over head of tatuls 2. Talar head denuded and becomes prominent anterolaterally 3. Medial and internal rotation of whole foot			
Severity grading (**Pirani** scoring)		Mild (0)	Moderate (0.5)	Severe (1)
	Posterior crease	Multiple fine creases	One or two deep creases	Deep creases changes the contour of arch
	Empty heel	Calcaneal tuberosity easily palpable	Difficult palpation of calcaneal tuberosity	Calcaneal tuberosity not palpable
	Equinus rigidity	Normal ankle dorsiflexion	Ankle dorsiflexion beyond normal but not fully	Can not dorsiflex up to neutral
	Lateral border	Straight	Mild distal curve	Proximal curve (calcaneocuboid joint)
	Head of talus	Lateral talar head can not felt	Lateral head less palpable	Lateral talar head easily palpable

Contd...

Contd...

	Medial crease	Multiple fine creases	One or two deep creases	Deep creases changes the contour of arches
	Foot should be kept in maximum correction during assessment of posteromedial creases			
Radiological angles	Angle	Normal value	Change in CTEV	Inference
	Tibiocalcaneal angle: Lateral view	10–40°	Decreased	Equinus
	Talocalcaneal angle: AP view Lateral view	30–55° 25–50°	Decreased	Varus
	Talo-first metatarsal angle: Lateral view	5–15°	Negative	Forefoot adduction
Surgical treatment indication	If deformities are not correctable with serial manipulation and casting.			
Soft tissue release surgery: Turco procedure Age: 1–3 years		Posterior structures	Medial structures	
	Joint	Ankle joint capsule Subtalar joint capsule Tibiofibular joint	Ankle joint capsule Subtalar joint capsule Talonavicular joint capsule	
	Tendon	Tendoachilles Z-plasty	Tibialis posterior lengthening FDL lengthening FHL lengthening	
	Ligaments	Deltoid ligament Talonavicular (spring ligament)	Posterior talofibular Calcaneofibular	
Osteotomy Age: After 4 years, because at this age talar bones are almost cartilaginous, hence hamper the growth of bones	1. **Dwyer** osteotomy: Lateral closed wedge calcaneal osteotomy for heel varus 2. **Dillwyn Evans** osteotomy: Calcaneocuboid fusion for correction of forefoot adduction 3. **Davis** wedge tarsectomy: Anterolateral dorsal wedge osteotomy of tarsal bones for correction of forefoot adduction. Preferred age is in between 8 years and 11 years			
Arthrodesis Age: After 13 year, because at this period maturation of tarsals started. Hence, chances of nonunion are minimal	Joint arthrodesis are: 1. Talocalcaneal 2. Talonavicular 3. Calcaneocuboid			
JESS and Ilizarov	Joshi external stabilization system (JESS) are used mainly in less sever deformity where Ilizarov should apply in severe deformity.			

Chapter

10

Genu Varus Deformity at Knee (Osteoarthritis Knee)

CASE PRESENTATION

- **History**: My patient, a 50-year-old man presented with complaint of pain in his both knees from last 10 years. Pain is of gradual onset, that aggravates with prolonged walking, squatting and stairs riding. It relieves with rest and some analgesics. Pain is associated with a progressive deformity so much so that his right leg is bowing towards midline of the body. There is no history of any previous trauma, fever, weight loss, multiple joints pain, and morning stiffness.
- **Examination**: Patient is of heavy built. His general physical and systemic examination is within normal limit. Local examination revealed a mild genu varus deformity in right knee. There are bilateral joint line tenderness, synovial thickening, and crepitus in both knees. The range of motion of both knee are decreased terminally but painful throughout the movement. There is no mediolateral instability. There is no limb length discrepancy. Distal neurovascular examination is also normal.

VIVA VOCE FROM CASE

Q. What is your diagnosis?

Ans. This is a case of genu varus deformity of knee due to osteoarthritis of knee (Fig. 10.1).

Q. What do you mean by genu varus?

Ans. Genu varus is defined as inward deviation of long axis of leg in relation to thigh when knee is fully extended (Table 10.1).

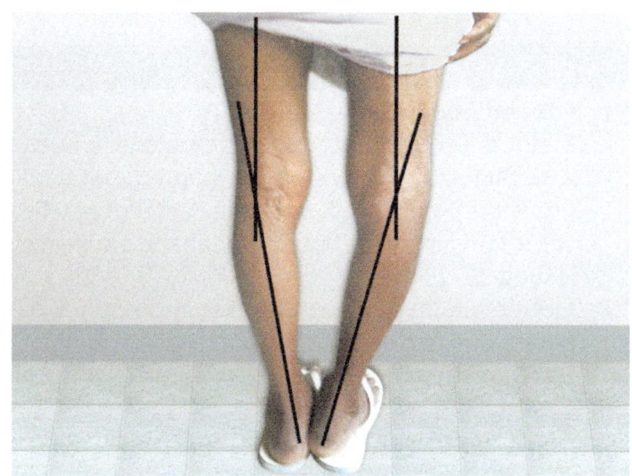

Fig. 10.1: A case of genu varus deformity in osteoarthritis knee.

Table 10.1: Causes of genu varus deformity.

Unilateral	Bilateral
• Growth anomaly • Trauma • Infection • Tumor	• Physiological (up to 3 years) • Congenital (tibia vara) • Idiopathic • Metabolic (rickets and Paget diseases) • Degenerative arthritis • Inflammatory arthritis

Q. Why you say that this genu varus deformity is due to osteoarthritis of knee?

Ans. The reasons are as follows:
- Elderly patient with heavy built.
- History of insidious onset pain which increases with loading of joint.
- Joint line tenderness and crepitus (shows joint irregularity).
- Synovial thickening present (superomedial aspect of knee).
- Range of motion restricted and painful.

Q. Any other associative finding you like to search in this case?

Ans. Yes sir, I will look for:
- Joint effusion in suprapatellar pouch (patellar tap) (Fig. 10.2)
- Baker's cyst in popliteal fossa
- Assessment of varus deformity by tibiofemoral axis (Chapter 11) and intercondylar distance measurement (Fig. 10.3).

Patellar tap test
- Position: Supine
- Method: First squeeze the suprapatellar pouch with thumb and fingers of one hand to get fluid under the patella. Now press the center of patella vertically with finger tips of other hand and leave it suddenly (Fig. 10.2).
- Interpretation: Now feel the sink and bounce of patella due to displacement and repositioning of fluid underlying the patella.

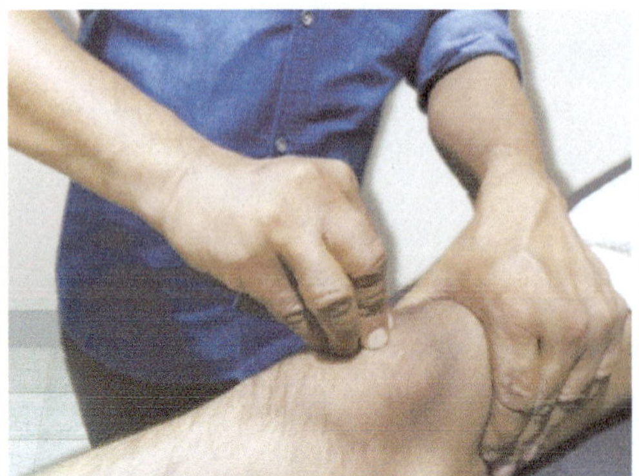

Fig. 10.2: Patellar tap for knee effusion.

Intercondylar distance measurement.
- Position of patient: Standing position
- Measurement: Measure the distance between two medial epicondyle of femur with a measuring tape.
- Interpretation: Normally this distance is 1 cm but if this distance is more than 3 cm it is significant and shows varus deformity

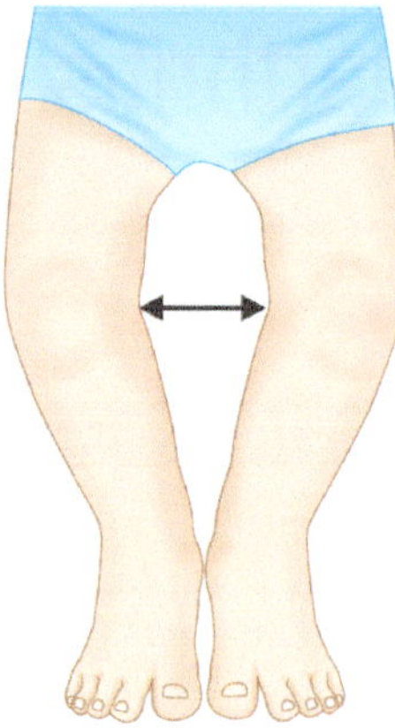

Fig. 10.3: Intercondylar distance measurement.

Q. What investigation you like to get in this case?

Ans. X-ray of the knee, both AP and lateral view, in **standing position** (Fig. 10.4). Because loading of joint reveals the deformity maximally.

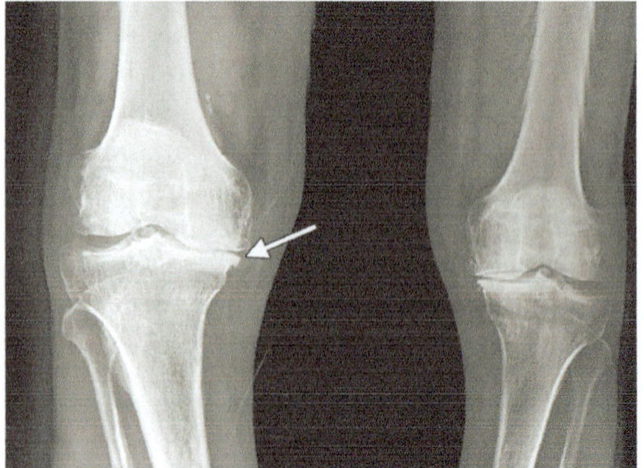

Fig. 10.4: X-ray of osteoarthritis knee.

- Decreased joint space
- Subchondral sclerosis
- Osteophytes formation
- Subchondral cyst
- Subchondral sclerosis
- Varus deformity.

Q. What treatment you like to offer for your case?

Ans. These are as:

- Analgesics: NSAIDs and opioids
- Cartilage supporting agents: Glucosamine, chondroitin sulfate, collagen peptides, and vitamin C preparations
- Viscosupplement: Intra-articular injection of hyaluronic acid (some time steroid also)
- Aspiration of joint if effusion present
- Physiotherapy: Static quadriceps exercises
- Electrotherapy: Infrared and ultrasonic therapy
- Orthosis: Lateral shoe raising or varus correcting orthosis at knee
- Habit changes: No squatting, minimal stairs riding use of western style toilet seats, etc. for off loading of joint
- General measures: For weight loss in obese patient.

Q. What are the surgical methods to deal with osteoarthritis knee?

Ans. These are:

- Joint debridement: Nowadays arthroscopy is being used for this purpose.
- High tibial osteotomy: Lateral closed wedge or medial open wedge osteotomy to realign the axis of lower limb. Commonly used in younger patient with varus deformity (Fig. 10.5A).
- Total knee arthroplasty: Replacement of natural knee with an artificial one. Reserved for severe cases of osteoarthritis as a last and best option (Fig. 10.5B).

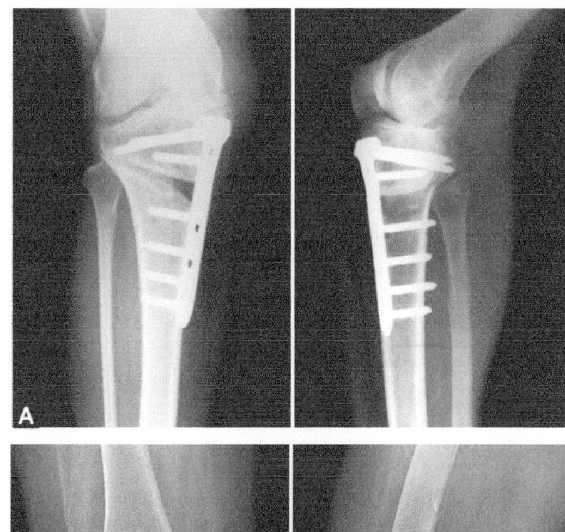

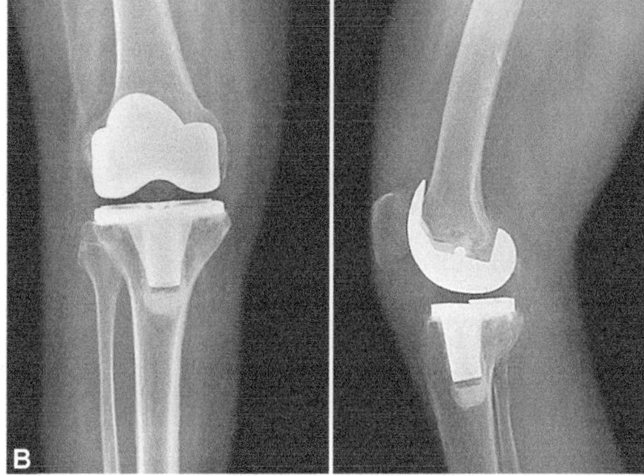

Figs. 10.5A and B: X-ray: A. high tibial osteotomy and; B. total knee replacement.

Q. What complication will develop if osteoarthritis knee left untreated?

Ans. These are as:

- Stiffness
- Baker cyst (outpouching of synovial membrane from posterior knee capsule)
- Deformity (varus is commonest)
- Instability (due to collateral ligament laxity).

Q. Define arthritis?

Ans. Inflammation of joint is called arthritis; here joint is painful throughout the range of motion. But in synovitis range of motion is only terminally painful.

Q. What are the most common sites for primary and secondary osteoarthritis?

Ans. Theses are as:
- For primary arthritis: Knee
- For secondary arthritis: Hip joint.

Q. What are the risk factors for primary osteoarthritis?

Ans. Risk factors for primary osteoarthritis are:
- Elderly persons
- Obesity and sedentary habits
- Hereditary
- Smoking
- Nutritional habits.

Q. What is secondary arthritis?

Ans. Osteoarthritis following some pre-existing disease in joint is called secondary osteoarthritis.

Causes of secondary osteoarthritis.
- Congenital anomalies in joint
- Intra-articular fracture
- Deformity at joint
- Metabolic diseases
- Avascular necrosis in joint
- Inflammatory arthropathy
- Postinfective

Q. What is the basic pathology behind osteoarthritis?

Ans. The loss of proteoglycan in joint cartilage (hyaline) leading to wear and tear of joint and resulting into sclerosis and osteophyte formation.

Q. How you can grade the severity of osteoarthritis?

Ans. On the basis of **Kellgren** and **Lawrence** radiological grading scale:
- Grade I (doubtful): Doubtful narrowing of joint space and possible osteophytic limping
- Grade II (mild): Definite osteophytes and definite narrowing of joint space
- Grade III (Moderate): Moderate multiple osteophyte, definite narrowing of joint space, some sclerosis, and possible deformity of bone contour
- Grade IV (severe): Large osteophytes, marked narrowing of joint space, severe sclerosis, and definite deformity of bone contour.

COMPARISON OF TUBERCULOUS, RHEUMATOID, AND GOUTY ARTHRITIS (TABLE 10.2.)

Table 10.2: Comparison of tuberculous, rheumatoid, and gouty arthritis.

	Tubercular arthritis (Fig. 10.6)	Rheumatoid arthritis (Fig. 10.7)	Gouty arthritis (Fig. 10.8)
Age/sex	Any age and sex	Elderly women	Middle age men
Risk factors	• Poor nutrition • Low socioeconomic status • History of pulmonary tuberculosis (primary)	Family history	• Obese • Alcoholic • Using rich protein diet • Hypertensive
Basic pathology	• For bone and joint always secondary • Agent: *Mycobacterium tuberculosis* • Tubercle formation in synovial and adjacent bone • Caseous necrosis • Staging: Synovitis-arthritis-erosion or deformity	• Autoimmune disease • HLA DR4, Dw4 association • Antibodies against IgM • Hyperplasia of synovium leading to pannus formation • Stage of synovitis-arthritis and deformity	Hyperuricemia and deposition of uric acid crystals in tendon, ligament, subcutaneous tissue, bursae, synovium, cartilage, and kidney

Contd...

Contd...

	Tubercular arthritis	Rheumatoid arthritis	Gouty arthritis
Presentation	• Constitutional symptoms: Evening fever, weight loss, appetite loss, perspiration • Solitary and unilateral joint involvement is the most common presentation • Local features: Typical attitude of joint, night pain, boggy swelling, deformity in late stage	• Multiple joint pain and swelling • Morning stiffness that relieves in afternoon • Deformities in late stages e.g. rheumatoid hand • Subcutaneous nodule formation	• Common site: Great toe MTP joint, ankle, knee, shoulder, hand • Pain and swelling • Redness and warmth in acute cases • Deformity e.g. (podagra) in late stage
X-ray	• Osteopenia • Joint space narrowing • Multiple erosion and lytic-lesion(cotton wool appearance • Knee deformity: Triple deformity (Knee flexion, lateral sublaxation, external rotation of tibia)	• Soft tissue swelling • Juxta-articular osteopenia • Morning stiffness • Marginal erosion • Joint space narrowing	• Soft tissue swelling • Joint space narrowing • Tophi (deposition of urate crystals) • Punched out deep erosive hanging lesion over joint edges (**Marotel sign**)
Other investigations	• TC, DC (lymphocyte) raised • ESR and CRP raised • Z/N staining and culture of aspirate • CBNAT • Biopsy of synovium	TC, DC (neutrophil) raised ESR and CRP raised RA factor (prognostic) Anti-CCP most sensitive	• Serum uric acid • Synovial fluid analysis—negative birefringence in polarizing microscope
Diagnosis	No investigation is confirmatory hence diagnosis is made on basis of clinical suspicion, radiology and blood investigations	**1987 New York criteria** • Morning stiffness > 1 hour • Symmetrical joint involvement • More than 3 pairs of large joint • Small joint of hand involvement • Radiographic changes • Soft tissue swelling • Rheumatoid factor • Rheumatoid nodule ➢ Above four must be more than 6 week duration ➢ Four out of seven is diagnostic *Note:* EULAR criteria is commonly used nowadays	• Clinical examination and fluctuation in serum uric acid level in high risk patient is diagnostic

Contd...

Contd...

	Tubercular arthritis	Rheumatoid arthritis	Gouty arthritis
Treatment	• Antitubercular drug treatment • Rest and splintage followed by mobilization • Protein rich nutrition • Aspiration/drainage of pus • Joint debridement • Osteotomy if joint is fused in unacceptable position • Arthroplasty in cases of painful arthritis	• Analgesics (NSAID/ opioids) • DMARD; disease modifying drugs like methotrexate, sulfasalazine, hydroxychloroquine • Steroids • Biologics like infliximab, adalimumab, etc. • Physiotherapy: Joint mobilizing exercises • Electrotherapy: Heat and ultrasonic	• In acute attack: NSAID, colchicine and steroids • In chronic gout: Allopurinol and febuxostat • Restricted protein diet

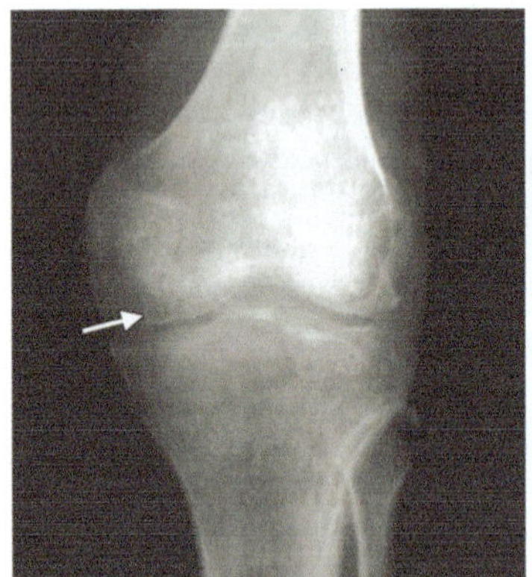

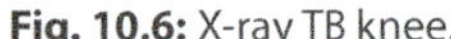

Fig. 10.6: X-ray TB knee.

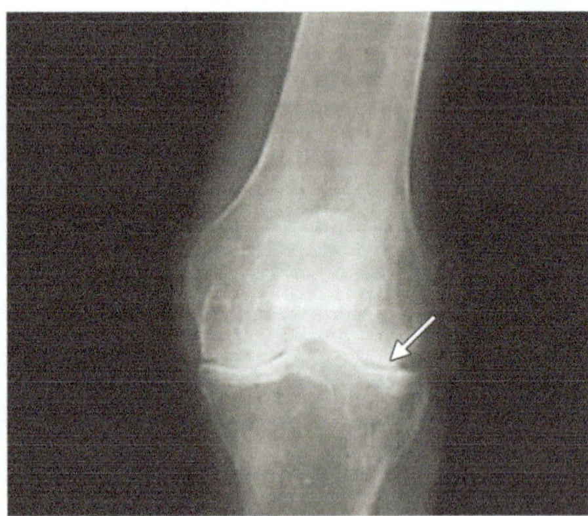

Fig. 10.7: X-ray RA knee.

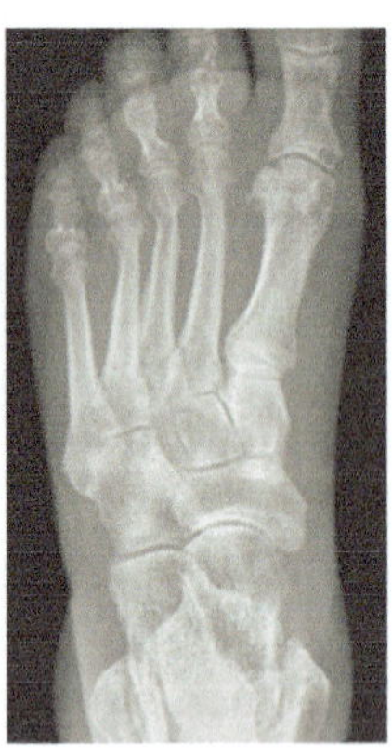

Fig. 10.8: Gout great toe.

Chapter

11

Genu Valgus Deformity at Knee (Rickets)

CASE PRESENTATION

- **History**: The parents of a 8-year-old girl presented with a complaint that both the legs of their daughter are deviating away from his body for last 5 years. The deformity is of gradual onset, painless, and progressive. Parents were also concerned about her protruded abdomen and widening of wrist. There is also a history of physical weakness. There is no history of any previous trauma, fever, weight loss, multiple joints pain, and morning stiffness.
- **Examination**: Patient is of poor built and poor nutrition. Her systemic examination is within normal limit. The local examination revealed a genu valgus deformity at both knees. There is no tenderness at joint line. The range of motion of both knees is normal. Intermalleolar distance is increased. There is no limb length discrepancy. Distal neurovascular examination is also normal.

VIVA VOCE FROM CASE

Q. What is your diagnosis?

Ans. This is a case of genu valgus deformity of knee most likely due to rickets (Fig. 11.1).

Q. Define genu valgus?

Ans. It is defined as abnormal outward deviation of long axis of leg in relation to thigh when knee is fully extended. Normal valgus is 5–7° (Table 11.1).

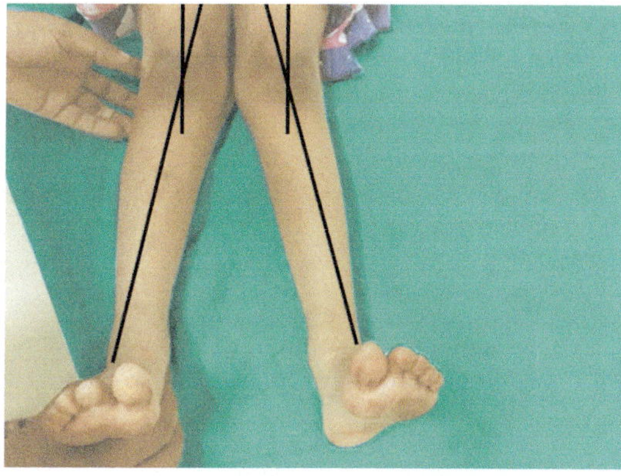

Fig. 11.1: A case of genu valgus deformity in rachitic knee.

Table 11.1: Causes of genu valgus deformity.

Unilateral	Bilateral
• Growth anomaly • Trauma • Infection • Tumor	• Physiological (normalized up to 7 years) • Congenital • Idiopathic (most common) • Metabolic (rickets and Paget) • Degenerative arthritis • Inflammatory arthritis

Q. Why you say that this genu valgus deformity is due to rickets?

Ans. The reasons are as follows:

- Age: Growing age
- Poor nourishment (dietary deficiency)
- Stigmata of rickets like progressive knee deformity, pot belly, and wrist widening.

Q. Any other associative finding you like to search in this case?

Ans. Yes sir, I will look for:

- History of bowel disorder, any liver disease or any chronic kidney disease.
- Assessment of valgus deformity by tibiofemoral axis (Fig. 11.2) and intermalleolar distance measurement (Fig. 11.3).

Tibiofemoral axis measurement.

- Position of patient: Standing
- Measurement: Draw a long axis along femur and long axis of tibia and measure the tibiofemoral axis (Fig. 11.2)
- Interpretation: (1) Normal: 5–7°. (2) If this angle decreases, neutral or negative condition is called genu varum. (3) If this angle increases condition is called genu valgus.

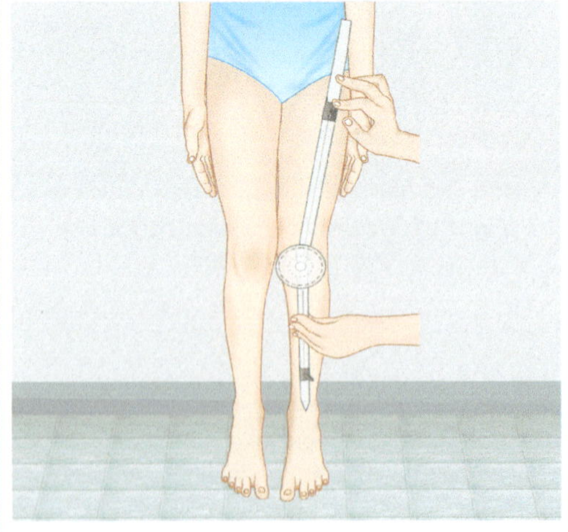

Fig. 11.2: Tibiofemoral axis measurement.

Intermalleolar distance measurement.

- Position of patient: Standing position
- Measurement: Measure the distance between two medial malleoli of tibia with a measuring tape.
- Interpretation: Normally this distance is 4–5 cm but if this distance is more than 8–10 cm it is significant.

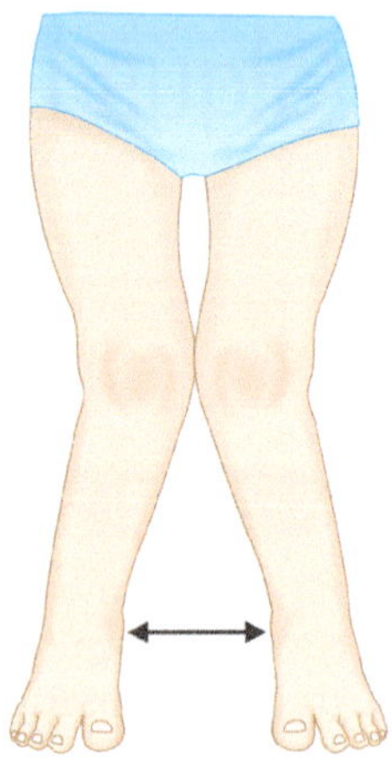

Fig. 11.3: Intercondylar distance measurement.

Q. What investigation you like to get in this case?

Ans. X-ray of AP view of the knee including full thigh and full leg in **standing position** (Fig. 11.4) because loading of joint

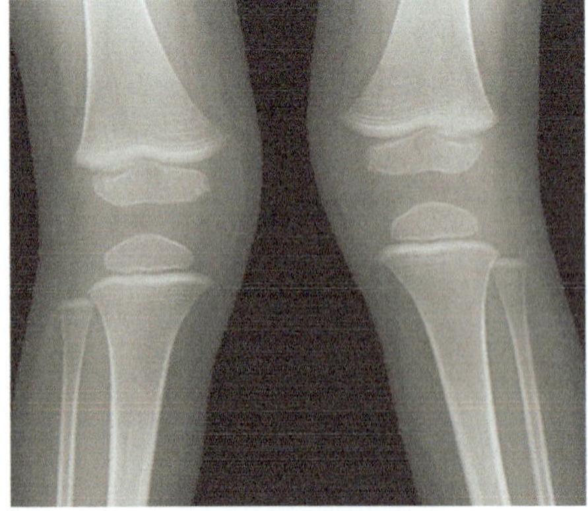

Fig. 11.4: X-ray of rachitic knee.

reveals the deformity maximally. Side by side I will also get X-ray of both wrists in AP view (Fig. 11.5).

- Osteopenia
- Metaphyseal widening
- Physical changes: Cupping, fraying, and splaying
- Genu valgus deformity.

Q. What other investigation you like to do in your case?

Ans. I will do some more investigation to search the cause of rickets like:

- Serum calcium: Decreased (normal: 8.5–10.5 mg/dL)
- Serum phosphate: Decreased (normal: 2.5–4.5 mg/dL)
- Serum alkaline phosphatase: Increased (normal: 44–177 IU/L)
- Serum vitamin D3 level: May altered (<20 ng/mL: deficient, 20–30 ng/mL: insufficient, >30–110 ng/mL: sufficient, >110 ng/mL: toxicity)
- Hb level decreased
- If needed, GI, liver, and kidney function tests.

Q. With these investigation what type of rickets it appears to be?

Ans. The picture of investigation goes in favor of nutritional deficiency rickets.

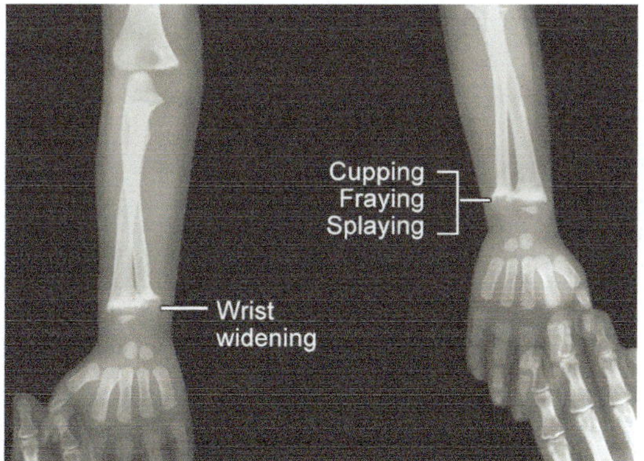

Fig. 11.5: X-ray of rachitic wrist.

Q. What is nutritional rickets?

Ans. This is due to dietary deficiency of vitamin D. Common in children below 4 years of age.

Q. How will you treat a case of nutritional rickets?

Ans. These are as:

- Vitamin D treatment: 6 lakhs IU of vitamin D stat by intramuscular or oral route along with other supportive measure mentioned as below. After 1 month, get an X-ray of joint and look for a healing line as sclerosis in physeal region. If yes, then start a maintenance dose 3,000–4,000 IU of vitamin D for 3–4 months. If not, then give another dose of 6 lakhs IU of vitamin D and search for healing line again in X-ray after another 1 month. This time if you get healing line then start maintenance dose as earlier and if there is no healing line again then investigate for vitamin D resistant rickets or some other causes of rickets.
- Calcium supplements
- Diet rich in calcium, protein, and fat like milk, egg, etc.
- Bracing: Valgus correcting orthosis (if valgus is less than 15°), e.g. mermaid splints (Fig. 11.6).

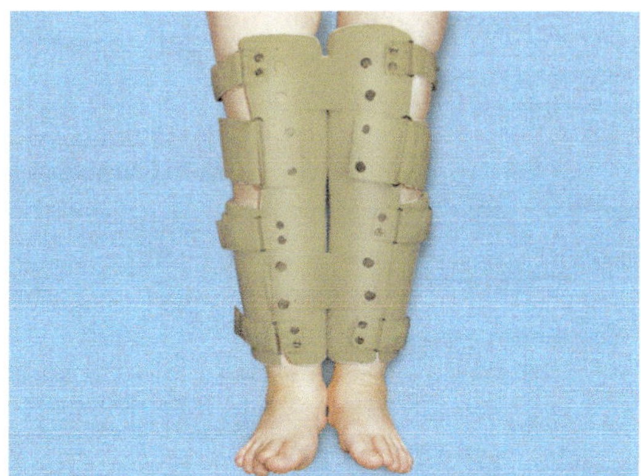

Fig. 11.6: Mermaid splint for valgus correction in children.

Q. What is the prerequisite of surgery for rachitic genu valgum deformity?

Ans. These are:
- Healing of disease as evident in radiograph and normalization of alkaline phosphatase level.
- Identification of contributory bone for deformity, i.e. distal femur or proximal tibia.

Q. How you can detect that deformity is contributed by either femur or tibia?

Ans. Knee flexion test:
- If deformity appears in knee extension and disappears on flexion then this is due to disease in femur (distal part).
- If deformity appears in knee extension and persists on flexing the knee then pathology is in tibia (proximal part).
- If deformity appears in knee extension and partially corrects on flexion then both femur and tibia are contributors.
- Reason: Because in extended knee anterior aspect of femoral condyle comes in contact of tibial plateau and in flexed knee posterior aspect of condyle comes in contact with plateau. As we know pathological site in femur is anterior condyle.

Q. What are the surgical methods to correct the genu valgus deformity?

Ans. If valgus is significant, i.e. more than 15°, one should plan for some surgery.
- Epiphysiodesis: A growth modulation technique as it arrests the growth one side of physis leaving opposite physis intact; hence, correcting the deformity. It is indicated in immature skeletal having sufficient time before maturity for correction due to growth modulation. Best for children age around 7–10 years (Fig. 11.7).
- Osteotomy: Lateral open wedge or medial closed wedge osteotomy in affected bone to restore the normal tibiofemoral axis. It is indicated in matured skeleton.

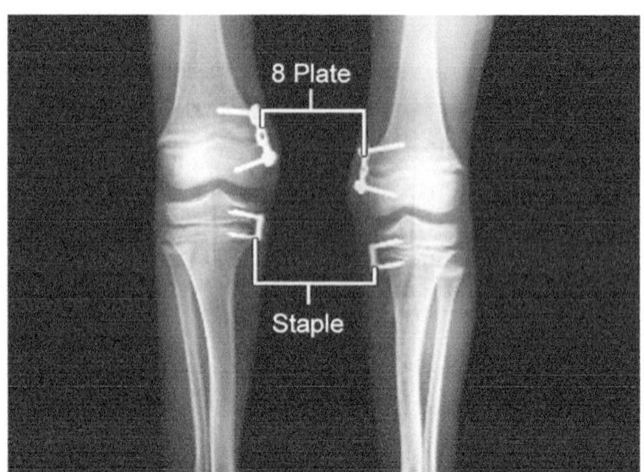

Fig. 11.7: X-ray of epiphysiodesis around knee fixed with figure 8 plate and Blount staple.

Q. What complication will develop if rachitic knee left untreated?

Ans. These are as:
- Severe valgus deformity
- Early arthritis
- Instability (due to collateral ligament laxity).

Q. Define rickets.

Ans. Failure of mineralization of osteoid matrix in immature skeletal is called rickets.

Q. What are the etiological factors of rickets development?

Ans. These are as:
- Nutritional deficiency
- Gastrointestinal absorption defect, e.g. gluten sensitivity
- Renal defect like enzyme 1-α-hydroxylase deficiency and end-organ resistance to vitamin D3, and renal tubular acidosis
- Hepatic factor: Microsomal enzyme stimulation following anticonvulsant tt.
- Other factor; like hypophosphatasia and heavy metal intoxication (Table 11.2).

Q. What is mode of action of vitamin D3 (calcitriol) in rickets?

Ans. The regulator of calcitriol is low serum calcium; vitamin D3 affects the following site and maintains serum calcium level:

- Gut: It increases the intestinal absorption of calcium and phosphate.
- Bone: It increases resorption of bone and increases serum calcium and phosphate level.
- Kidney: It increases renal tubular reabsorption of calcium.

Table 11.2: Clinical presentation of rickets.

General	• Hypotonia, lethargy, irritability, and weakness
Skull	• Craniotabes: Softening of skull bone • Skull bossing of frontal and parietal bone
Teeth	• Delayed dental eruption
Chest	• Pigeon chest: Protrusion of chest like pigeon keel • Rachitic rosary: Prominent costochondral Junction • Harrison sulcus: Horizontal indrawing in subcostal area due to softening of bone
Spine	• Kyphoscoliosis
Pelvis	• Bilateral coxa vara
Wrist	• Widening of wrist
Knee	• Genu valgus (knock knee) • Genu varum • Wind swept deformity (valgus in one and varus in another)

Q. What do you mean by osteomalacia, osteoporosis, osteosclerosis, and osteopenia?

Ans. Their definitions are as follows:

- Osteomalacia: Failure of mineralization of osteoid matrix in mature skeleton (adult) is called osteomalacia.
- Osteoporosis: Reduction of bone mass or matrix per unit volume along with normal mineralization is called osteoporosis. It may be postmenopausal and senile.
- Osteosclerosis: Increase in bone mass is called osteosclerosis, e.g. Paget disease and osteopetrosis.
- Osteopenia: It is clinical term used for bone mass deficient disease like osteoporosis.

DIFFERENT TYPES OF RICKETS (TABLE 11.3)

Table 11.3: Types of rickets with their features and treatment.

Rickets type	Features	Treatment
Gluten enteropathy induced rickets	• Gluten sensitive enteropathy leads to malabsorption of fat. Hence, there is excessive excretion of Ca^{++} leading to rickets	• Gluten free diet • Calcium and vitamin D supplement
Vitamin D dependent rickets	• Type I: 1-α-hydroxylase deficiency (kidney) • Type II: End-organ resistance to vitamin D3 (kidney) • In type I, there is deficiency or defective vitamin D3 and in type II there is enteric insensitivity of vitamin D3. Both factors lead to development of rickets of serious variety	• High doses of vitamin D3 administration (up to 1 lakh IU daily)

Contd...

Contd...

Rickets type	Features	Treatment
X-linked hypophosphatemic rickets (vitamin D resistant rickets)/ phosphate diabetes	• X-linked dominant disease (*PHEX* gene). Alteration phosphate reabsorption in renal tubule leading to phosphaturia. Hence, deficient mineralization leading to rickets • Special features are: (1) short stature; (2) craniosynostosis, dental delaying, and deafness; and (3) extraskeletal calcification in tendon or ligament	• Phosphate replacement (1–4 g daily) along with vitamin D3 • **Joule** solution (dibasic sodium phosphate)
Renal tubular acidosis induced rickets (congenital or chronic kidney diseases)	• In such diseases there is loss of fixed bases from renal tubule making an acidic environment leading to acidosis. This situation is neutralized by chelation of Ca^{++} from bones and rachitic features develop	• Administration of alkaline solution (bicarbonate and phosphate) to correct acidosis • **Shohl** solution (citric acid and sod citrate)
Hypophosphatasia	• The lack of alkaline phosphatase leading to impaired synthesis of inorganic phosphate hence defective mineralization • Low serum alkaline phosphatase and increased urinary phosphoethanolamine	Phosphate therapy

Chapter

12

Nonunion Fracture Neck of Femur

CASE PRESENTATION

- **History**: My patient, a 60-year-old male, presented with complaint of inability to bear weight on his right lower limb from last 6 months. Six months back he slipped at his home and sustained an injury at his right hip. Following this he could not stand himself (significant trauma) and carried by attendants to a local bone setter. There, treatment was given in the form of some traction with rope and straps. With this treatment his pain was relieved but unable to bear weight even with some support. There is no history of any fever, weight loss, morning stiffness or multiple joint pain.
- **Examination**: Patient is of average built and average nutrition. His general and systemic examination is within normal limit. He lies comfortably on bed with his right lower limb in external rotation attitude. His both ASIS (anterior superior iliac spine) are at same level. Right-sided GT (greater trochanter) at higher level which is smooth, not broadened and nontender. There is absence of tenderness in Scarpa's triangle also. Right-sided femoral pulse is feeble compared to left side. There is no fixed deformity and range of motion is increased in all planes. The apparent and true shortening is same (say 2 cm) which is supratrochanteric and confirmed by Bryant measurement. The Trendelenburg test (supported) and telescopy test positive. Examination of opposite hip and spine appears to be normal. The distal neurovascular status is also intact.

VIVA VOCE FROM CASE

Q. What is your diagnosis?

Ans. This is a case of nonunion fracture neck of femur (Fig. 12.1).

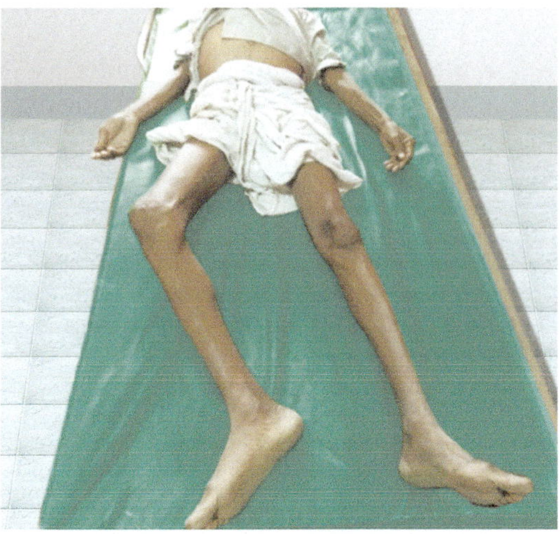

Fig. 12.1: A case of nonunion fracture neck of femur.

Q. What is time limit to say a fracture neck of femur as nonunion?

Ans. 3 months (after 3 weeks it is called neglected fracture).

Factors promoting nonunion fracture neck of femur.

- Poor blood supply
- Washing of hematoma with synovial fluid
- Absent of cambium layer in periosteum that produces callus
- Continuous shearing forces at fracture site
- Varied degree of communication on posterior surface

Q. What are the points favoring your diagnosis?

Ans. The reasons are as follows:

- History of trauma and inability to bear weight
- External rotation attitude of lower limb
- No tenderness in inguinal region (Scarpa's triangle) (Fig. 12.2). It might be tender sometime
- Right-sided femoral pulse is feeble (vascular sign of **Narath** positive)
- Increased range of motion which is painless
- Shortening of affected limb (supratrochanteric shortening, (Fig. 12.3) Bryant's triangle)
- Straight leg raising not possible
- Assisted **Trendelenburg** test positive
- Telescopy test positive.

Scarpa's triangle (femoral triangle) (Fig. 12.2).

The Scarpa's triangle is another name for femoral triangle situated in upper anterior aspect of thigh. It contains femoral nerve, femoral artery, femoral vein, and lymph nodes. The boundaries of triangle is as follows:

- Superiorly: Inguinal ligament
- Medially: Medial border of adductor longus
- Laterally: Medial border of sartorius
- Floor: Iliopsoas and pectineus

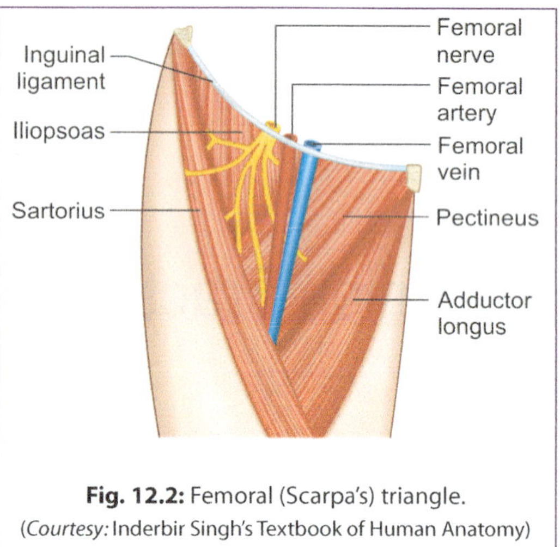

Fig. 12.2: Femoral (Scarpa's) triangle.
(*Courtesy:* Inderbir Singh's Textbook of Human Anatomy)

Q. What is vascular sign of Narath and what is it significant?

Ans. If the femoral pulse is less prominent or absent in comparison to normal side, this is called vascular sign of Narath. The causes for positive vascular sign of Narath are:

- Posterior dislocation of hip
- Developmental dysplasia of hip
- Peripheral vascular diseases.

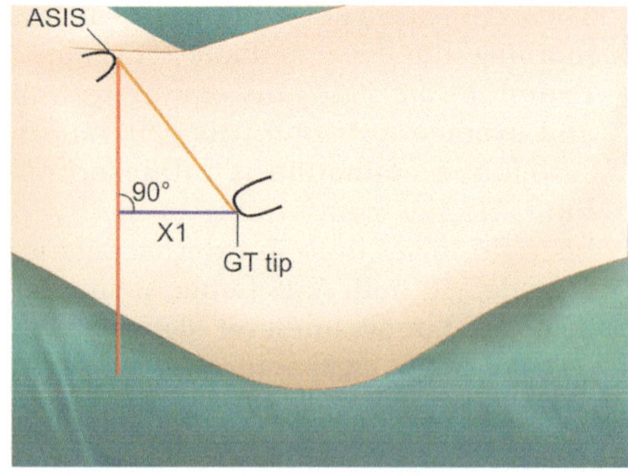

Fig. 12.3: Bryant's triangle.

Normal range of motion at hip.

- Flexion: 0–120°
- Extension: 0–15°
- Abduction: 0–450°
- Adduction: 0–30°
- External rotation: 0–450°
- Internal rotation: 0–30°

Q. What is meant by fixed deformity?

Ans. Due to pathological process at a particular joint, only some degree of its movement is allowed in a particular direction but its opposite movement is not possible. This is called fixed deformity. For example, in fixed flexion deformity of hip, the limb lies in attitude of flexion and we can do further flexion up to its range but no extension at all.

Q. What is Thomas test?

Ans. It is a historical test designed by **Huge Owen Thomas** to elicit the fixed flexion deformity of hip (Figs. 12.4A and B).

- Position of patient: Patient lies in supine position on a hard couch. He is asked to straighten his leg and patient is able to do this by producing excessive lumbar lordosis which is easily detected by insinuating a hand in between couch and back of the patient.
- Method: Now slowly bend the normal thigh in flexed knee position till the lumbar lordosis is totally disappeared. In this situation examiner cannot insinuate his hand in between couch and back of patient. In this process the affected thigh automatically comes in a position of fixed flexion.
- Inference: The angle between couch and affected thigh shows the degree of fixed flexion.

Bryant's triangle (Fig. 12.4).

- Prerequisite: Supine position, both ASIS at same level and limb in identical position. Draw it in both sides.
- Drawing: (1) ASIS and GT are joined by straight line. (2) A vertical line is drawn from ASIS towards couch. (3) A perpendicular line is drawn from GT to the vertical line. This line is parallel to couch and shows the base of triangle.
- Interpretation: The difference between the bases of the both sides of triangle shown the supratrochanteric shortening of limb.

Q. How will you measure the apparent length and true length?

Ans. Limb length is measured with the help of a measuring tape. During apparent length measurement both limbs must lie parallel to midline but in true length measurement both ASIS (squaring of pelvis) must lies at same level and both limbs should be in identical position.

- Apparent length measurement: It is measured from xiphisternum or umbilicus to the tip of medial malleoli in both sides (Fig. 12.5A).

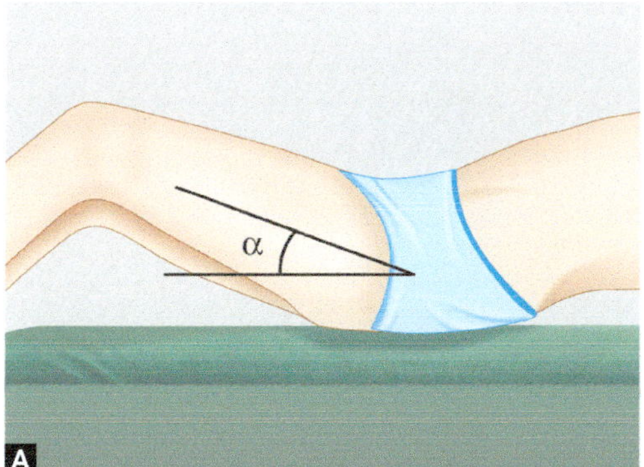

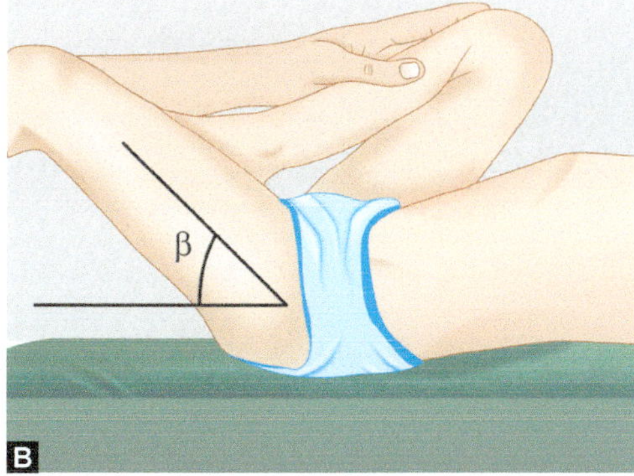

Figs. 12.4A and B: Thomas test.

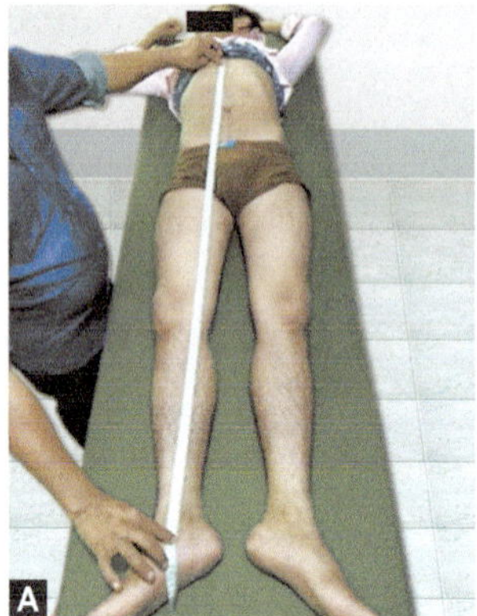

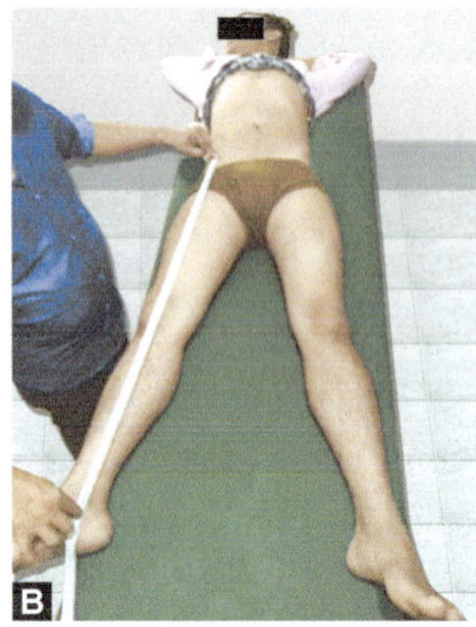

Figs. 12.5A and B: A. Apparent and; B. True measurement of lower limb.

- True length measurement: It is measured from ASIS (anterior superior iliac spine) to the tip of medial malleoli in both sides (Fig. 12.5B).

Q. What is Trendelenburg test and how will you do this?

Ans. It detects the integrity of lever arm/ abductor mechanism of hip. In this mechanism power is supplied by gluteus medius and minimus, hip joint acts as fulcrum, neck of femur act as lever arm, and weight is itself the lower limb (Figs. 12.6A and B). It should be done only in those patients who can stand on their affected limb for at least 30 seconds; otherwise assisted Trendelenburg test is performed. Mark the posterior superior iliac spine (PSIS) and anterior superior iliac spine (ASIS) of patient with a marker after proper exposure of pelvic area. Examiner should kneel down either in back (to look over PSIS) or in front (to look over ASIS) of the patient.

- Method: Ask the patient to stand over his normal limb by flexing his opposite knee but not at hip to clear the ground. The opposite pelvis tilts up due to abductor pull of normal hip. Now ask the patient to stand on affected limb, the drooping of pelvis of normal side is noticed due to insufficiency of abductor pull on affected hip, i.e. sound side sink.
- Interpretation: The lifting and drooping of pelvis is appreciated by excursion of marked bony points as PSIS.

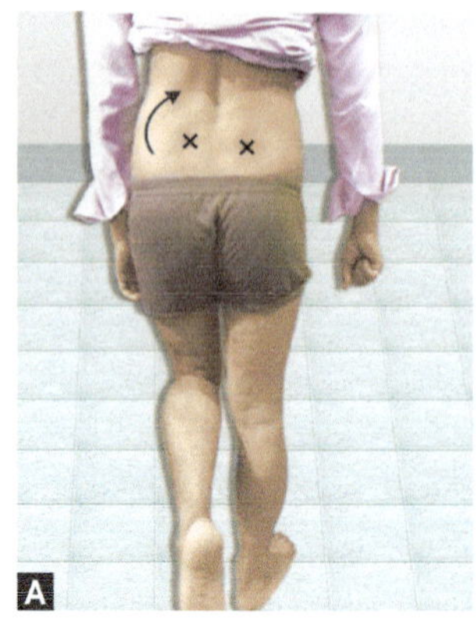

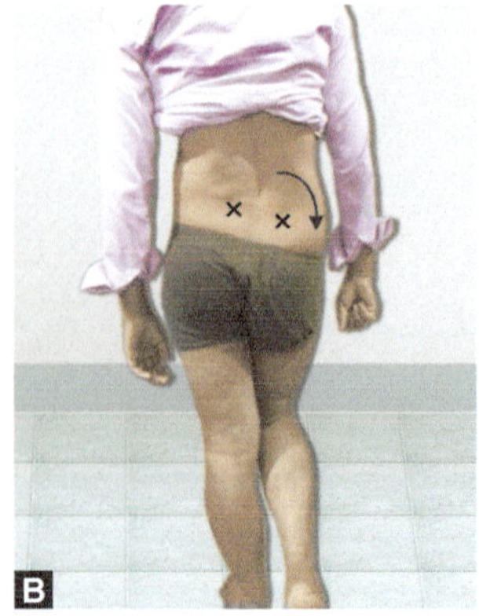

Figs. 12.6A and B: Trendelenburg test: A. Standing on normal limb (RT) and; B. standing on affected limb (LT).

Q. How will you perform telescopy test?

Ans. As telescopy test confirms nonunion. (Fig. 12.7). This test is performed as follows:

- Position of patient: Patient lies in supine position on a hard couch with affected hip in 90° flexion and slight adduction (to clear the acetabular margin during excursion of trochanter).
- Method: Examiner holds the pelvis by one hand in such a way that his thumb lies on ASIS and rest four fingers touches the greater trochanter. Now flexed knee of affected side is grasped with another hand and a downward force (push-pull) is applied in line of long axis of femur and simultaneously the motion of greater trochanter is felt by fingers kept on it. Compare it with normal side.
- Interpretation: This is found positive in (1) nonunion fracture neck of femur, (2) posterior dislocation of hip, and (3) developmental dysplasia of hip, etc.

Q. What investigation you like to get in this case?

Ans. X-ray of pelvis AP view showing both hip joint and lateral view of affected hip (Fig. 12.8).

- Discontinuity in neck (fracture neck)
- Fracture line (oblique or vertical)
- Proximal migration of greater trochanter
- Shenton like broken
- Lesser trochanter more prominent
- Also comment on density of head (vascularity), hip joint congruity, and acetabular surface.

Note: Shenton line is a continuous line formed along lower border of sup. pubic rammi and inferior margin of femur neck in AP X-ray of internally rotated hips.

Q. Any other investigation you like to get in this case?

Ans. Yes, MRI of hip to see the vascularity of femur head.

Q. How will you treat a case of nonunion fracture neck of femur?

Ans. I will follow this simple guideline:

- Neck preservation technique: It gives stable hip
  - Indication: If age < 60 years
  - Modality of treatment: Valgus osteotomy, neck reconstruction with muscle pedicle graft
- Neck and head sacrificing technique: It gives a stable hip
  - Indication: If age > 60 years or avascular necrosis of hip

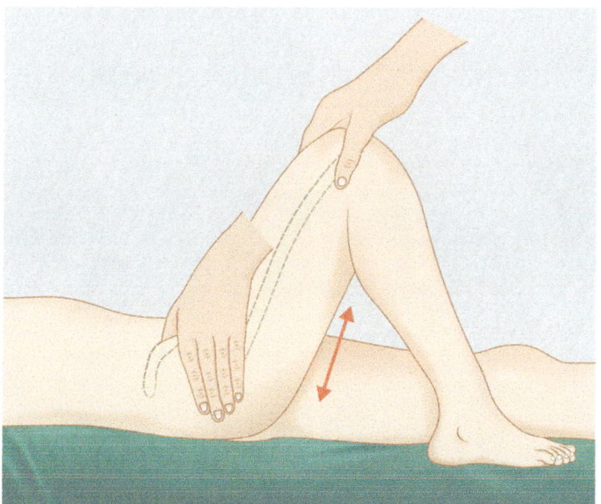

Fig. 12.7: Telescopy test.

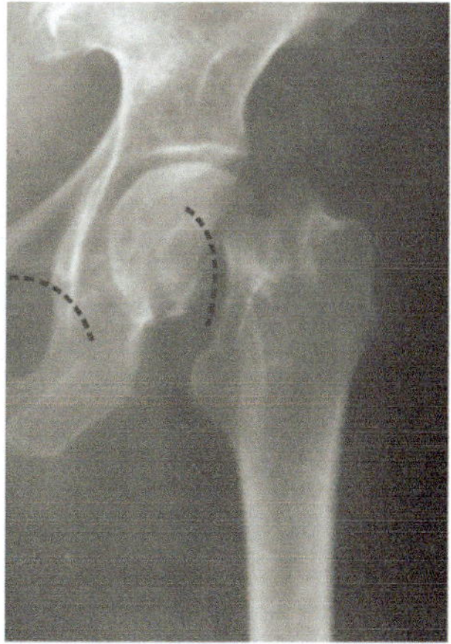

Fig. 12.8: Nonunion fracture neck of femur (Shenton's line broken).

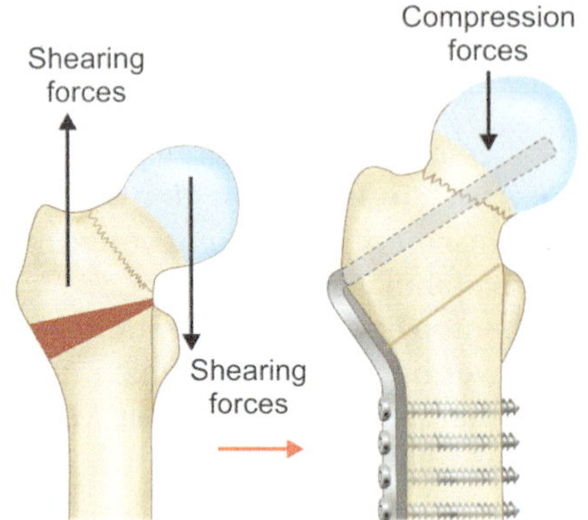

Fig. 12.9: Valgus osteotomy for nonunion fracture neck of femur.

- Modality of treatment: Hip arthroplasty
- Salvage technique: It gives a unstable hip
  - Indication: Any age with failure of above technique
  e.g. McMurray osteotomy.

Q. What is principle of valgus osteotomy?

Ans. It is a lateral closed wedge osteotomy in peritrochanteric area. It converts a relatively vertical fracture line into horizontal one so much so that shearing forces acting on fracture site must be converted into compressive forces that enhances union; e.g. Pauwel osteotomy (Fig. 12.9).

Q. Give an example of muscle pedicle graft for neck reconstruction?

Ans. Meyers procedure (Fig. 12.10): Here a vascularized muscle pedicle graft of quadratus femoris is used in neck reconstruction procedure. Dr DP Bakshi from Kolkata also popularized such technique in which he used muscle pedicle graft of tensor fascia lata. This procedure is famously known as Bakshi procedure.

Q. What is hip arthroplasty?

Ans. Replacement of natural hip with some artificial hip is called hip arthroplasty. It is of two types:

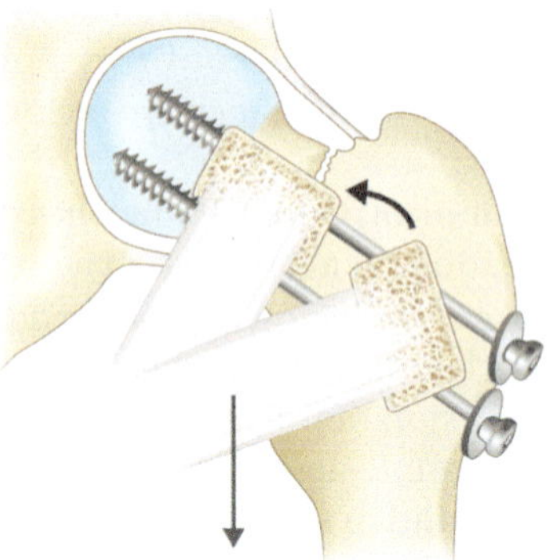

Fig. 12.10: Meyers procedure.

- Hemiarthroplasty: When only it femoral component (head of femur) is replaced it is called hemiarthroplasty (Fig. 12.11A).
- Total hip arthroplasty: When both femoral and acetabular component are replaced then it is called total hip arthroplasty (Fig. 12.11B).

Q. What is McMurray's osteotomy?

Ans. It acts on the principle of arm-chair effect and directly transfers the body weight to the shaft of femur (Fig. 12.12). Procedure wise it is an oblique osteotomy done at lesser trochanter level followed by medialization of distal segment and fixed with some

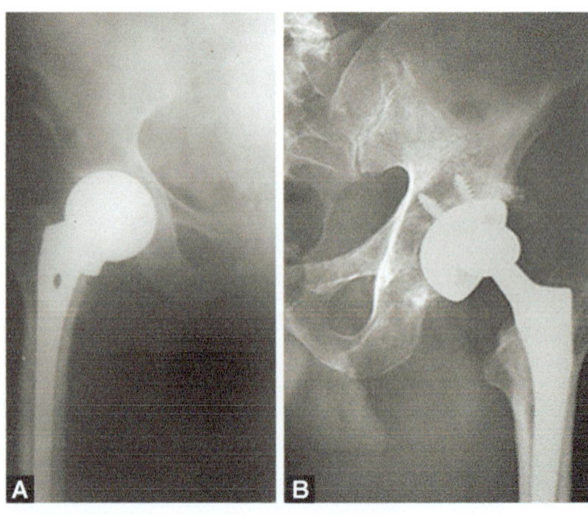

Figs. 12.11A and B: X-ray: A. hemiarthroplasty and; B. total hip arthroplasty.

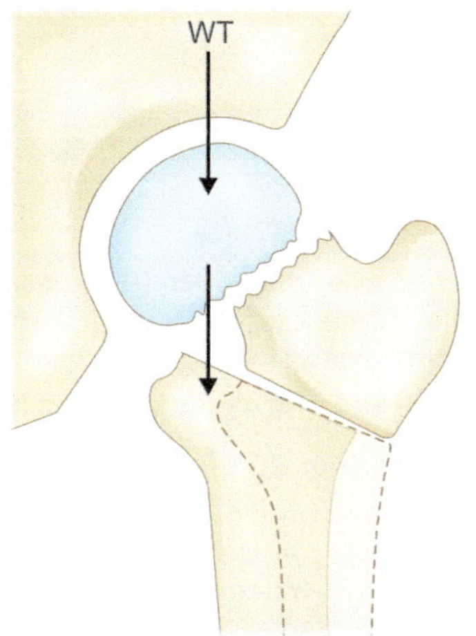

Fig. 12.12: McMurray osteotomy for nonunion fracture neck of femur.

implant like Wainwright plate. Note that originally osteotomy was not fixed rather than maintained in cast.

Q. Do you know any condition where fracture neck of femur can be treated conservatively in adult?

Ans. Yes, valgus-impacted fracture neck of femur.

Q. What is the flood supply of femur head and neck?

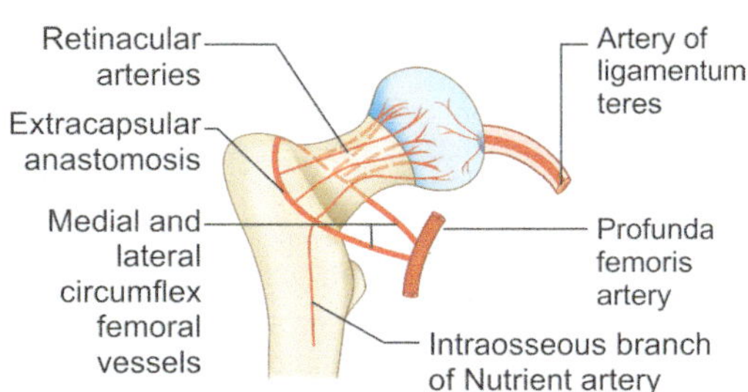

Fig. 12.13: Blood supply of head and neck of femur.

Ans. These are as (Fig. 12.13):

- Retinacular supply: From medial and lateral circumflex femoral branches
- Artery to ligamentum teres: Foveal vessels from obturator artery
- Intraosseous blood supply: From nutrient vessels.

Q. How will you treat a fracture neck of femur in children?

Ans. As follows:

- Conservative: Close reduction and immobilization in hip spica
- Surgical: Closed or open reduction and fixation with Moores pin or 4 mm cannulated cancellous screw.

Delbet classification for pediatric fracture neck of femur is shown in Figure 12.14.

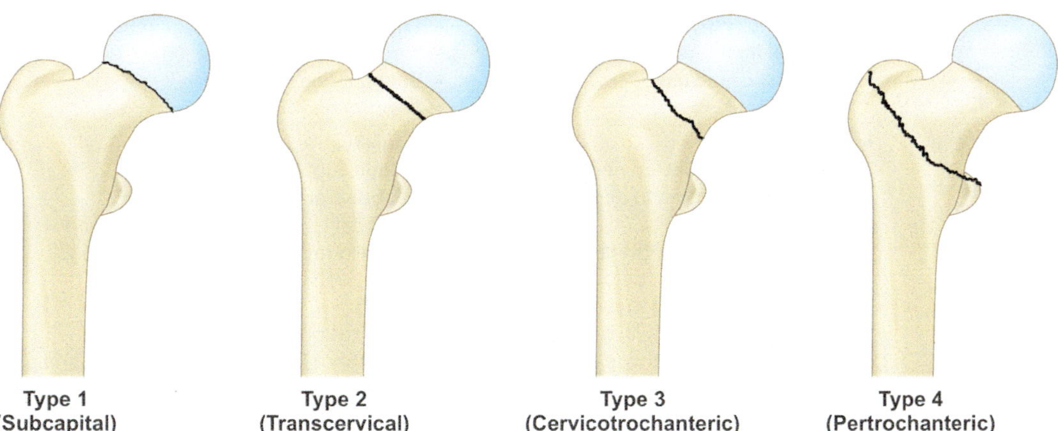

Fig. 12.14: Delbet classification for pediatric fracture neck of femur.

FRACTURE NECK OF FEMUR VS FRACTURE TROCHANTER (TABLE 12.1.)

Table 12.1: Difference between fracture neck of femur and fracture trochanter.

	Fracture neck of femur	Fracture trochanter
• Age	More than 50 years	More than 60 years
• Sex	Female preponderance	Common in female
• Mechanism of injury	Trivial trauma as fall due to slip. It might be extracapsular or intracapsular. Fracture line may be subcapital, cervical, and basal	Fracture may lie in trochanteric region or subtrochanteric (from lesser trochanter to 5 cm distal up to isthmus)
• Classification	• **Pauwel classification (Fig. 12.15)**: On the basis of angle formed between fracture line and horizontal ➢ Type I —upto 30° ➢ Type II— 30°–50° ➢ Type III— > 50° • **Gardens classification (Fig. 12.16)**: On the basis of breach and displacement of trabeculae ➢ Garden I: Incomplete fracture of the femoral neck ➢ Garden II: Complete fracture without Displacement ➢ Garden III: Complete fracture with partial displacement ➢ Garden IV: Complete fracture with full displacement	• **Boyd and Griffith classification (Fig. 12.17)**: ➢ Type I – Stable two part ➢ Type II – Unstable comminuted ➢ Type III – Unstable reverse oblique ➢ Type IV – Intertrochanteric subtrochanteric with two planes of fracture • **Evans classification:** ➢ Type I: Stable fracture ➢ Type II: Unstable fracture The factors of instability are: • Posteromedial comminution • Posterolateral comminution • Reverse obliquity • Subtrochanteric extension
• Clinical Presentation		
Attitude	External rotation < 45°	External rotation > 45°
Tenderness	Present in Scarpa's triangle	Present at GT
Swelling	Present in Scarpa's triangle	Present at GT
Broadening	Absent	Present at GT
Ecchymosis	Absent	Present at GT
Shortening	Less	More
• X-ray	• Discontinuity in neck • Proximal migration of trochanter • Shenton line broken • LT prominent	• Fracture line in trochanteric region • Neck shaft angle decreased • Shenton line broken • LT prominent
• Treatment	• Conservative: ➢ Indication: Impacted neck fracture ➢ Modality: Bed rest in derotation bar • Surgical: ➢ Indication: All neck fracture in adult ➢ Method: In patient below 60 years of age: Close or open reduction and fixation with multiple hip screws (Fig. 12.18). In patient above 60 years: Arthroplasty	• Conservative: ➢ Indication: Medically unfit or undisplaced fracture ➢ Modality: Continuous traction for 6 weeks in abducted hip positioning followed by weight-bearing. • Surgical: ➢ Indication: All displaced fractures ➢ Method: Close or open reduction and fixation with dynamic hip screw (DHS) (Fig. 12.19A) and barrel plate or proximal femoral nail (PFN) (Fig. 12.19B)
• Complication	• Nonunion • Avascular necrosis of head • Hip arthritis	• Malunion (coxa vara) • Hip arthritis

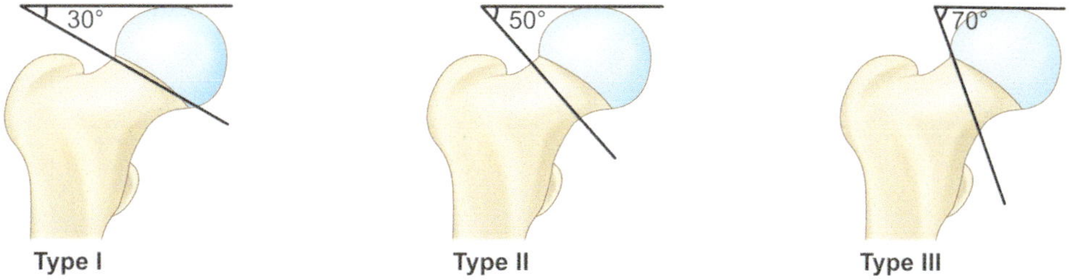

30° 50° 70°

Type I Type II Type III

Fig. 12.15: Pauwel classification.

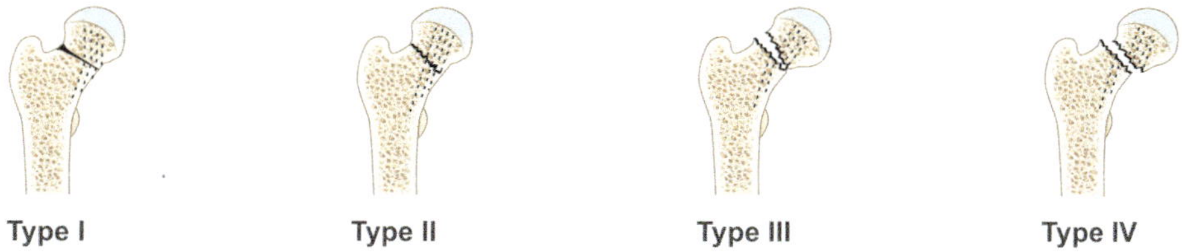

Type I Type II Type III Type IV

Fig. 12.16: Garden classification.

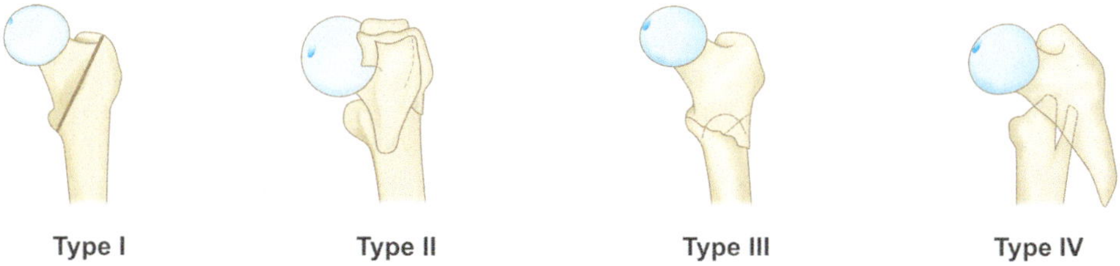

Type I Type II Type III Type IV

Fig. 12.17: Boyd and **Griffith** classification.

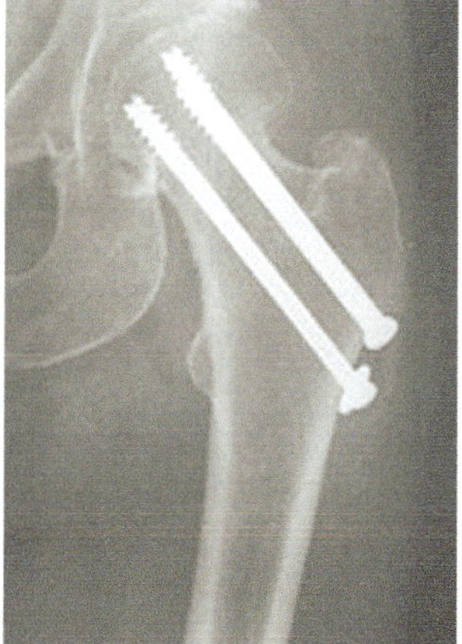

Fig. 12.18: Fixation with multiple hip screw.

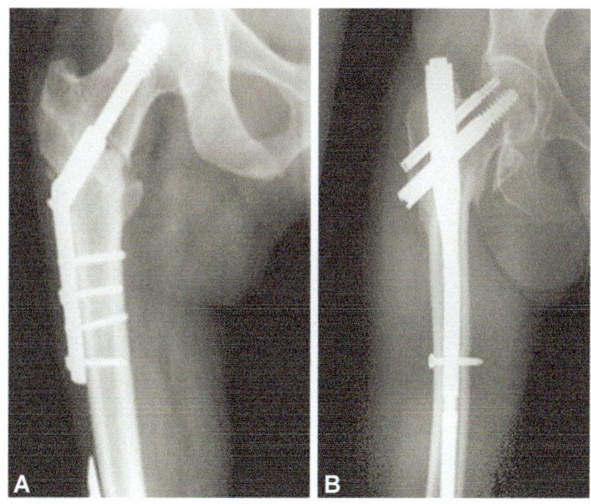

Figs. 12.19A and B: Fixation with: A. Dynamic hip screw (DHS) and; B. Proximal femoral nail (PFN).

2

Section

Some Orthopedic Appliances

- Plaster of Paris and Different Types of Cast
- Review of Orthopedic Tractions
- Some Orthosis and Prosthesis

Chapter

13

Plaster of Paris and Different Types of Casts

PLASTER OF PARIS BANDAGE (FIG. 13.1)

- First used by Matthysen Dutch military surgeon in year 1852.
- *Characteristics*:
  - Plaster of Paris (POP) impregnated bandage
  - *Setting time:* 4–5 minutes
  - Full strength of cast is achieved in 24–48 hours
  - Chemical reaction: Plaster of Paris (calcium sulfate hemihydrate) is obtained by heating gypsum (calcium sulfate dihydrate). And again when plaster of Paris comes in contact of water, gypsum reappears with release of some heat (exothermic).

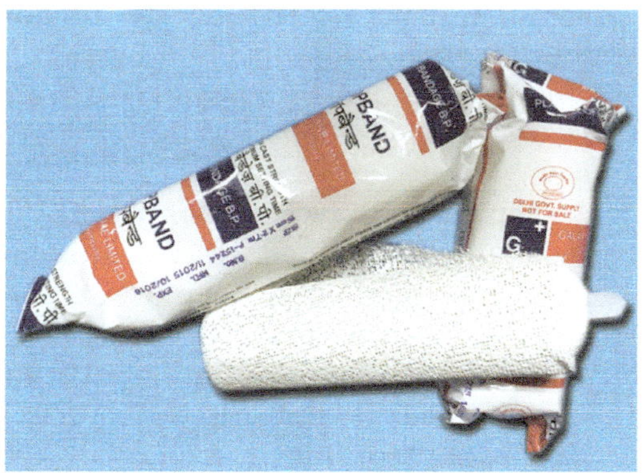

Fig. 13.1: Plaster of Paris bandage.

$$2(CaSO_4.2H_2O) + \text{heat}—2(CaSO_4.1/2\,H_2O) + 3H_2O$$

$$2(CaSO_4.1/2H_2O) + 3H_2O—2(CaSO_4.2H_2O) + \text{heat}$$

  - Water resistant cast is prepared when melamine resin is mixed with plaster of Paris.
- Commonly available sizes: 4 inch, 6 inch × 2.7 meter.
- *Factors affecting setting time:*
  - Temperature of water
  - Manufacturers setting time
  - Impurities in plaster
  - Water condition (hard and soft)
  - Humidity
  - Room temperature.
- *Uses of POP bandage:*
  - As a slab for immobilization:
    - Extent of slab coverage: 50–70% circumference (2/3rd) of limb.
    - For upper limb: 6–8 layers and for lower limb: 10–12 layers.
    - Volar surface in upper limb and dorsal surface in lower limb is preferred. Why? Molding is easier against splint and also helps in reduction maintenance.
  - *As definitive casting:*
    - Wrapped around whole circumference of limb or part involved.
    - The overlapping of bandage is 1/3rd to 1/2 of previous turn.

  - Thickness of cast varies according to nature of fracture, limb type (upper or lower), and age of patient.
- Functional cast bracing.
- Deformity correction by serial casting.
- Partial weight relieving orthosis.
- Spica.

- *Complications with POP bandage:*
  - Neurovascular compromise
  - Compartment syndrome
  - Pressure sore
  - Purulent dermatitis
  - Reactionary edema
  - Fracture disease
  - Wasting of limb
  - Joint stiffness
  - Loss of reduction.

Fracture disease

- It occurs as a result of prolonged immobilization of a fracture leading to:
  - Pain
  - Swelling
  - Stiffness
  - Osteopenia

- *Care of a limb in plaster:*
  - Constant movements of finger or toes.
  - Keep limb elevated.
  - Do not bring the plaster in contact with water.
  - Report immediately if any swelling, color changes, numbness or excess pain.

PRINCIPLE OF REDUCTION AND CASTING

- For fracture reduction appropriate amount of traction and countertraction is applied in proper direction.
- Reduction is achieved by manipulation of distal fragment.
- A perfect reduction is said when all cortices are in contact at fracture site or reduction is said to be acceptable when both fragments have at least 50% contact both in AP and lateral views.
- Even minimal rotation at fracture site is hardly accepted.
- Appropriate padding should be done around fractured limb, especially over bony prominence.
- Reduced position of limb should maintain before, during, and after casting.
- Any indentation during molding and wrinkles should be avoided during cast application.
- A reduced fracture is maintained in such a way that one joint above and one joint below is fully immobilized. But exceptions are Colles' fracture, fracture around ankle, etc.
- The position of limb should be maintained in functional position or position of immobilization. For most of the joint these two are the same but for wrist and hand these stands differently.
  - *Functional position:* The position in which limb can be maximally utilized even after its stiffness, e.g. glass holding position of wrist. This position is used for arthrodesis of a joint.
  - *Position of immobilization:* The position in which the ligaments and tendons around joints remains maximally stretched, so that the contracture of joint could be prevented, e.g. James position of hand (lumbrical plus hand posture).
- The fracture reduction and maintenance under cast also follows the "three-point molding principle of **Charnley's**". Out of these three points, two points lies proximal and distal to fracture site. The third point lies at the site of fracture site but the direction of molding force working here is apposite to the above two points (Fig. 13.2).
- *Ask the patient to follow the instructions like:*
  - Keep the limb elevated. Why we ask the patient lying on bed with a cast in his either of the limb to keep over pillow or hang it with some cord or bandage? Just to maintain the limb above the patient heart level to ensure easy venous drainage and this act minimizes the swelling.

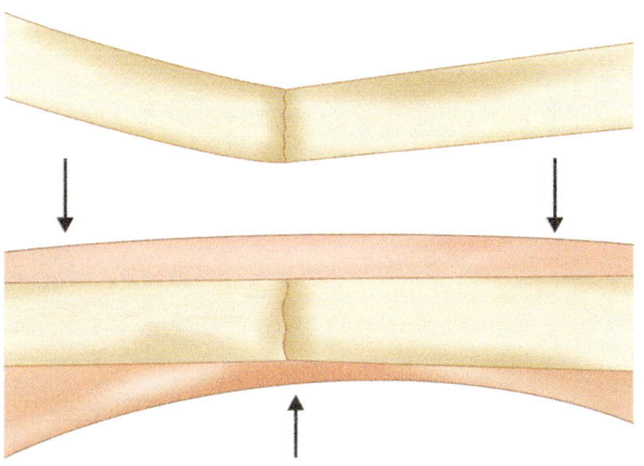

Fig. 13.2: Three-point molding principle of Charnley's.

- Ask the patient to do finger or toe movement—this improves the circulation in the respective limb and side-by-side keep the muscle active and finally minimize postcast stiffness.
- Removal of cast is done immediately if any sign of cast tightness develops in the limb—like continuous pain, discoloration of finger, etc.

SOME COMMON PLASTER SPLINTAGE AND CAST

CASTING IN JAME'S POSITION: RADIAL GUTTER, ULNAR GUTTER, AND VOLAR SPLINTAGE WITH POP (FIGS. 13.3A TO C)

It maintains the wrist in functional position. Its indications are—metacarpals fractures, proximal phalanx fracture of fingers, metacarpophalangeal joint injury, for prevention of clawing, after tendon repair and transfer.

SCAPHOID CAST (FIG. 13.4)

It maintains the thumb in slight abduction. It is also called glass holding position. At its name suggest it is used for scaphoid fracture.

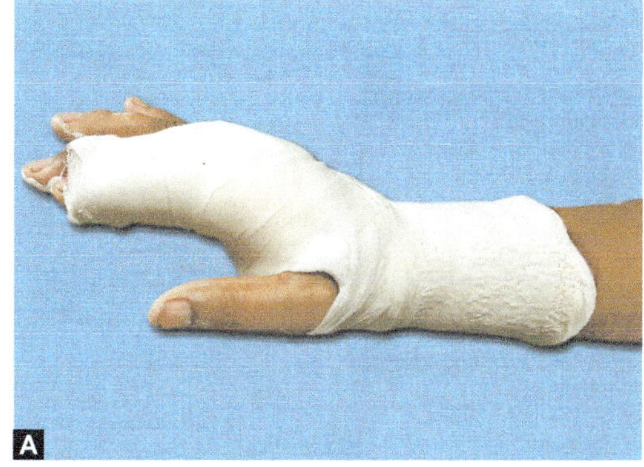

Fig. 13.3A: Radial gutter in Jame's position.

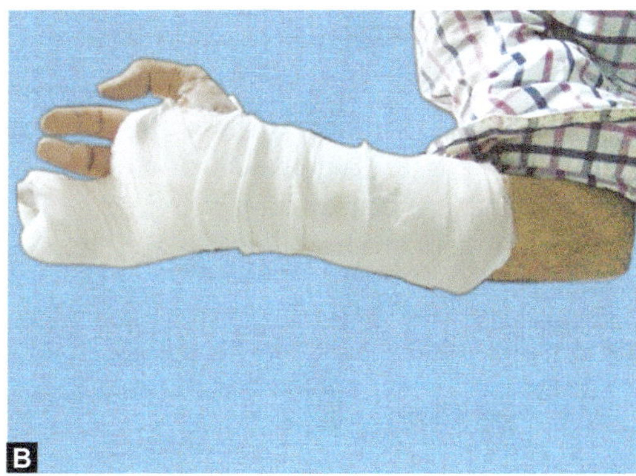

Fig. 13.3B: Ulnar gutter in Jame's position.

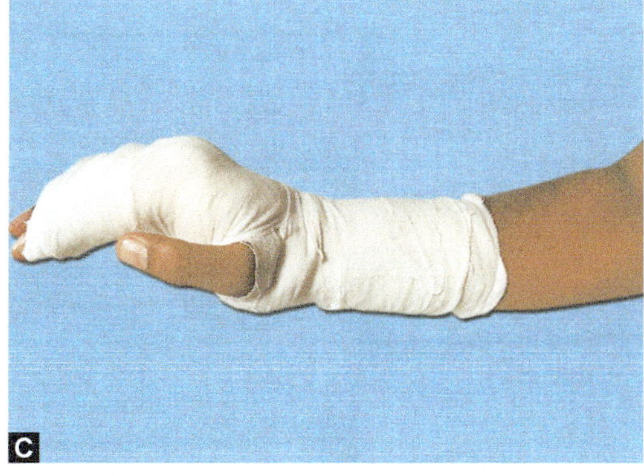

Fig. 13.3C: Volar splint in Jame's position.

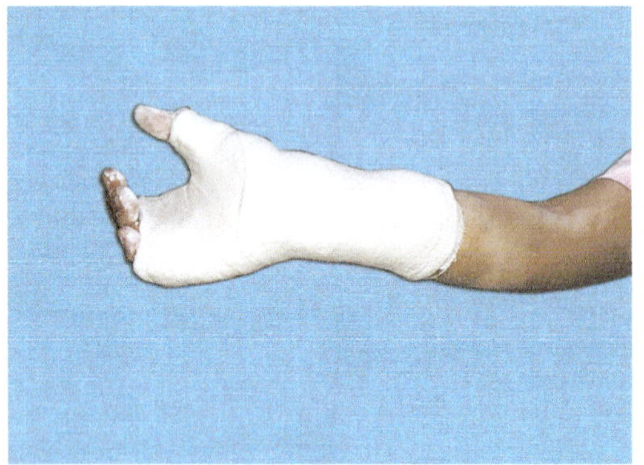

Fig. 13.4: Scaphoid cast.

THUMB SPICA (FIG. 13.5)

Here limb is incorporated with thumb. It is commonly used for immobilization of thumb injuries around first carpometacarpal joint, metacarpophalangeal joint and interphalangeal joint.

COLLES' CAST (FIG. 13.6)

It maintains the wrist in palmar flexed position and slightly ulnarward deviated to counter the deformity of Colles, fracture. As name suggest suggests it is used for Colles's fracture of distal radius.

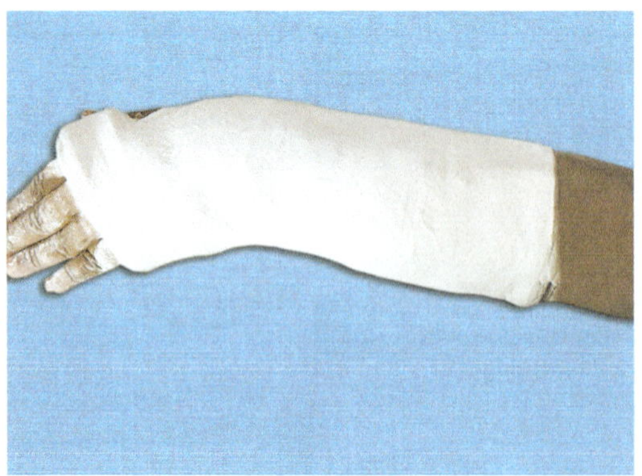

Fig. 13.6: Colles' cast.

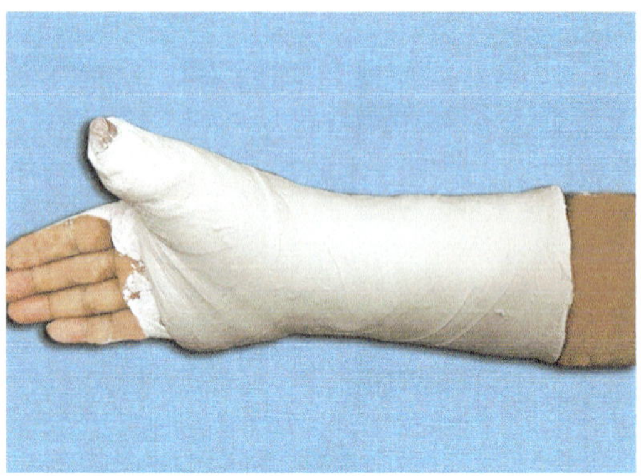

Fig. 13.5: Thumb spica.

U-SLAB/CAST (FIG. 13.7)

It incorporates outer and inner arm and extends upto junction of shoulder and neck. It is used for fracture shaft humerus and sometimes for proximal humerus too.

ABOVE ELBOW POP CAST (FIGS. 13.8A TO C)

It extends from wrist to mid arm. This is indicated for both bone radius and ulna fracture: (i) For proximal 1/3 fracture in supinated position; (ii) For middle 1/3rd

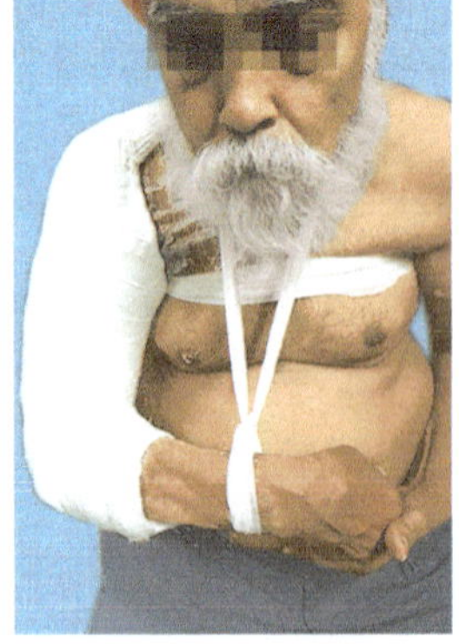

Fig. 13.7: U-cast.

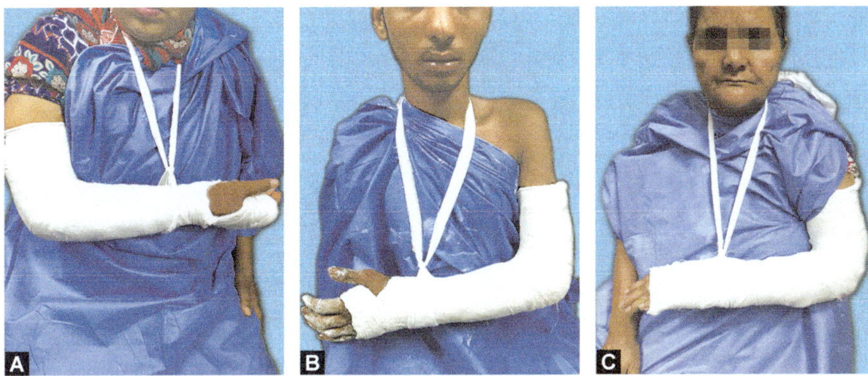

Figs. 13.8A to C: Above elbow cast: A. Supinated forearm; B. Midprone forearm; C. Pronated forearm.

fracture in mid prone position; (iii) For lower 1/3rd fracture in pronated position.

SHOULDER SPICA (FIG. 13.9)

This incorporates trunk with upper limb. It is not very common now a days. Indicated for brachial palsy and selected cases of proximal humerus fractures.

BELOW KNEE CAST AND BOOT CAST (FIG. 13.10A AND B)

It extends from just below the knee (above calf bulk) to the toes. Commonly used: (i) For fracture tarsals as talus, calcaneum; (ii) For fracture metatarsals; (iii) For fracture dislocation around ankle sometimes. When below knee cast is limited distal to the calf bulk, it is called boot cast as it looks like military boot.

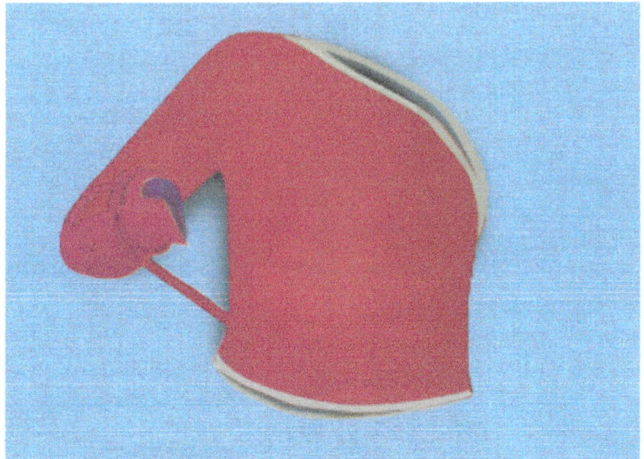

Fig. 13.9: Shoulder spica.

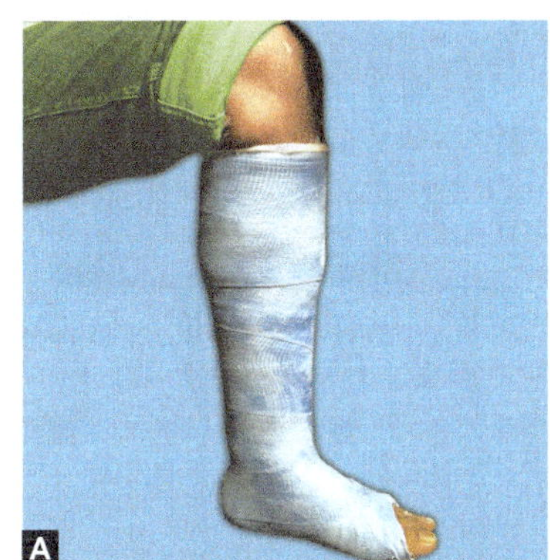

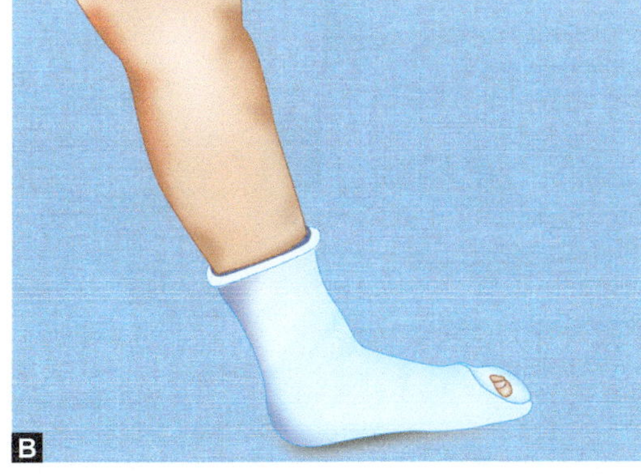

Figs. 13.10A and B: A. Below knee cast; B. Boot cast.

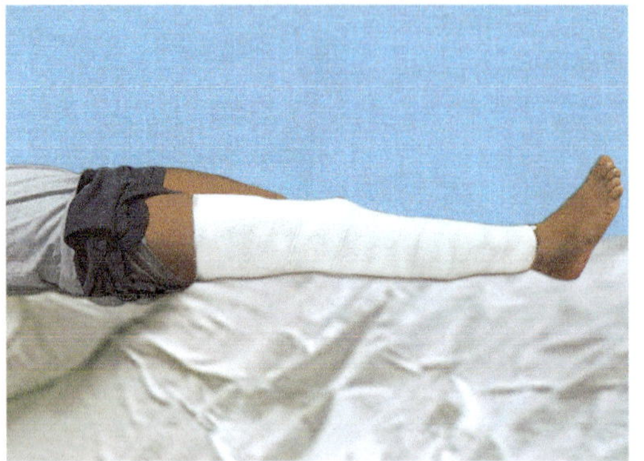

Fig. 13.11: Cylindrical cast.

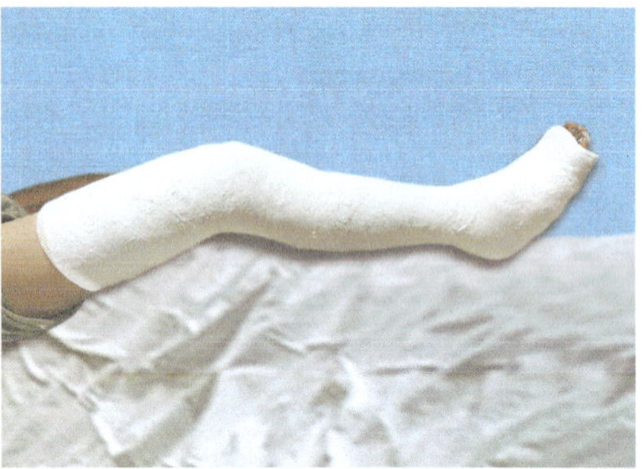

Fig. 13.12: Above knee cast.

CYLINDRICAL CAST (FIG. 13.11)

It extends from groin to just above ankle. Commonly indicated for: (i) injuries around knee; (ii) For fracture patella.

ABOVE KNEE CAST (FIG. 13.12)

It extends from mid thigh to short of metatarsophalangeal joint. It is commonly indicated for: (i) Fracture tibial platue and fracture dislocation around knee; (ii) Fracture shaft tibia and fibula; (iii) For fracture tibial pilon and ankle fracture dislocation. CTEV cast (Fig. 13.13) is a special type of above knee cast used for serial casting in congenital club foot cases.

PATELLAR TENDON BEARING (PTB) CAST (FIG. 13.14)

It acts on the principle of Pascal's Law which enhances osteosynthesis at fracture site

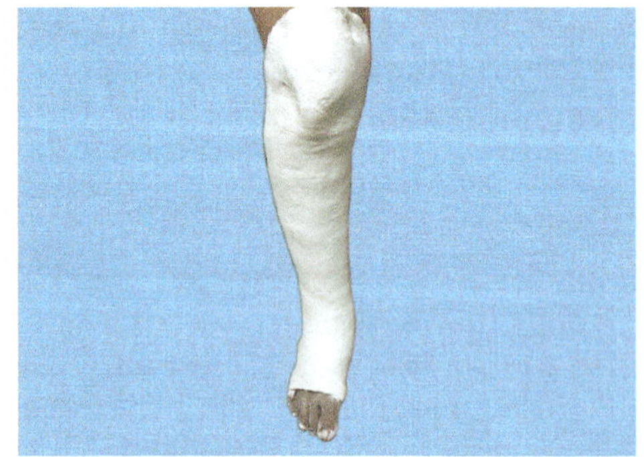

Fig. 13.14: PTB cast—a functional cast bracing.

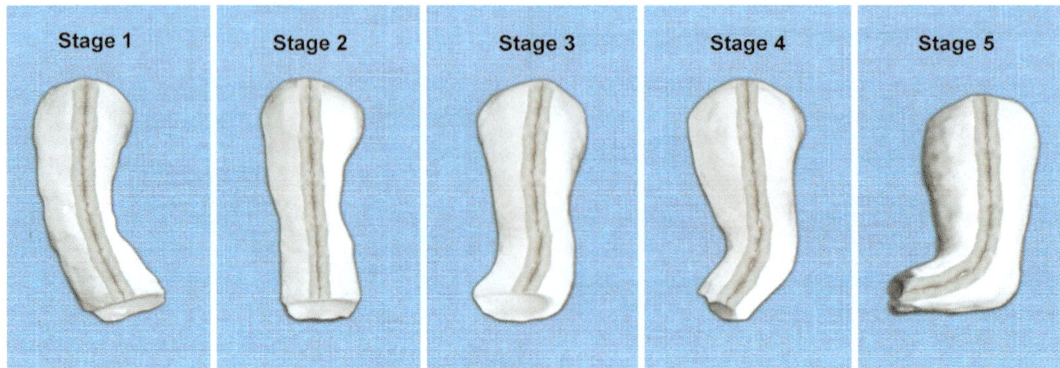

Fig. 13.13: CTEV cast, a special type of AK cast.

during limb loading, i.e. during functioning. Its most common indication is fracture tibia and fibula after removal of conventional above knee cast.

HIP SPICA (FIGS. 13.14A TO D)

It incorporates lower trunk with lower limb. On the basis its extent it may be of three types as under. This cast is commonly practised for: (i) For fracture emur in children; (ii) after pediatric hip surgeries; (iii) After close reduction in development dysplasia of hip.

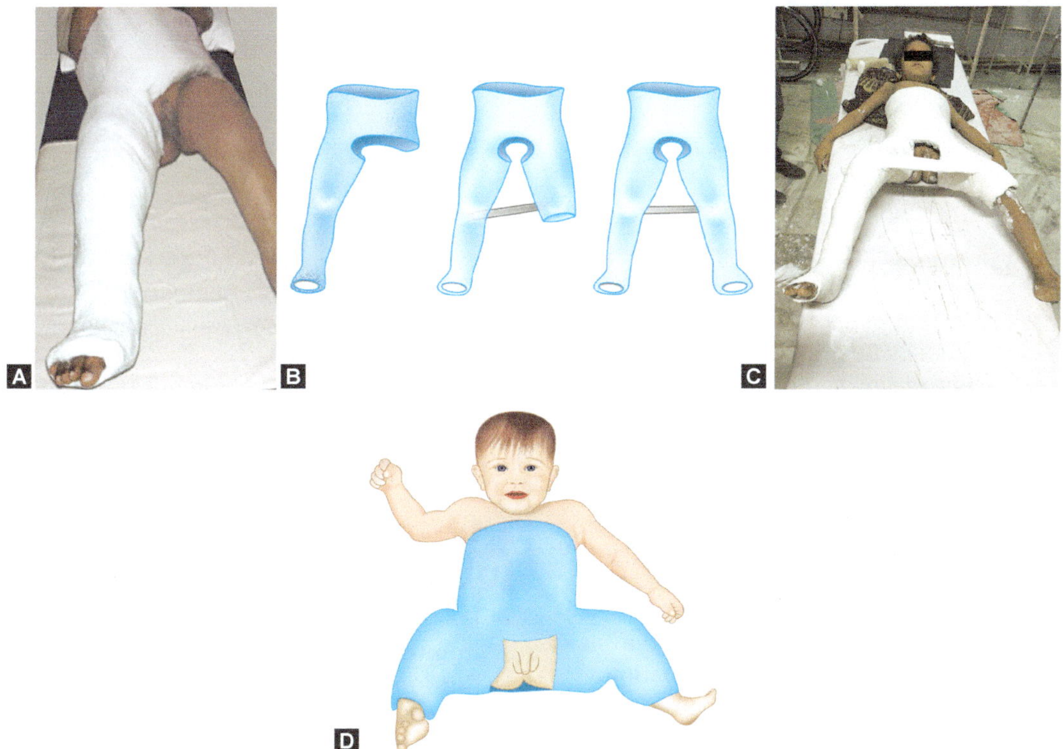

Figs. 13.14A to D: Hip spica: A. Single hip spica; B. Types of hip spica; C. One and half spica; D. Hip spica in human position for developmental dysplasia of the hip (DDH). Spica, when limb is incorporated with its appendages such plaster system is called spica.

Chapter 14

Review of Orthopedic Tractions

BOHLER BRAUN SPLINT (BOHLER: AN AUSTRIAN SURGEON) (FIG. 14.1)

- Designed by **Braun**, modified by **Bohler**.
  - Only one lower most pulley was there in Braun's design.
  - Bohler added two more pulleys.
  - Four pulleys set also available.
- *Uses of pulleys*:
  - 1st pulley in the line of leg—for calcaneum and distal tibial traction.
  - 2nd pulley:
    - In line of supracondylar area of femur—for upper tibial traction.
    - In the line of femur shaft—for distal femoral traction.

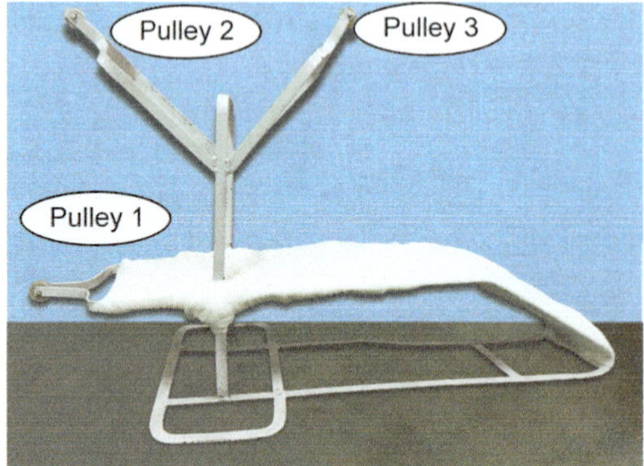

Fig. 14.1: Bohler Braun splint.

  - 3rd pulley—to change the angle of traction and prevent equinus deformity at ankle.
- *Advantages*:
  - Changing the angle of traction as required.
  - Multiple traction can be given simultaneously.

THOMAS SPLINT (ROBERT JONES) (FIGS. 14.2A AND B)

- Designed by **Robert Jones** for immobilization of tuberculosis of knee, but Jones proposed its name as Thomas splint in honor of his maternal uncle **Hugh Owen Thomas**. This splint is also known as Thomas bed knee splint.
- *Components of splint*:
  - Well padded circular or oval ring.
  - Outer bar with proximal angulation-angulation clears the greater trochanter.
  - Inner bar.
  - W-shaped joint of two bars.
- *Measurement of splint*:
  - *Length of splint (inner bar)*: Length between crotch to heel and add 6–9" to it.
  - For circumference of splint:
    - Oblique circumference is taken below gluteal fold and ischial tuberosity.
    - *With normal thigh*: Oblique circumference of thigh and add 2" to it.

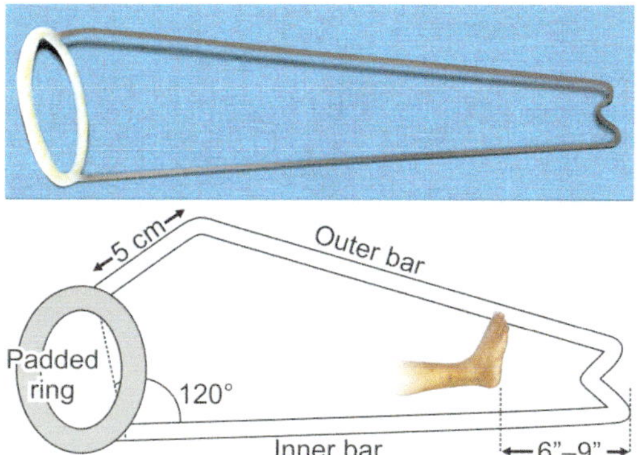

Fig. 14.2A: Thomas splint.

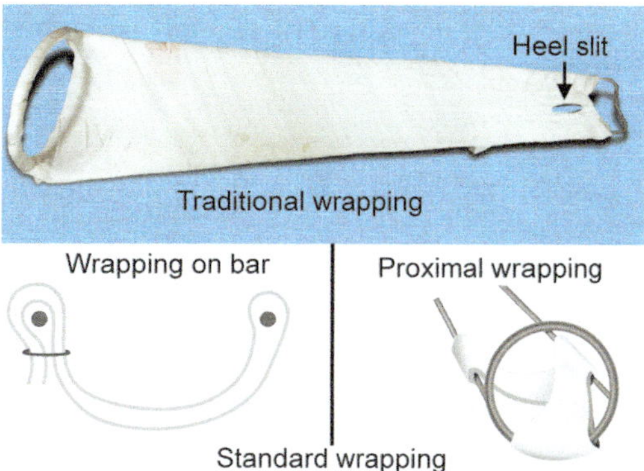

Fig. 14.2B: Thomas splint padding.

  - *With affected thigh*: Oblique circumference equal to internal circumference of padded ring.
- Angle between plane of ring and inner bar—120°.
- Proximal angulation in outer bar is at 5 cm from ring.

- *Wrapping and padding of splint*:
  - Wrapping of splints in U manner with 6" roller bandage
- *Uses:*
  - For transportation of fractured lower limb.
  - For traction (fixed or sliding) in pediatric fracture shaft femur.

BOHLER'S STIRRUP (FIG. 14.3)

- *Components of Bohler's stirrup*:
  - Loop for traction cord.
  - Screw securing Steinmann pin.
  - Side limbs.

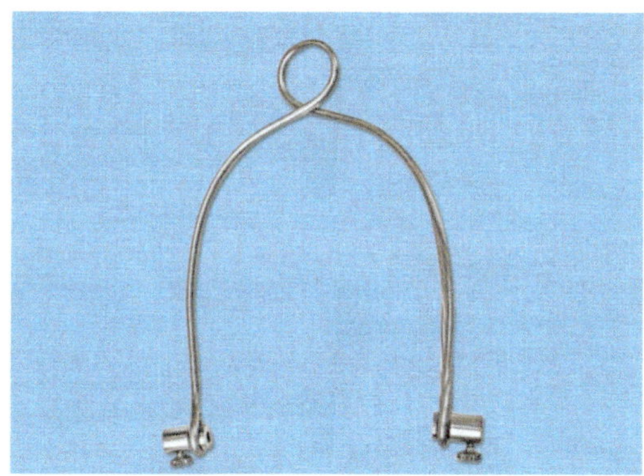

Fig. 14.3: Bohler's stirrup.

- *Used as a* component of skeletal traction.
- *Advantage:* Traction can be applied in any direction without rotating the pin.

STEINMANN PIN AND DENHAM PIN (FIGS. 14.4 A AND B) (TABLE 14.1)

Table 14.1: Difference between Steinmann pin and Denham pin.

	Steinman pin	Denham pin
Parts	• Trocar tip. • Smooth and rounded shaft. • Quadrangular top—to hold firmly in T-handle.	• Trocar tip. • Threaded (32 mm) midportion, thread diameter 0.5 mm more than shaft. • Quadrangular top—to hold firmly in T-handle.
Sizes	Diameter 3–6 mm (interval 0.5 mm), length 15–30 cm (interval 5 cm).	Diameter 3–6 mm (interval 0.5 mm), length 15–30 cm (interval 5 cm).
Uses	For skeletal traction in good quality bone.	For skeletal traction in osteoporotic bone and fully cancellous bone like calcaneum.

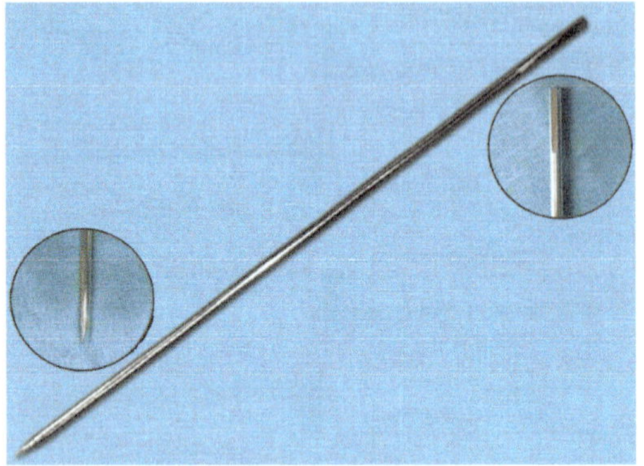

Fig. 14.4A: Steinmann pin.

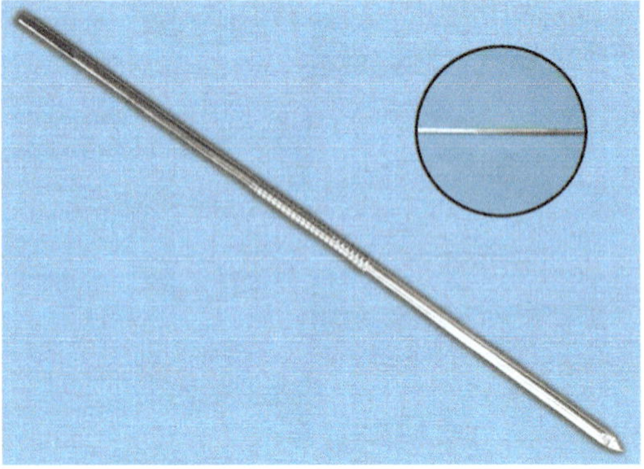

Fig. 14.4B: Denham pin.

BUCK'S PULLEY (FIG. 14.5)

- *Components*:
  - Three pulleys as upper, middle and lower.
  - Bed holding frame.

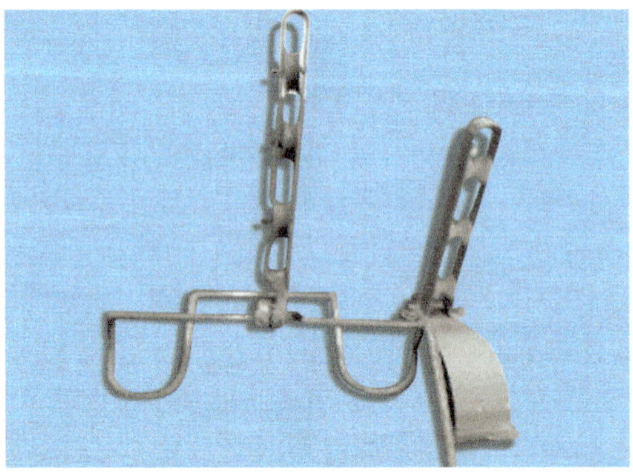

Fig. 14.5: Buck's pulley.

- *Preferred pulley wheels*:
  - *Wheel diameter*: 5-6.25 cm.
  - *Axel-diameter*: 6 mm.
- *Uses:* Different pulleys are used for alignment of distal fragment in relation to proximal fragment by adjusting traction cord on at different heights.

TRACTION (FIGS. 14.6A AND B)

- A mechanical force applied against a resistance to overcome deforming forces on a fractured fragment or pathologic joint.
- *Benefits of traction*:
  - Relives spasm and pain.
  - Fracture reduction and maintenance.
  - Deformity prevention and correction.
  - Controls movement at fracture site which promotes healing.

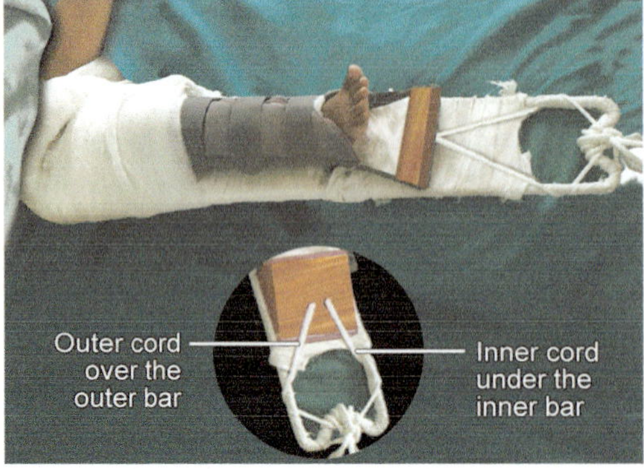

Fig. 14.6A: Fixed traction.

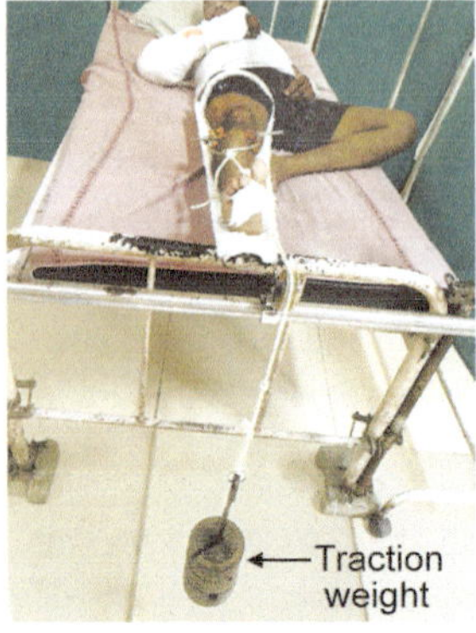

Fig. 14.6B: Sliding traction.

Table 14.2: Types of traction.

	Fixed traction (Fig. 14.6A)	Sliding traction (Fig. 14.6B)
Definition	When counter traction obtained by an appliance which takes the purchase on a part of body, arrangement is called fixed traction.	When counter traction obtained by weight of all or part of body under influence of gravity, it is called sliding traction.
Characteristics	• Given through skin traction (mainly). • *Traction weight*: 2.3 kg. • Cord is fixed to splint. • Part of the couch is not elevated.	• It can be given by both skin and skeletal traction. • A traction cord runs over the pulley system. • The traction weight is fastened with traction cord. • Here counter traction is achieved by elevating the side of couch from where traction weight is passing, e.g. lower limb traction—foot end of couch is elevated.
Uses	• Maintain undisplaced fractures. • Used for transportation.	• For fracture reduction. • For pathological joint immobilization.
Wooden blocks: Standard height—9″ (6″ blocks are also available); 1″ elevation of couch corresponds to 0.46 kg CT force.		

- *Traction weight*: On an average, traction weight is equivalent to 10% of body weight but it depends upon following factors (Fig. 14.6B):
  - Site of fracture.
  - Skin condition of limb.
  - Bulk and power of muscle.
  - Age and body weight of patient.
  - Friction and mechanical advantage of system.
- *Counter traction (CT)*: A force applied apposite to traction force is called counter traction. On the basis of counter traction, traction can be divided into two broad groups, (Table 14.2).

Skin Traction (Figs. 14.7A and B)

- Traction force applied over large area of skin called skin traction.
- Features:
  - Apply distal to fracture site; do not extend it too proximal or too distal to fracture site otherwise traction will be inefficient.
  - Two types of skin traction are commonly used:
    - Adhesive (maximum weight—6.7 kg)
    - Nonadhesive (maximum weight—4.5 kg) and used for:
      - Allergic skin from adhesive traction
      - Thin and atrophic skin.
- Skin traction kit contains:
  - *Skin strap*: Recommended length of strap is approximately 15-20 cm and add 5 cm to it that loops beyond the distal most part of the limb; loop ensures free movement of toes or fingers.
  - Crepe bandage.
  - Spreader (wooden or metallic)—7.5 cm.
  - Cotton roll.
  - Tincture benzoin.
- How to apply skin traction:
  - Do shaving of skin hairs.
  - Apply tincture benzoin in nonadhesive type.
  - Do padding over bony prominences if any.
  - Apply strapping by the side of limb.
  - Apply crepe bandage around the limb.
- *Complications*:
  - Skin allergy due to adhesive material.
  - Pressure sore due to inadequate padding over bony prominences.

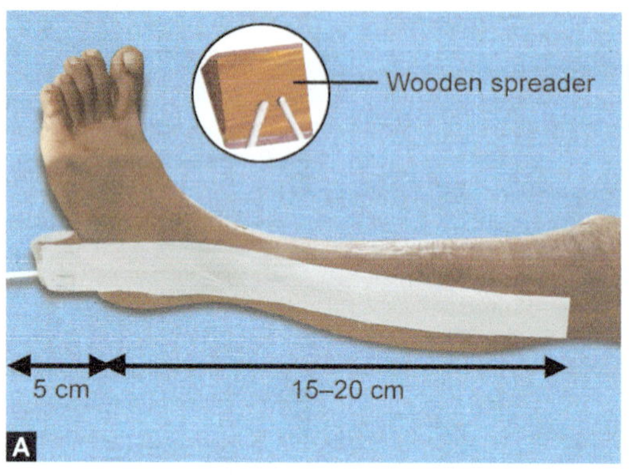

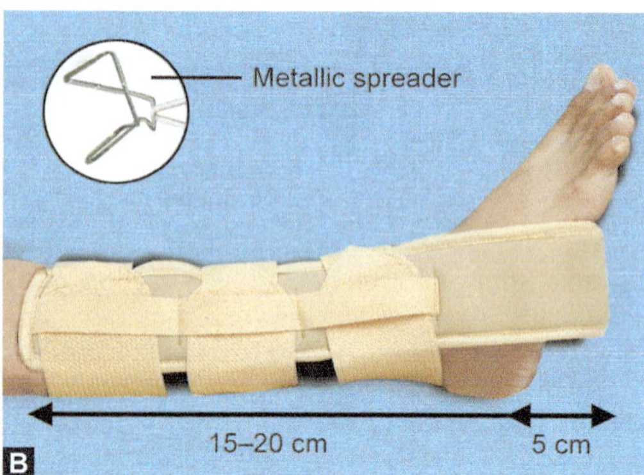

Figs. 14.7A and B: Skin traction: A. Adhesive type; B. Nonadhesive type.

- *Common peroneal nerve palsy*:
  - Due to lateral rotation of limb.
  - Direct compression by splint.
  - Sliding skin traction compressing over fibular head.
- *Contraindications*:
  - Injured skin (abrasion, severe bruise or laceration).
  - Skin disease like dermatitis.
  - Gangrene or varicose ulcer following impaired circulation.
  - Overriding of fracture fragment where skeletal traction is needed.

Skeleton Traction

- Traction forces acting directly through a part of a bone are called skeleton traction.
- *Features*:
  - It is also applied distal to the fracture site.
  - Applied through a pin or K-wire.
  - More traction weight can be given.
- *Equipment for skeletal traction*:
  - Steinmann pin.
  - T-handle with Jacob's chuck.
  - Surgical blade.
  - Xylocaine injection.
  - Syringe with needle.
  - Surgical gloves.
- *Steps of traction application*:
  - Stab incision.
  - Secure underlying structures.
  - Keep the limb in position of 15° external rotation (lower limb).
  - Penetrate horizontally.
  - Apply tincture benzoin soaked 2 separate gauze over pin-skin interface.
- *Direction of entry of pin*: Always keep the entry point of pin through the side where there is any neurovascular bundle because there is control over pin at entry point but not at exit point.
- *Complications*:
  - Pin track infection (ring sequestrum).
  - Physeal injury in children.
  - Ligamentous injury if heavy traction for prolonged periods.
  - Distraction of fracture site.
  - Neurovascular injury.
  - Splintering of cortex (due to hammering).
  - Incorrect placement of pin leading to:
    - Altered direction of traction.
    - Rotation of limb.
    - Make splint application difficult.
- *Care of pin tract*:
  - Daily dressing is preferred.
  - Two step dressing:
    - First wipe the pin-skin interface with spirit (some prefer normal saline).
    - Then apply cotton gauze soaked with betadine or chlorhexidine solution.
  - Do not apply pressure bandage around the limb adjacent to Steinmann pin due to risk of local edema or pressure sore.

- Do local examination for any pin-tract infection. Tenderness, warmth, pus, loosening of pin, etc. If so remove skeletal traction and apply some other modality of traction.
- Prophylactic antibiotic is also preferred in systemically ill patient.

SOME COMMON ORTHOPEDIC TRACTIONS

BRYANT'S/GALLOW'S TRACTION (FIG. 14.8)

Indication

(1) For fracture femur in children below 2 years; (2) After pediatric hip surgeries, and; (3) After close reduction in development dysplasia of hip.

UPPER TIBIAL TRACTION (FIGS. 14.9A AND B)

Indication

(1) For fracture neck femur; (2) For fracture trochanter of femur; (3) For fracture shaft femur; (4) For supra condylar fracture of femur,

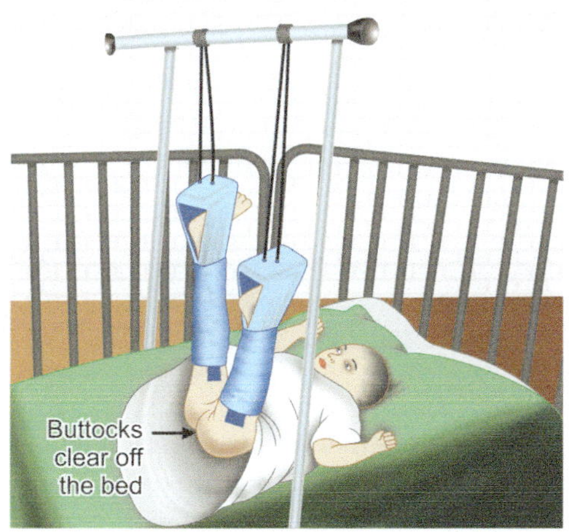

Fig. 14.8: Bryant's/Gallow's traction.

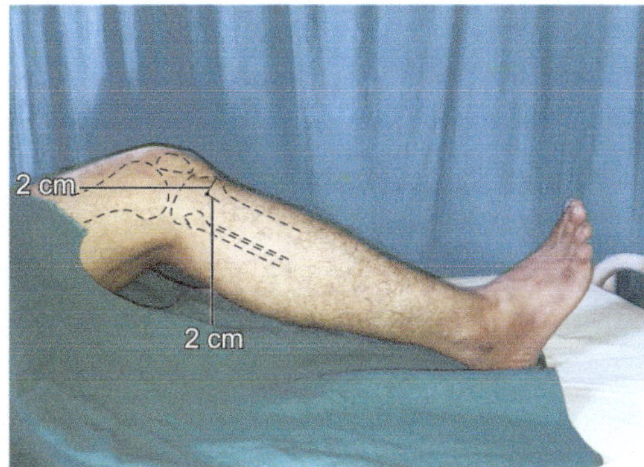

Fig. 14.9A: Site for upper tibial traction application.

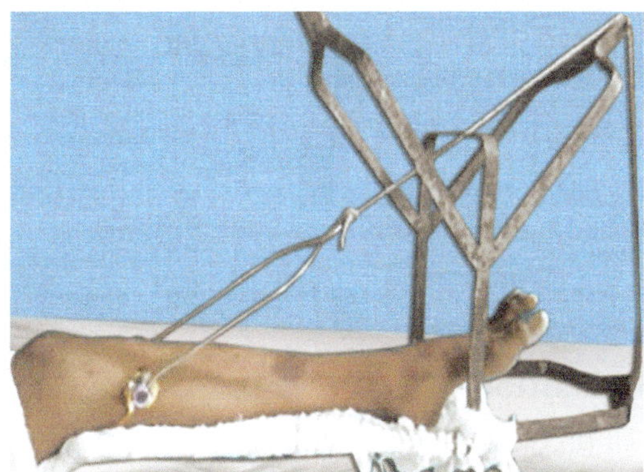

Fig. 14.9B: Upper tibial traction on Bohler-Braun splint.

and; (5) For maintenance after reduction of hip dislocation.

DISTAL TIBIAL TRACTION (FIG. 14.10)

Indication

(1) For proximal tibial fracture and; (2) For knee fracture dislocation.

CALCANEAL TRACTION (FIG. 14.11)

Indication

(1) For distal tibial fracture and; (2) For ankle fracture dislocation.

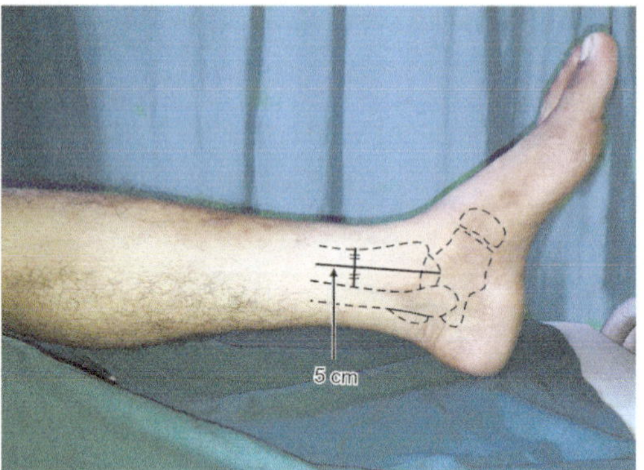

Fig. 14.10: Site for distal tibial traction application.

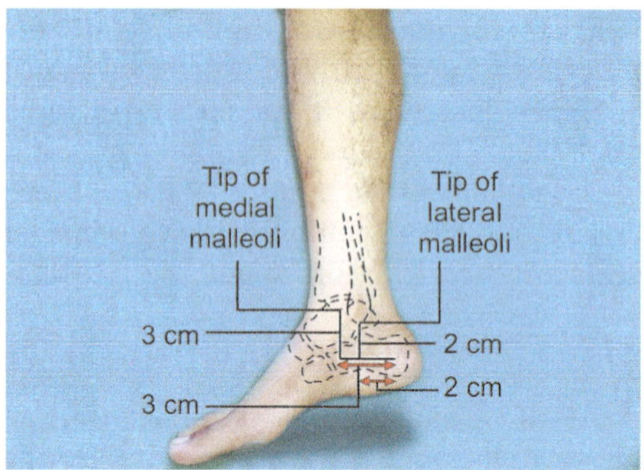

Fig. 14.11: Site for calcaneal traction application.

HEAD HALTER TRACTION (FIG. 14.12)

Indication

(1) For cervical spine fracture dislocation and;
(2) For cervical spondylosis treatment.

PELVIC TRACTION (FIG. 14.13)

Indication

For prolapsed intervertebral disk diseases.

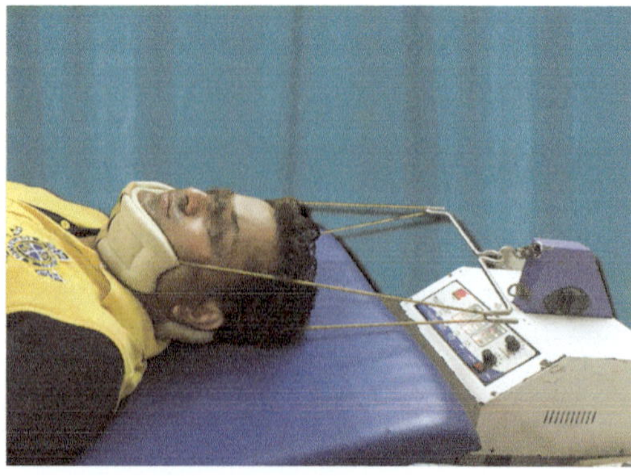

Fig. 14.12: Head halter traction.

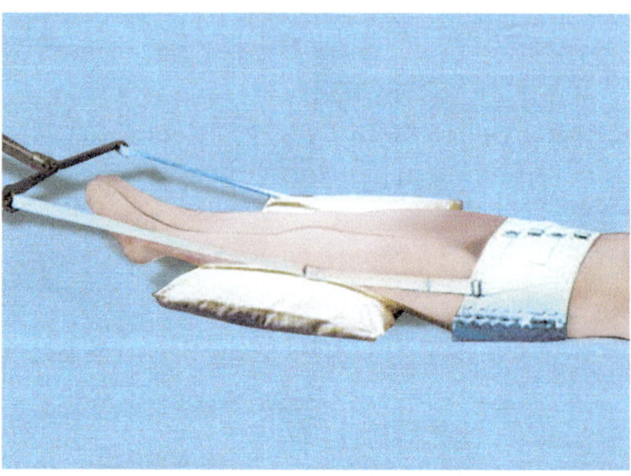

Fig. 14.13: Pelvic traction.

CERVICAL TRACTION BY CRUTCH-FIELD TONG (FIGS. 14.14A AND B)

Indication

(1) For cervical spine fracture dislocation and;
(2) For cervical spondylosis with severe nerve compression.

BOOT AND BAR/DEROTATION BAR/ FLAPPER (FIG. 14.15)

Indication

For conservative treatment of intertrochanteric fracture and impacted fracture neck femur.

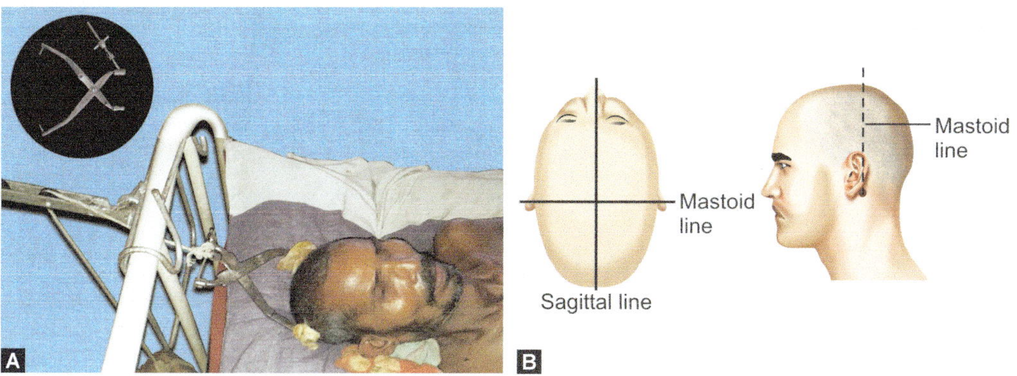

Figs. 14.14A and B: A. Cervical traction; B. Site for Crutchfield tong application.

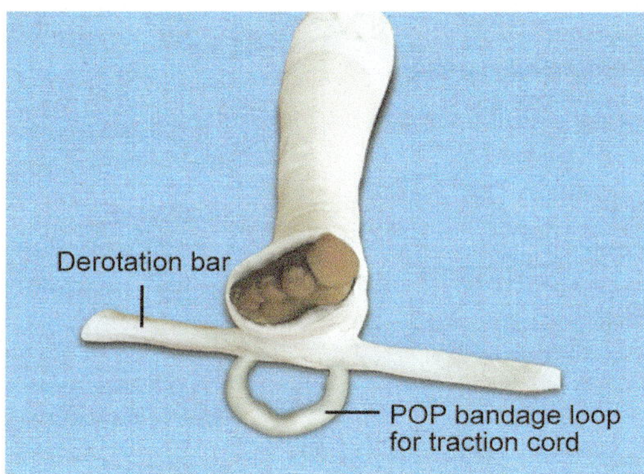

Fig. 14.15: Boot and bar.

Chapter

15

Some Orthosis and Prosthesis

BASICS OF ORTHOSIS

- An orthosis is an orthopedic appliance used to modify the structural and functional characteristics of body parts. Its functions are as follows:
  - To control, limit or guide an extremity or joints
  - To correct deformity of body or body parts
  - To assist weaker segment of body
  - To enforce specific directional control to joint
  - To keep the joints or body parts in functional position.
- Classification of orthosis (anatomical basis) (Table 15.1).
- Classification of orthosis (Functional basis):
  - *Dynamic orthosis*: These splints have some mobile unit and allow movement to splinted part (Fig. 15.1A).
  - *Static orthosis*: These splints have neither any mobile unit nor allow any motion to splinted part (Fig. 15.1B).
- Complications of orthosis:
  - Atrophy of the part
  - Neurovascular compromise
  - Joint stiffness
  - Skin complication.

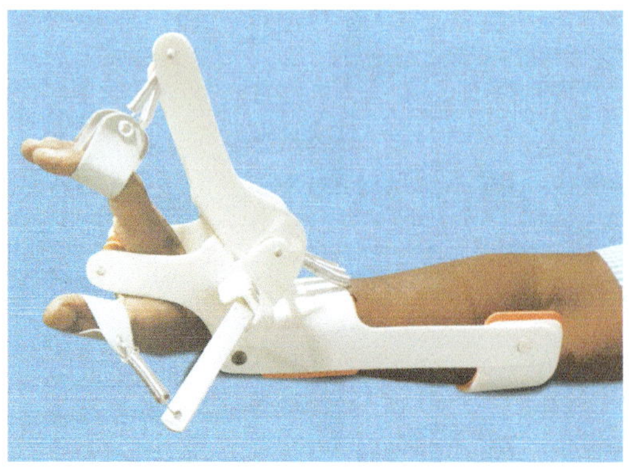

Fig. 15.1A: Dynamic orthosis.

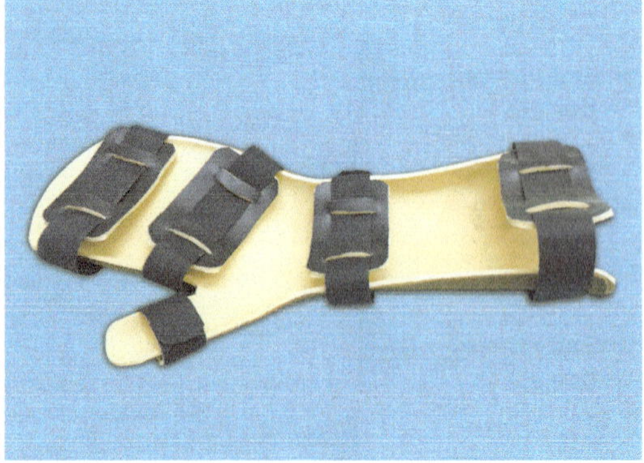

Fig. 15.1B: Static orthosis.

Table 15.1: Anatomical classification of orthosis.

Lower limb	Upper limb	Spine
• Hip knee ankle foot orthosis (HKAFO) • Knee ankle foot orthosis (KAFO) • Ankle foot orthosis (AFO) • Foot orthosis (FO)	• Shoulder orthosis (SO) • Elbow wrist hand orthosis (EWHO) • Wrist hand orthosis (WHO) • Hand orthosis (HO)	• Cervical orthosis (CO) • Cervico-thoraco-lumbo-sacral orthosis (CTLSO) • Thoraco-lumbo-sacral orthosis (TLSO) • Lumbo-sacral orthosis (LSO)

SOME COMMON ORTHOSIS

Conventional Type Ankle Foot Orthosis (AFO) (Figs. 15.2A and B)

- The components of conventional ankle foot orthosis is shown in Figure 15.2A. The moulded variety also called total contact AFO is very common nowadays. The function of orthosis are as follows:
  - Support the ankle and foot, e.g. foot drop
  - To maintain ankle stability, e.g. post-polio residual deformity, neuropathic feet.

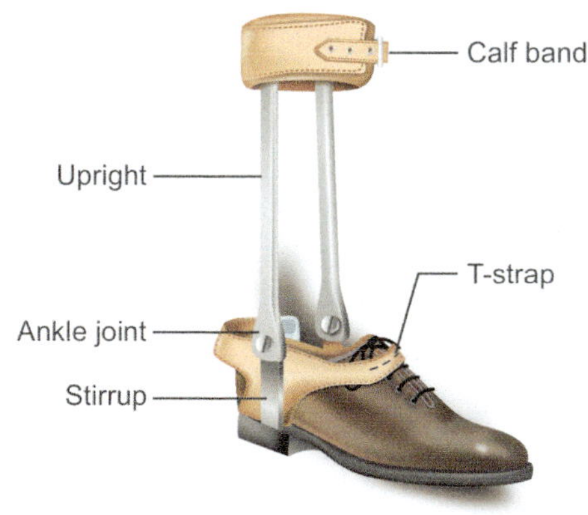

Fig. 15.2A: Conventional type AFO.

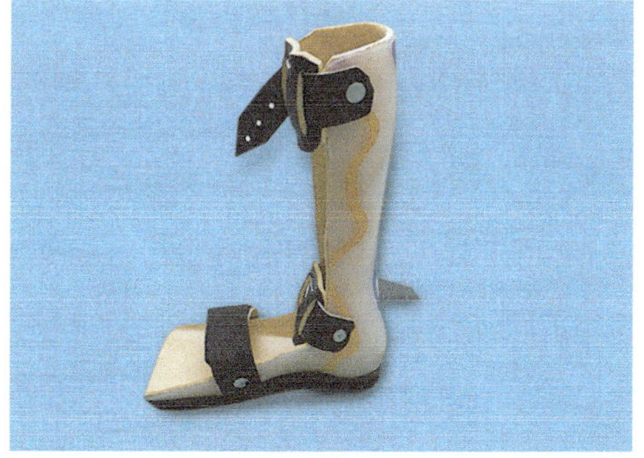

Fig. 15.2B: Total contact AFO.

Orthoses for Congenital Talipes Equinovarus (CTEV) (Figs. 15.3A to C)

CTEV Shoe

- *Characteristics of CTEV shoe are as*:
  - No heel
  - Straight medial border
  - Lateral sole wedge.

Dennis-Browne Splint

- This device is named after Australian borne **Dr John Dennis Wolko Browne** working in London (1934).

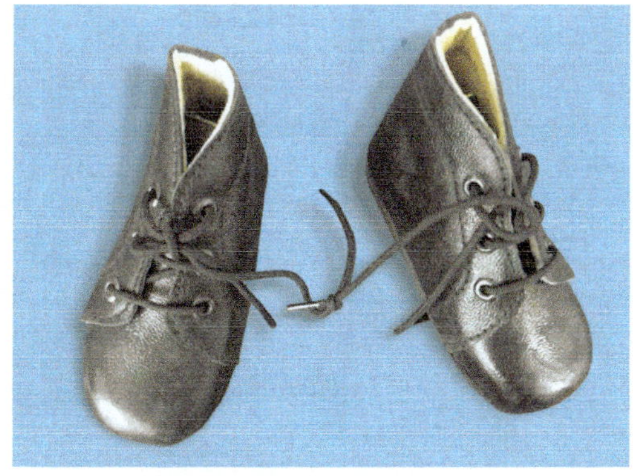

Fig. 15.3A: CTEV shoe.

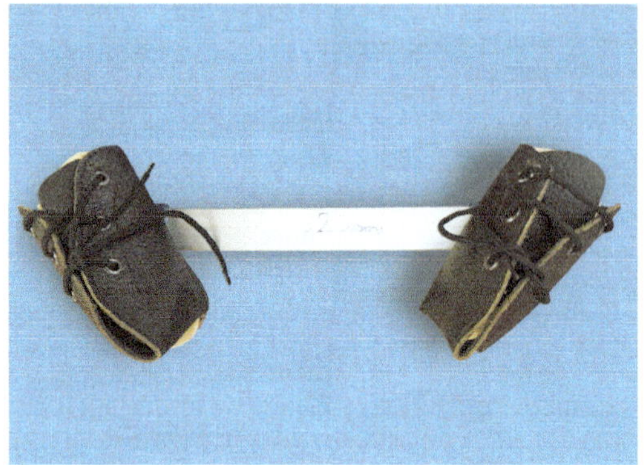

Fig. 15.3B: Dennis-Browne splint.

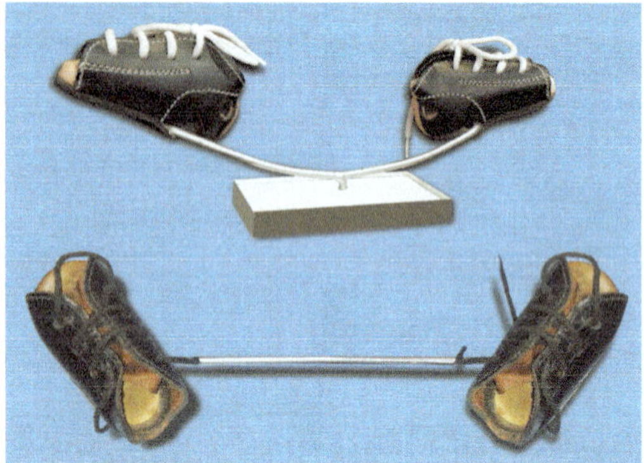

Fig. 15.3C: Steinbeck foot abduction brace.

Components and function:
- Curved bar (equal to width of shoulders) to maintain dorsiflexion at ankle
- Pair of CTEV shoes attached at ends of bar
- Winged nuts to allow abduction of each foot
- Commonly used in night.

Note: A similar orthosis called Steinbeck foot abduction brace is commonly used nowadays for maintenance of corrected club foot. It was designed in Uganda by **Michael Steinbeck** and endorsed by **Dr Ponsetti**. This is effective and low cost option for developing countries (Fig. 15.3C).

Cock-up Splints (Wrist Hand Orthosis) (Figs. 15.4A and B)

- It is a wrist hand orthosis and may be dynamic or static.
- *How it works:*
  The static cock-up splints act as a resting splint that maintain the wrist in extension position, but provide freedom for finger movement. On the other hand, its dynamic variant is a functional splint where wrist is maintained in almost 45° of extension and passive extension of fingers are performed by recoiling of actively flexed finger on rubber loop system, e.g. wrist drop.

Cervical Collar (Soft and Hard Variety) (Figs. 15.5A and B)

- Cervical collar extends superiorly from base of mandible and superior nuchal line to manubrium and C-7 spine inferiorly. On the basis of fabrication it may be of soft or rigid variety. It performs the following funtions:

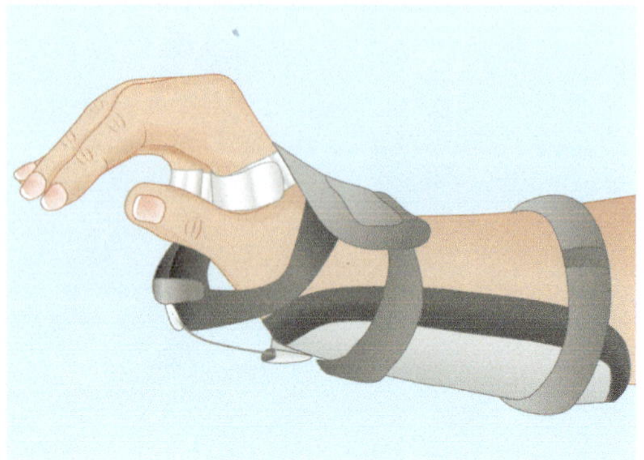

Fig. 15.4A: Static cock-up splints.

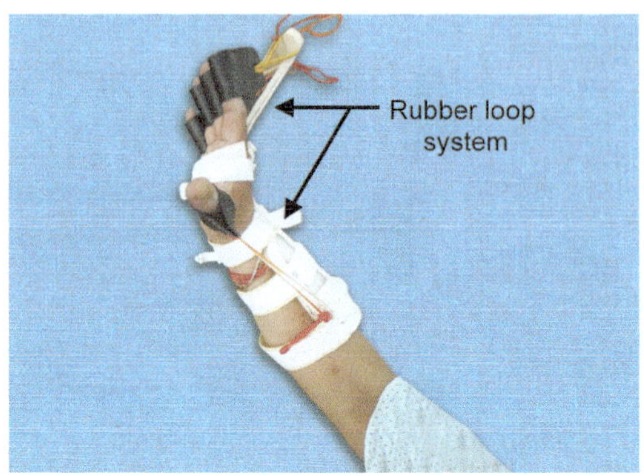

Fig. 15.4B: Dynamic cock-up splints.

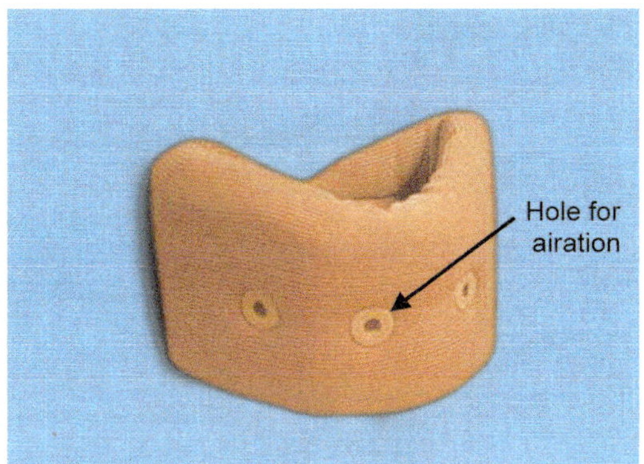

Fig. 15.5A: Soft cervical collar.

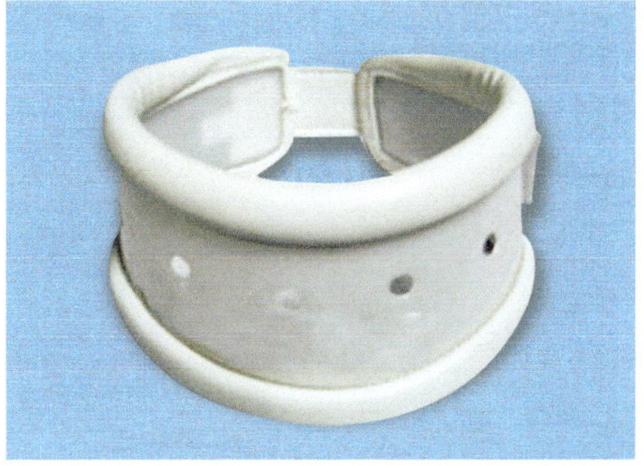

Fig. 15.5B: Hard cervical collar.

- Kinesthetic reminder to limit cervical motion—relieve inflammation.
- Heat retention for pain relief.
- Motion control: Rigid variety has more control over cervical motion than soft variety.

Indication: Commonly used for mild soft-tissue strain and sprain, spasm, spondylosis, disk diseases, etc. around neck.

Thoracolumbosacral Orthosis (TLSO) Taylor's Brace (Figs. 15.6A and B)

- **Taylor brace** is a semi-rigid design orthosis. It works in the following ways:
  - It acts on the principle of three point pressure (application of single main force against two already acting counter-forces) and limits flexion and extension movement of thoracolumbar spine.
  - It also increases intra-abdominal pressure and convert abdominal cavity into semi-rigid cylinder that helps spinal motion restriction.

  Indication: Commonly used for spinal pathology of level T4-L2.
  - Spinal osteoporosis
  - Spinal trauma
  - Degenerative disk disease
  - Pott's spine.

Note: An another semi-rigid frame orthosis, used for similar purpose, famously known as anterior spinal hyperextension (ASH) orthosis (Fig. 15.6B).

Lumbosacral Corset/Brace (Figs. 15.7A and B)

Comparision between lumbosacral corset and lumbosacral brace is shown in Table 15.2.

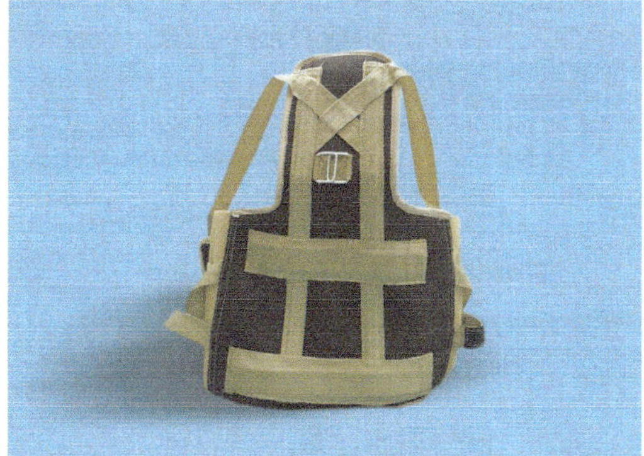

Fig. 15.6A: Taylor's brace.

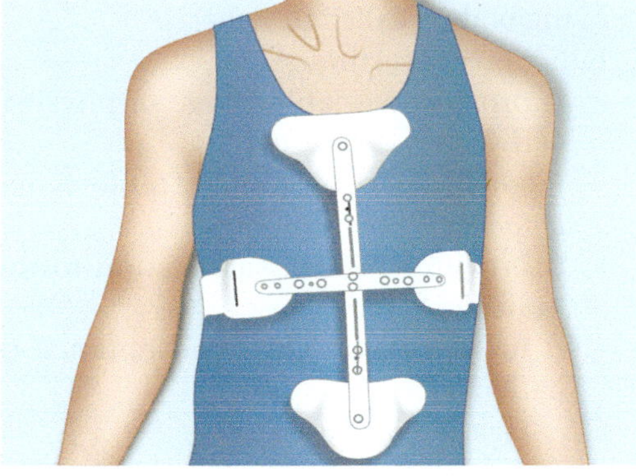

Fig. 15.6B: Anterior spinal hyperextension orthosis.

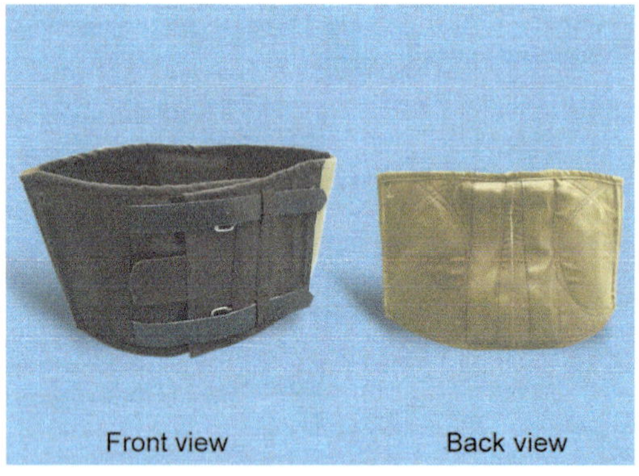

Fig. 15.7A: Lumbosacral corset.

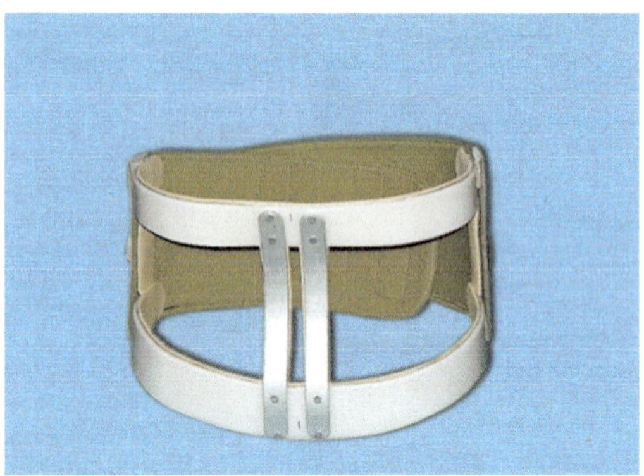

Fig. 15.7B: LS brace/frame.

Table 15.2: Difference between lumbosacral corset and lumbosacral brace.

	Lumbosacral corset	Lumbosacral brace/frame
Functions	• Corset is a fabric garment that encircle the part of body. • LS corset encompasses the abdomen and pelvis and support the lumbosacral spine. It acts as following ways: ➢ Kinesthetic reminder and restrict only terminal movement. ➢ It also increases intra-abdominal pressure and make spine rigid to some-extent.	• It is semi-rigid design orthosis. • It also encompasses the abdomen and pelvis and support the lumbosacral spine. It acts in following ways: ➢ Acts on the principle of 3 point pressure and restrict spinal motion more than the corset. ➢ Increases intra-abdominal pressure and contribute in segmental spinal rigidity.
Indications	Commonly used for spinal pathology level LI-L4 of lesser severity. • Spinal strain and sprain • Degenerative lumbar spine disk disease • Sciatica.	Commonly used for spinal pathology level L1-L4. • Spinal osteoporosis • Spinal trauma • Degenerative disk disease • Spondylosis • Lumbosacral strain • Sciatica.

BASICS OF PROSTHESIS

- Prosthesis: A replacement of missing part of the body is called prosthesis.
- Function of prosthesis:-
  - It provides variable range of physical activity.
  - It provides variable range of professional activities.
  - It provides mental satisfaction to the individual.
  - It increases the social acceptance of patient.
- Classification of prosthesis:
  - *Endoprosthesis:* A prosthesis that replaces internal body part is called endoprosthesis. For example; Austin Moore prosthesis replacement for fracture neck femur in elderly persons.
  - *Exoprosthesis:* A prosthesis that replaces external missing part of body is called exoprosthesis. For example; prosthesis used for amputees.
- Classification of prosthesis (anatomical basis) (Table 15.3):

Table 15.3: Anatomical classification of prosthesis.

Lower limb prosthesis	Upper limb prosthesis
• Above knee (AK) prosthesis • Below knee (BK) prosthesis	• Above elbow (AE) prosthesis • Below elbow (BE) prosthesis

- Complication of prosthesis:
  - Trophy of the part.
  - Skin complication

SOME COMMON PROSTHESIS

Exoskeletal and Endoskeletal Lower Limb Prosthesis (Figs. 15.8A and B)

On the basis of fabrication, the lower limb prosthesis may be of exoskeleton type or endoskeletal type.

- Exoskeletal prosthesis
  - Durable but not adjustable
  - *Parts of ESP*:
    - Socket
    - Shank
    - Foot and ankle assembly
- Endoskeletal prosthesis (ESP):
  - Cosmetic and adjustable
  - *Parts of ESP*:
    - Socket
    - Socket adapter
    - Pylon
    - Ankle adapter
    - Foot component

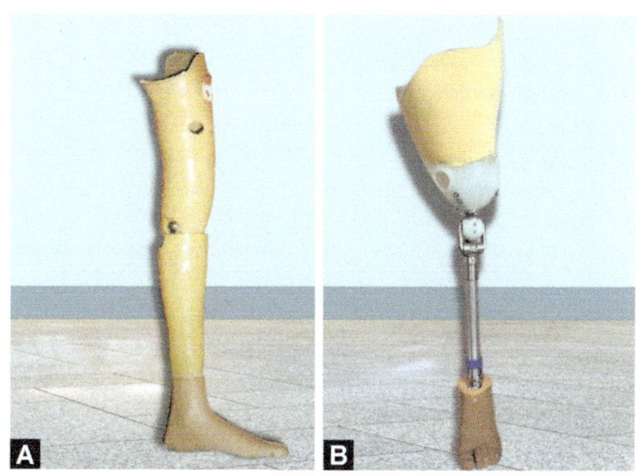

Figs. 15.8A and B: A. Exoskeleton prosthesis; B. Endoskeleton prosthesis.
(*Courtesy:* Sant Prakash Gautam MPO (NIOH), Kolkata)

Prosthetic Foot: Jaipur Foot and Sach Foot (Figs. 15.9A to C) (Table 15.4)

- *Madras foot*:
  - It is also a modification of SACH foot.
  - Crafted in Government Institute of Rehabilitation Medicine (GRIM), Chennai previously called Madras.
  - There are alternate layers of soft and hard rubber separated by 5 mm thick canvas rubber sheet.

Table 15.4: Comparison between Jaipur foot and SACH foot.

	Jaipur foot	SACH foot
Name	Made in Jaipur by Dr **PK Sethi**	Solid ankle cushion heel
Parts	Rubber core + wooden block + vulcanized rubber coating	Wooden keel+ rubber body + straps of hard and soft rubber in heel
Raw material availability	Easily available	Not easily available
Look	Like normal foot	Have to wear under shoes
Durability and water resistance	More	Lesser
Squatting and cross leg sitting	Possible	Possible
Ankle and foot movement like dorsi/plantar flexion + inversion/ eversion + rotation	All three possible	Limited but heel push off present
Walking on uneven surface and bare foot walking	Possible	Not possible
Fatigue resistance	More	Easily cracks
Maintenance	Minimum	More
Cost-effectiveness	More	Less in Indian scenario
Availability	Everywhere	Not everywhere

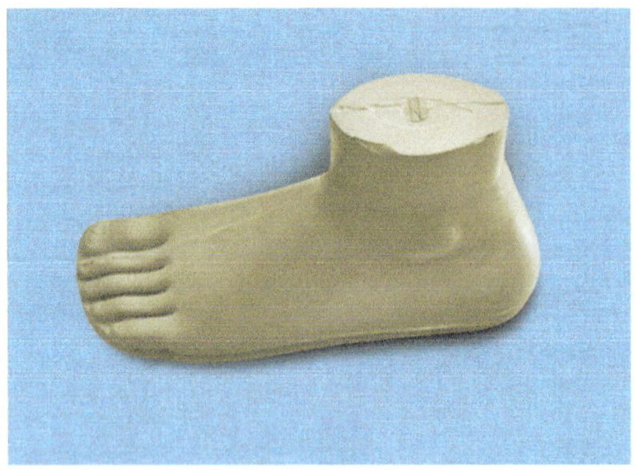

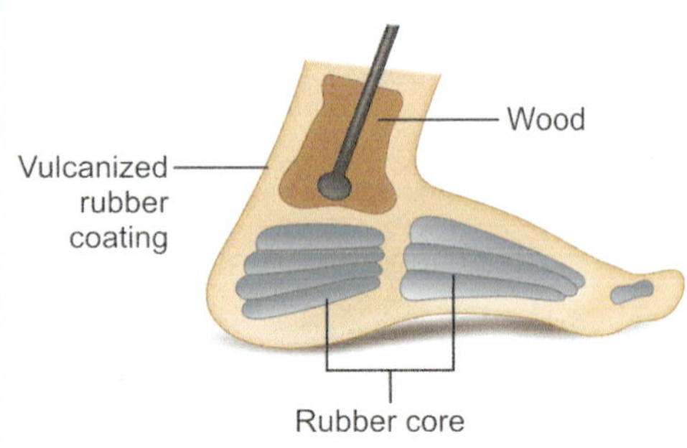

Fig. 15.9A: Jaipur foot.

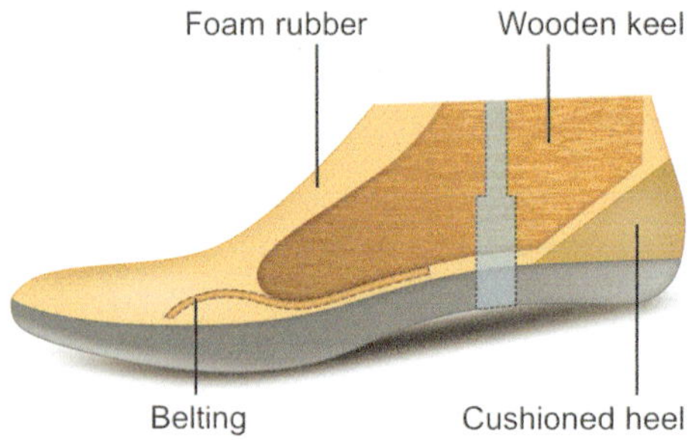

Fig. 15.9B: SACH (solid ankle cushion heel) foot.

- Normal looking dorsum, toes, and tendo-Achilles.
- Advantage of bare foot walking, durability, and cultural value like toe ring wearing, etc.

Upper Limb Prosthesis (Fig. 15.10)

The upper limb prosthesis have components like—power system(body powered, electrical or hybrid), terminal devices(cosmetic hand or functional hand), wrist and elbow section, arm and forearm system, and socket and suspension.

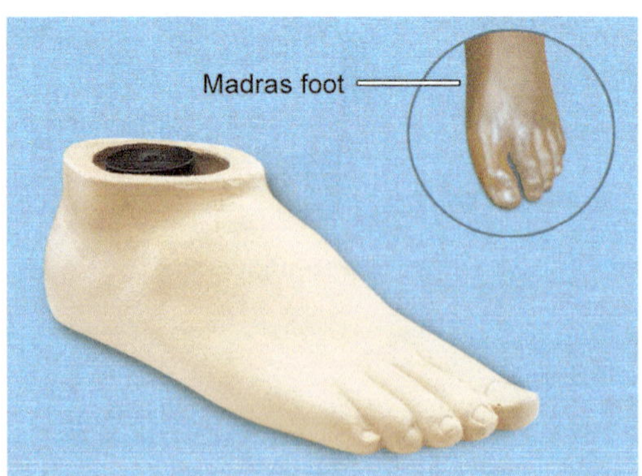

Fig. 15.9C: Madras foot.

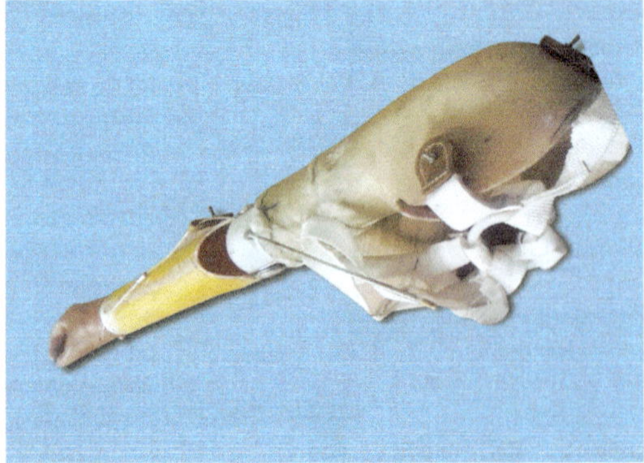

Fig. 15.10: Body powered upper limb prosthesis.
(*Courtesy*: Surjit Kumar, Patna)

3

Section

Some Orthopedic Instruments and Implants

Chapter

16

Some Common Orthopedic Instruments

PERIOSTEAL ELEVATOR (FIGS. 16.1A AND B)

Parts:

- Handle
- Thumb rest
- Sharp beveled curved tip.

Uses: For raising the periosteum from bone.

Why you elevate periosteum?

- Periosteum is tough and slippery structure hence any instrument may slip over it.
- Get a safer plane as neurovascular structures are retracted away along with periosteum.
- Helps in reduction of displaced fracture.

Note: **Jones** type periosteal elevator is not very common nowadays.

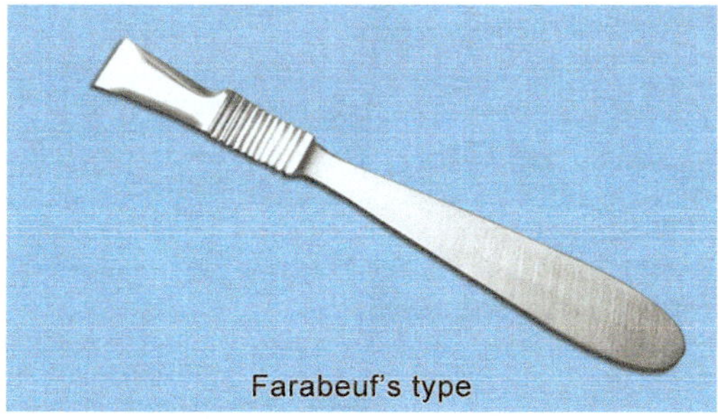

Fig. 16.1: Periosteal elevator.

BONE LEVER (FIGS. 16.2A AND B)

Parts:

- Handle with a ring
- A blade with variation like
  - *Straight or curved*: Curved levers confine the curvature of bone

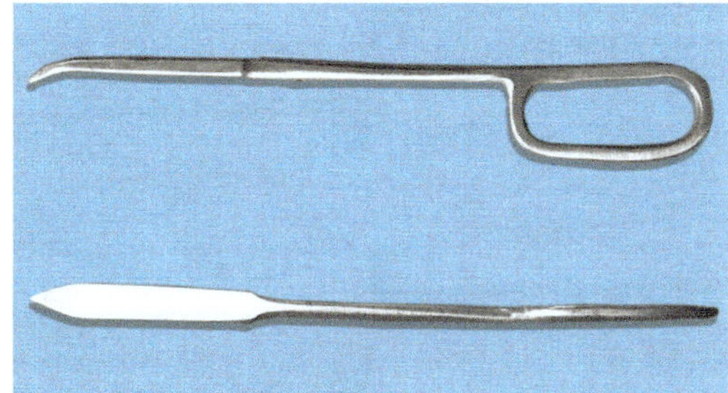

Fig. 16.2A: Lane bone lever.

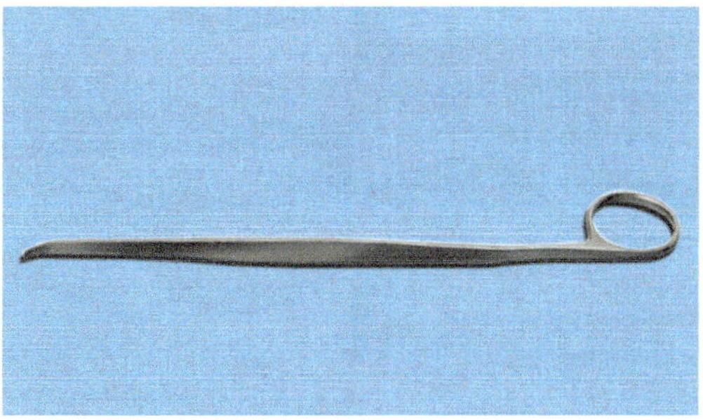

Fig. 16.2B: Trethowan bone lever (spike).

- *Smooth or serrated*: Serrated levers prevent the slippage over periosteum

Uses: Retraction of soft tissue during surgeries over long bone.

Trethowan bone lever (spike): It is similar to Lane bone lever, but having a long blade with a hook at one end and ring at another (Fig. 16.2B).

OSTEOTOME, CHISEL, AND GOUGE (STILLE TYPE) (FIGS. 16.3A TO C)

Comparison of osteotome, chisel, and gouge has been shown in Table 16.1.

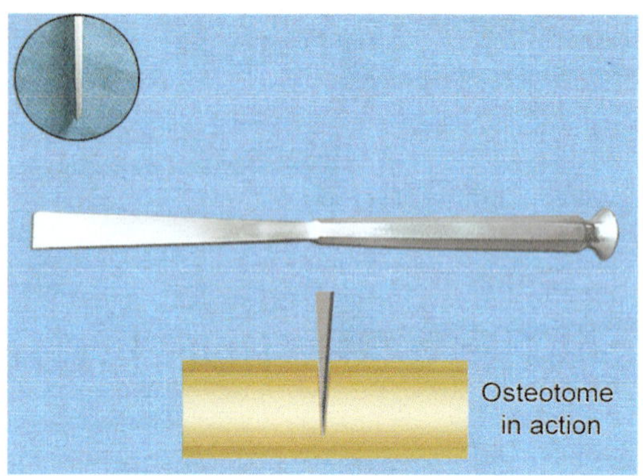

Fig. 16.3A: Osteotome (Stille type).

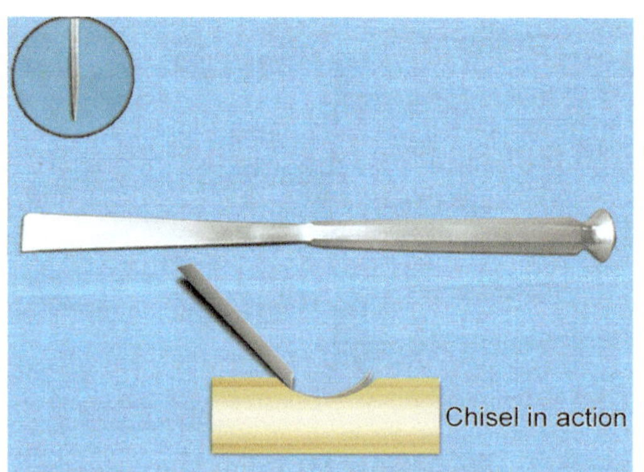

Fig. 16.3B: Bone chisel (Stille type).

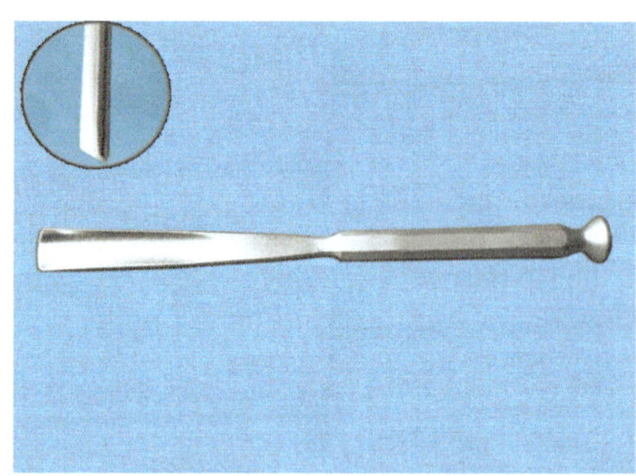

Fig. 16.3C: Bone gouge (Stille type).

Table 16.1: Comparison of osteotome, chisel, and gouge.

	Osteotome	Chisel	Bone gouge
Parts	• Blunt flat top • Handle • Quadrangular shaft—flattened and both edges beveled	• Blunt flat top • Handle • Quadrangular shaft—flattened and one edge beveled	• Blunt flat top • Handle • Curved blade with sharp end
Variations	Straight and curved	Straight and curved	Straight and curved
Uses	• For cutting of bone • For making osteoperiosteal flap and petalling.	• For removal of unwanted callus at nonunion site • For saucerization in chronic osteomyelitis. • Extraperiosteal resection of osteochondroma • For removal of excess bone over implant	• For harvesting bone graft
Note: Osteotome, chisel, and gouge are commonly available in fiber handle.			

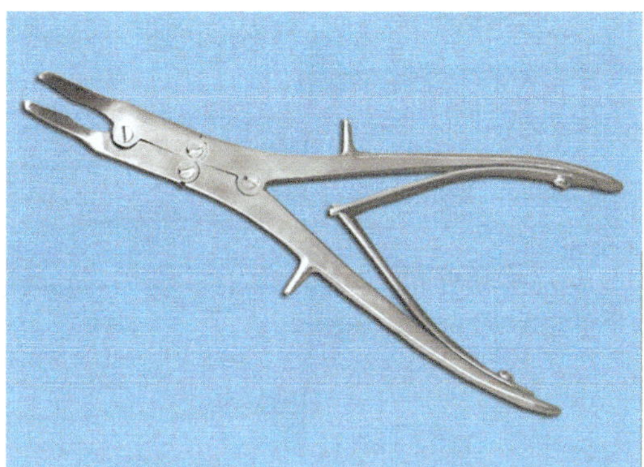

Fig. 16.4: Bone nibbler (Rongeur).

BONE NIBBLER (RONGEUR) (FIG. 16.4)

Parts:

- Hand piece with spring action
- Hinge—single or double action
- Cupped blades with sharp edges.

Variation: Straight or curved.

Uses:

- For smoothening the ends of bone.
- For biting of excess bone.
- For removal of unwanted fibrous tissue.

Stille-Horsley, Leksell, Sargent, and Duckbill are some famous Rongeurs.

SCOOP OR CURETTE (VOLKSMANN'S TYPE) (FIGS. 16.5A AND B)

Parts:

- Handle ribbed for good hold
- Sharp, edged, and trough like end (one or both end).

Uses:

- Scrapping the wall of cavities of benign bone tumor.
- Scrapping of osteomyelitis cavity.
- To remove immature callus or fibrous tissues from neglected fracture ends.
- Freshening of sinus or fistulous tracts.
- Freshening of fracture ends.

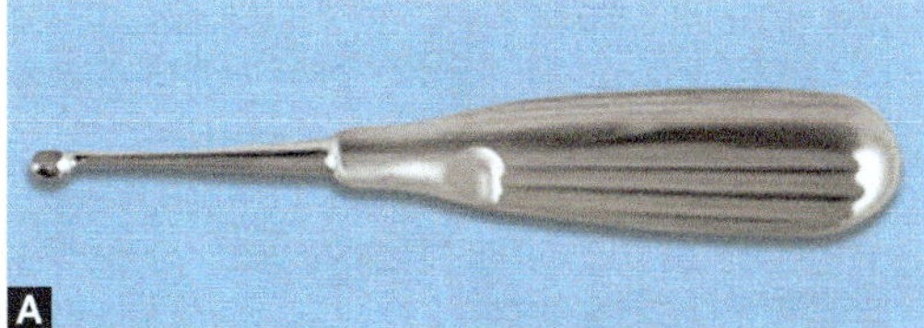

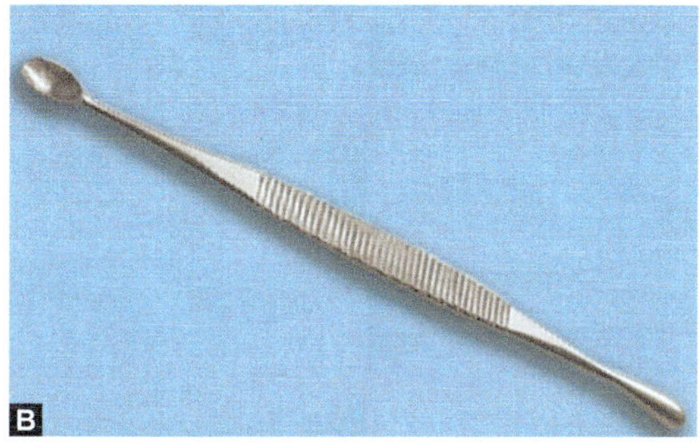

Figs. 16.5A and B: Scoop or curette (Volksmann's type).

BONE HOLDERS

Parts:

- Hand piece with or without locking system. Two types of locking system—(i) speed lock mechanism (ii) catch/rachet lock mechanism.
- Hinge
- Bone holding blades.

Uses:

- Holding the bone for manipulation during reduction.
- Steadies the bone during reaming, nibbling, drilling, etc.
- It steadies reduced bone with plate also.

Reduction Clamp/Forceps (Figs. 16.6A to C)

- Speed-lock or catch-lock mechanism in hand piece.
- Blades are curved.
- *Variations*: Pointed, serrated or ball tipped.

Heygroove's Bone Holders (Fig. 16.7)

- Speed lock mechanism is at top of hand piece.

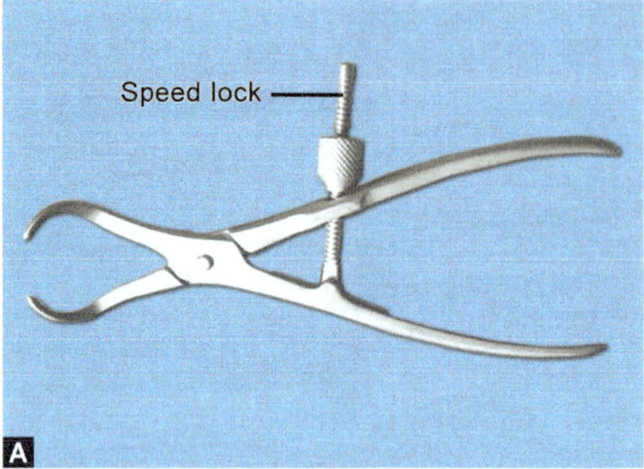

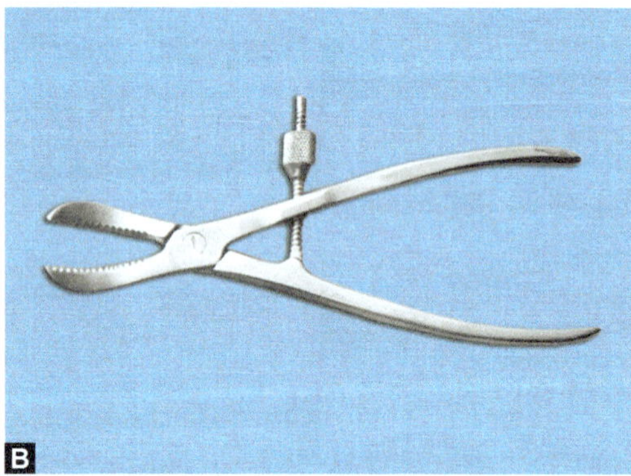

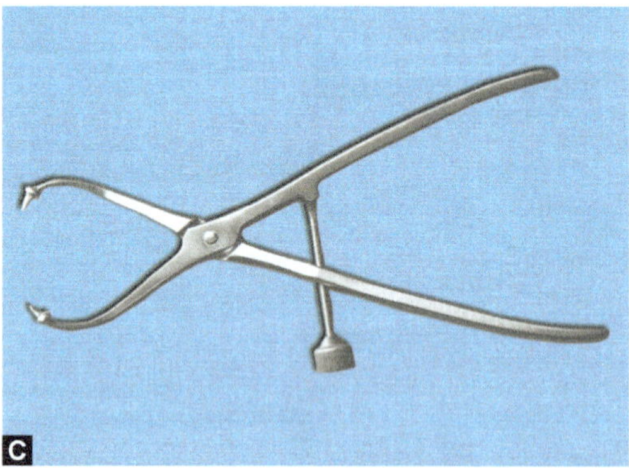

Figs. 16.6A to C: Reduction clamp/forceps.

- Bone holding blades are cylindrical, curved, and serrated to accommodate the convexity of bone and to make grip firm.

Lane's Bone Holders (Fig. 16.8)

- With or without locking system (rachet lock).
- Bone holding blades are rectangular, slightly curved, serrated, and toothed to make grip more firm.

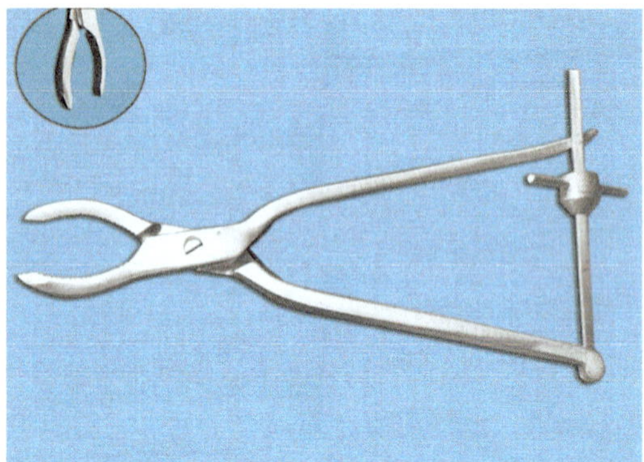

Fig. 16.7: Heygroove's bone holders.

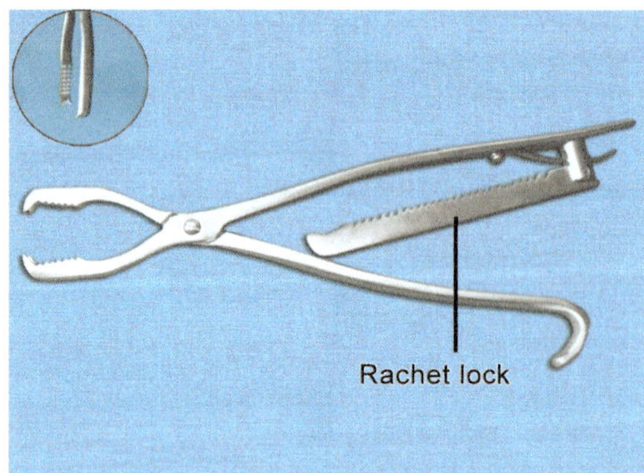

Fig. 16.8: Lane's bone holders.

Note: Bone holders, such as **Kern** (straight blade) type and **Ferguson** (double row of tooth) type.

Burn's Bone Holders (Fig. 16.9)

- Speed-lock mechanism for locking.
- Blades are triangular, curved, serrated, and with pointed tip having fenestration over it.
- Mainly used for radius, ulna, and fibula.

Lowman's Clamp (Fig. 16.10)

- Opposing sets of incurving claws which can be screwed into a tight position.
- May be two pronged, three pronged, and four pronged.

Verbrugge's Self-centering Bone Holding Forceps (Fig. 16.11)

- Speed-lock mechanism.
- Self-centering hinge.

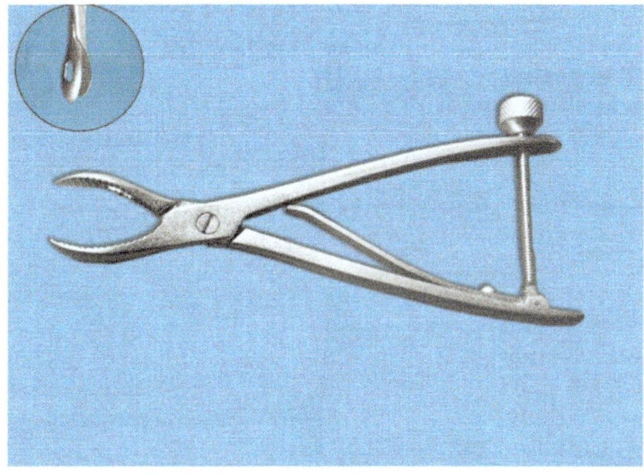

Fig. 16.9: Burn's bone holders.

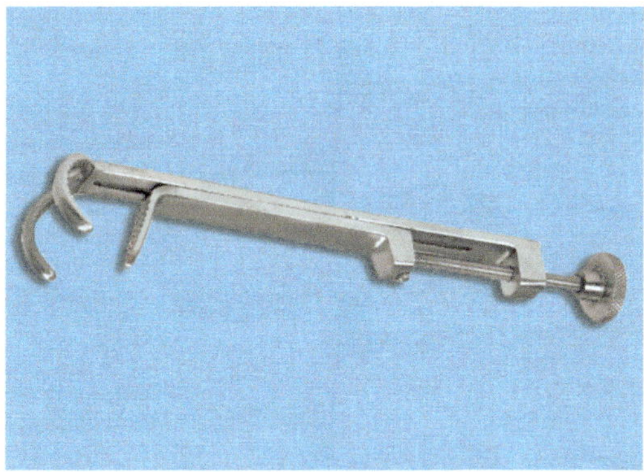

Fig. 16.10: Lowman's clamp.

- Out of two curved blades; one is flattened and serrated inner surface and other is pointed and smooth inner surface.

ORTHOPEDIC PLIERS (FIGS. 16.12A TO C)

- Plier is a gripping tool having a pair of hinged arm with serrated jaw.
- It is used for holding, bending, and cutting purposes.
- Some pliers (flat nose plier) are provided with small hole near the tip of its jaw that can be used as tensionier.

  Orthopedic pliers are mainly three types:

  1. Needle nose plier.
  2. Flat nose plier.
  3. English (parallel) plier.

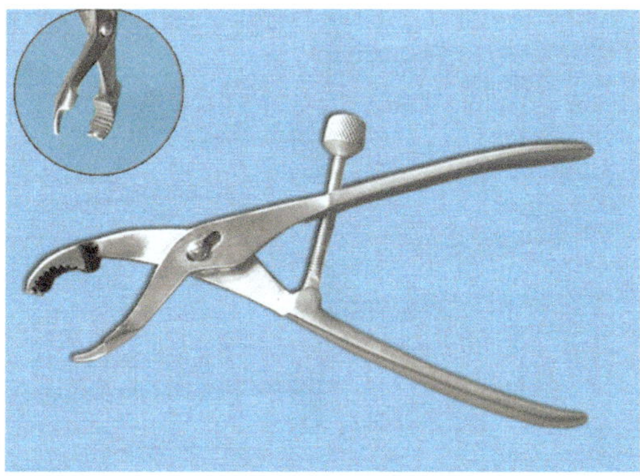

Fig. 16.11: Verbrugge's self-centering bone holding forceps.

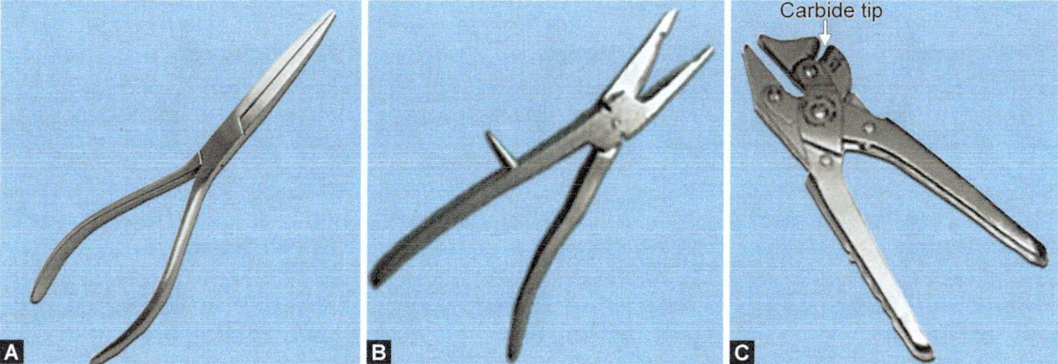

Figs. 16.12A to C: Orthopedic pliers: A. Needle nose plier; B. Flat nose plier; C. English (parallel) plier.

MALLET (FIG. 16.13)

- It is an orthopedic hammer with handle and cylindrical head.
- *Uses*:
  - It is a companion instrument of osteotome, chisel, gouge, etc.
  - Used for insertion of some implants such as nails (K-nail, V-nail, and Rush nail), plate (wein-wright plate), prosthesis (Austin Moore), Steinmann pins, thick K-wires, etc.

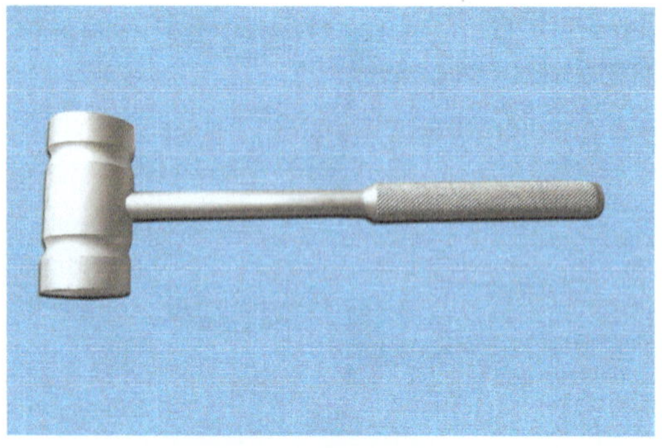

Fig. 16.13: Mallet.

Chapter

17

Some Common Orthopedic Implants

KIRSCHNER'S WIRE (FIG. 17.1)

- *Parts*:
  - Trocar tipped both ends.
  - Rounded shaft.
- *Variations*:
  - Smooth and threaded.
- *Size*: 1-3.5 mm; at interval of 0.5 mm.
- *Uses*:
  - For pediatric skeletal traction.
  - For fixation of pediatric fracture like supracondylar fracture, physeal injury, etc.
  - For fixation after correction of deformity like cubitus varus deformity at elbow (Chapter 6).
  - As a component of Joshi's external stabilizing system (JESS).
  - As a component of tension band wiring (TBW).
  - As a temporary scaffolding for fixation of periarticular fractures.

Note: End of K-wire protruding from skin is acutely bent and rest of the wire is cut down. Why so?
  - It prevents inward migration of wire in the bone and soft tissue.
  - It also facilitates its easy removal when purpose is solved.

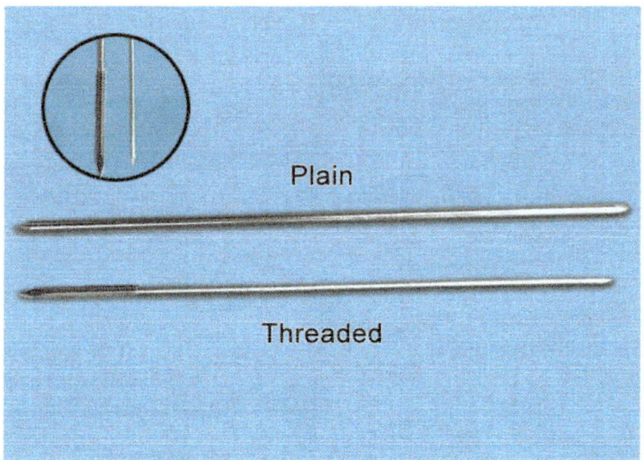

Fig. 17.1: Kirschner's wire.

STAINLESS STEEL WIRE (FIG. 17.2)

- These are stainless steel (SS) wires wrapped over wire spool.
- *Sizes*: 16 gauze (1.6 mm) to 30 gauze (0.3 mm).

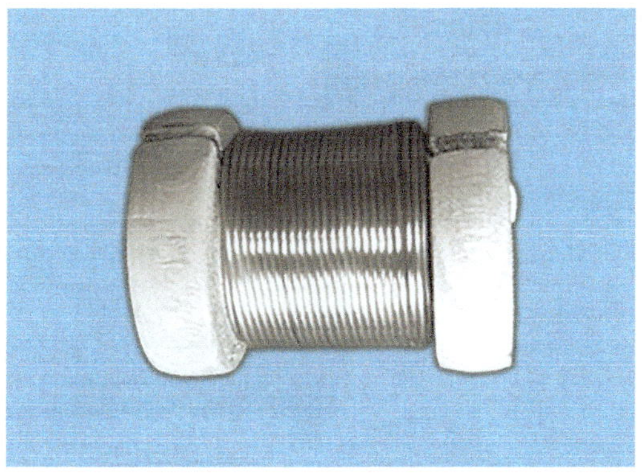

Fig. 17.2: Stainless steel wire over spool.

- *Uses*:
  - As a component of TBW.
  - To hold the comminuted fragment where screw fixation is not possible, e.g. during intramedullary nailing in long bone.
  - To encirclage the comminuted fracture patella.
  - For reconstruction of comminuted greater trochanter.

ORTHOPEDIC SCREW (FIG. 17.3)

- *Definition*: A screw is a mechanical device which converts the torsional forces into compressive force.
- *Parts of screw*:
  - *Head*: It has a recess for attachment to screwdriver. There is also a countersink for buttress which prevents sinking of head into bone.
  - *Shaft*: It links between head and thread.
  - *Run-out*: It is a zone of transition between shaft and thread. This is a point of stress concentration. Screw may break from this site on faulty application.
  - *Thread*: It makes purchase of screw with bone.
    - Thread diameter—it represents the diameter of screw.
    - Core diameter—it is narrowest diameter and weakest part of screw.
    - Pitch—distance between two adjacent threads.

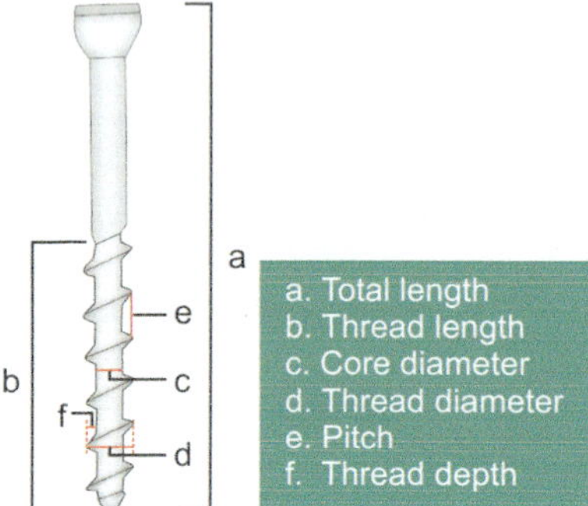

Fig. 17.3: Screw description.

    - Purchase—resistance between screw and bone interface.
    - Thread depth—half of difference between thread and core diameter.
    - Lead—distance traveled by screw in one turn.
  - *Tip of screw*:
    - Simple tip (nontapping)—smooth conical tip and needs tapping to make channel for passage of screw; cortical screw.
    - Self-tapping—having cutting flutes for creating a channel, e.g. locking screw.
    - Self-drilling and self-tapping—screw tip makes a drill hole and also cuts channel for passage of screw, e.g. locking screw.
    - Cork screw—e.g. cancellous screw.
- Factor affecting pull out strength of screw:
  - Number of thread engaging the cortex.
  - Type of screw; (thread depth µ pull out strength).
  - Bone quality.
  - Screw augmented with cement.
  - Hydroxyapatite coated screw.

Cortical and Cancellous Screw (Figs. 17.4A and B)

Comparison between cortical and cancellous screw has been shown in Table 17.1.

Table 17.1: Comparison between cortical and cancellous screw.

	Cortical screw	Cancellous screw
Modification of	Machine screw	Wood screw
Core diameter	More	Less
Thread depth	Lesser	More
Pitch	Lesser	More
Tip	Simple	Cork screw
Cutting flutes	Absent	Present
Solid or cannulated	Mainly solid	Both

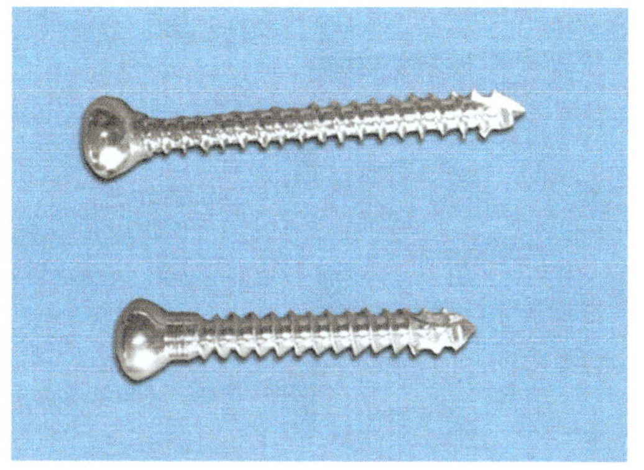
Fig. 17.4A: Cortical screw.

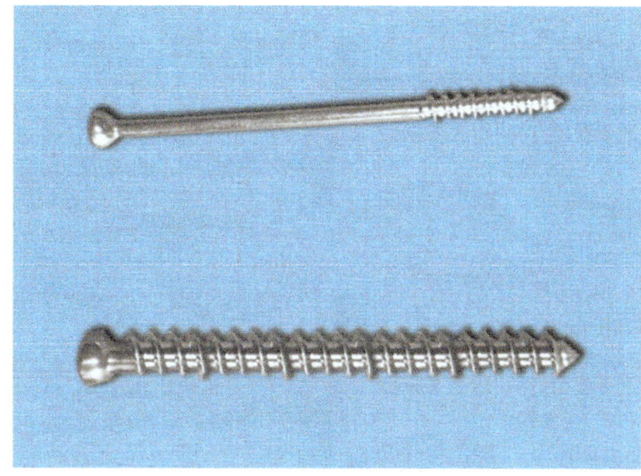
Fig. 17.4B: Cancellous screw.

BONE PLATES (FIGS. 17.5A TO D)

- **Sherman** plate is supposed to the first scientific plate in the history of orthopedic hardware.
- *Definition*: A flat internal splints with holes that hold together the fracture end of bone.
- What does a plate do?
  - Maintain alignment of bone.
  - Transfer forces from one end of bone to other end.
- *Functional classification of plating*:
  - *Bridging mode (Fig. 17.5A)*: For comminuted fractures.
  - *Neutralization mode (Fig. 17.5B)*: For oblique fractures.
  - *Buttress mode (Fig. 17.5C)*: For periarticular or intra-articular metaphyseal fracture.
  - *Compression mode (Fig. 17.5D)*: Used for transverse and short oblique fractures.

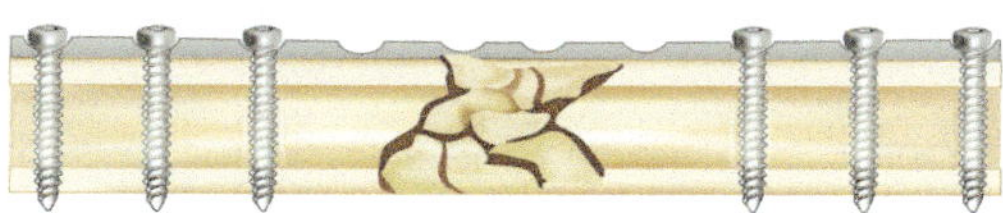
Fig. 17.5A: Bridging mode of plating.

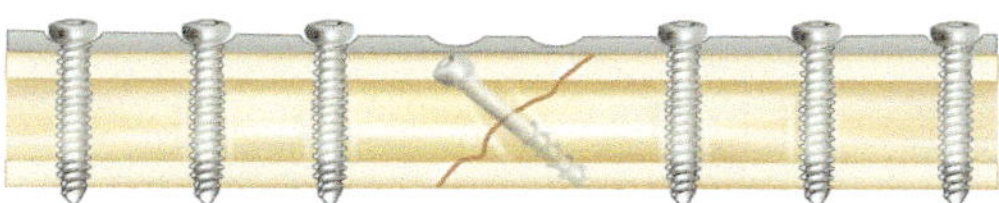
Fig. 17.5B: Neutralization mode of plating.

Dynamic Compression Plates: (Allgower 1960) (Fig. 17.6)

Classification of dynamic compression plates has been shown in Table 17.2.

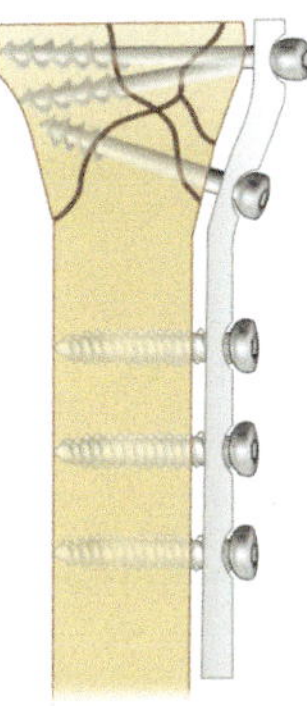
Fig. 17.5C: Buttress mode of plating.

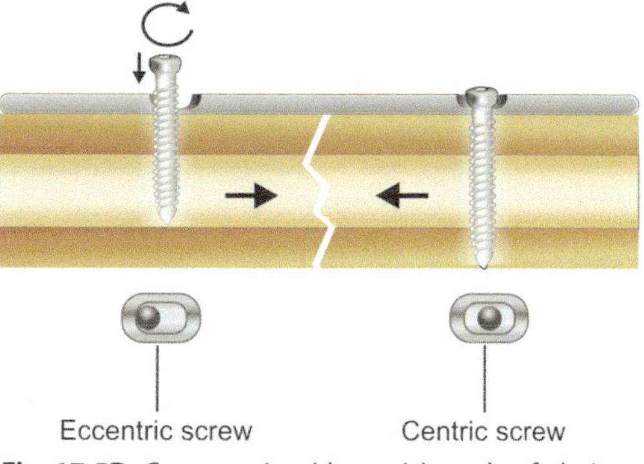

Fig. 17.5D: Compression (dynamic) mode of plating.

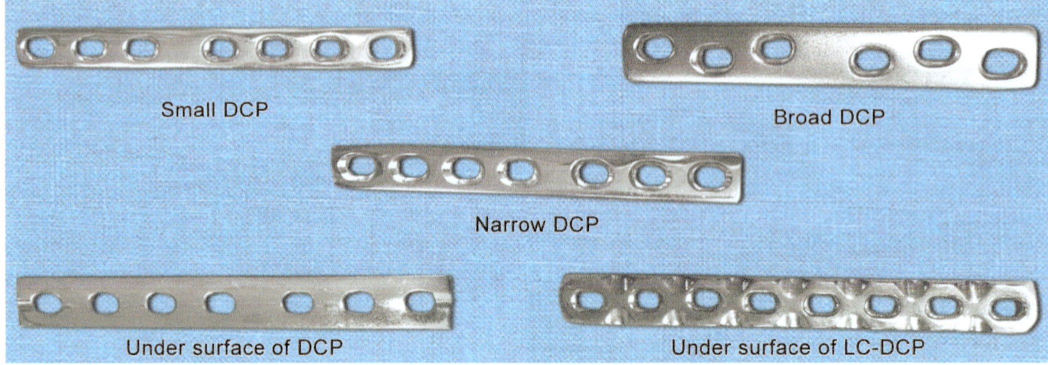

Fig. 17.6: Dynamic compression plates (DCP).

Table 17.2: Classification of dynamic compression plates.

DCP type	Width of plate	Screw diameter	Commonly used for
Small DCP	10 mm	3.5 mm	Radius and ulna
Narrow DCP	12 mm	4.5 mm	Humerus and tibia
Broad DCP	16 mm	4.5 mm	Femur

Tubular Plates (Figs. 17.7A to C)

- These plates are actually part of a metallic cylindrical tube.
- Mainly used in bridging and neutralization mode.

Classification of tubular plates has been shown in Table 17.3.

Table 17.3: Classification of tubular plates.

Plate type	Circumference	Screw diameter
Quarter tubular	1/4th circumference of cylinder	2.7 mm
One-third tubular	l/3rd circumference of cylinder	3.5 mm
Semi-tubular	1/2 circumference of cylinder	4.5 mm

INTRAMEDULLARY NAILS

- *Definition*: Nail is an internal splint that allows axial forces to be transmitted from on end of bone to other. This is a load sharing implant.
- *Cross section of nail (Fig. 17.8)*: Different nail has different cross section; e.g.

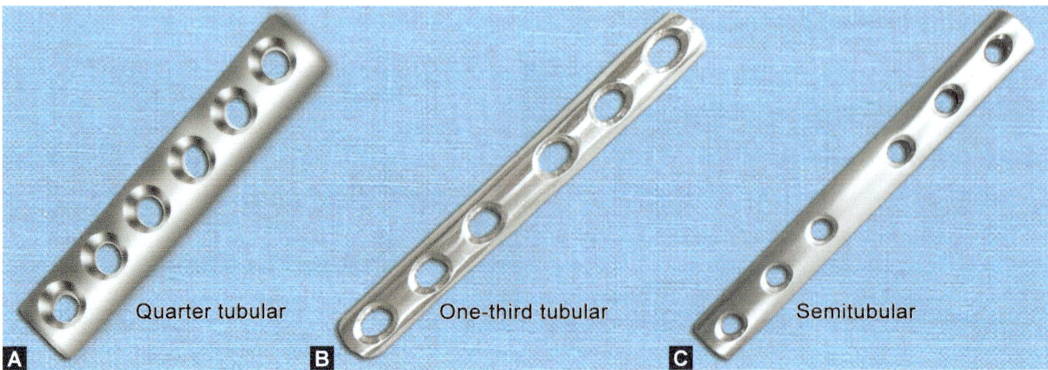

Figs. 17.7A to C: Tubular plates.

Fig. 17.8: Cross section of different nails.

K-nail—clover leaf transection, V-nail—V-shape transection, Talwalkar's square nail—square-shaped transection, Ender's or rush nail—solid circular transection, interlocking nail—circular ring transection. Diamond-shaped transection has maximum bending strength.

- *Three point fixation*: The two ends of nail hold at metaphyseal area of the bone and one point of nail lies against the insthmus the narrowest area of medullary cavity.

Rush Nail (Fig. 17.9)

- *Parts of nail*:
  - *One end having beveled tip*: For easy migration in medullary cavity.
  - *Another end having hook*: Prevent inward migration of nail in medullary cavity and for easy extraction.
  - *Cylindrical shaft*: No rotational stability.
- *Principle*: Three point fixation.
- *Uses*: For fracture fibula, fracture both bone forearm, and fracture humerus.
- *Disadvantages*:
  - No rotational stability.
  - No locking mechanism.
- Commonly available in 2-4 mm diameter (variation 0.5 mm) of various length.

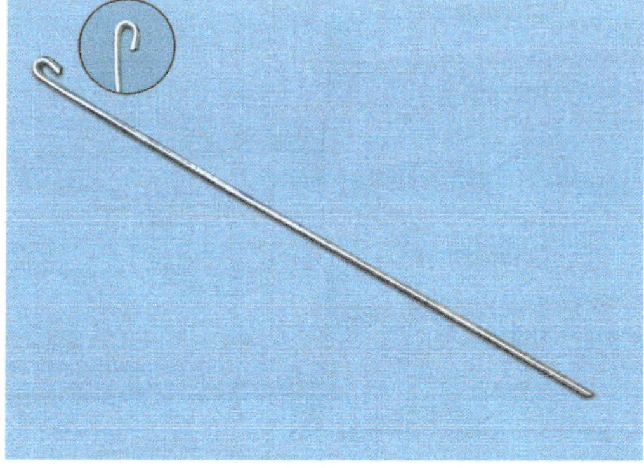

Fig. 17.9: Rush nail.

Talwalkar's Square Nail (Fig. 17.10)

- *Parts of nail*:
  - *One end threaded*: For insertion and extraction of nail.
  - *Another end*: Tongue shaped (radius square nail) and trocar tipped (ulnar square nail).
  - *Square-shaped shaft (transection)*: Provide minimal rotational stability.
- *Principle*: Three point fixation.
- *Uses*: For fracture both bone forearm, fracture fibula, and fracture humerus
- *Disadvantages*:
  - Do not provide complete rotational stability.
  - No locking mechanism.
- Commonly available in 1.5-6.5 mm diameter (0.5 mm variation) of various length.

Ender's Nail (Fig. 17.11)

- *Parts of nail*:
  - *One end flattened with an eye*: For insertion and extraction of nail.
  - Another end blunt.
  - *Cylindrical shaft (transection)*: No rotational stability.
- *Principle*: Three point fixation.
- *Uses*:
  - For fracture shaft of femur, for fracture tibia, and fracture humerus.

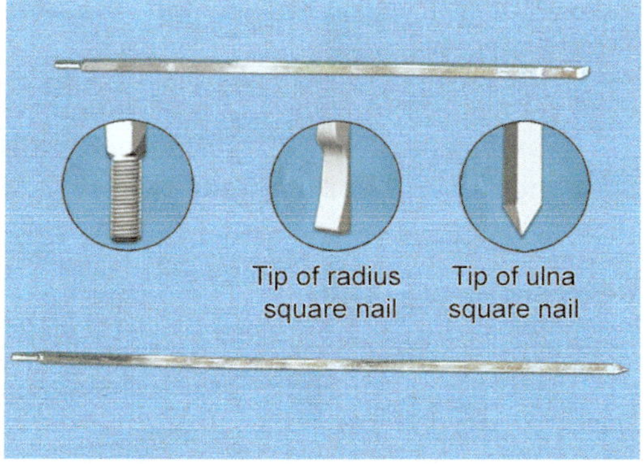

Fig. 17.10: Talwalkar's square nail.

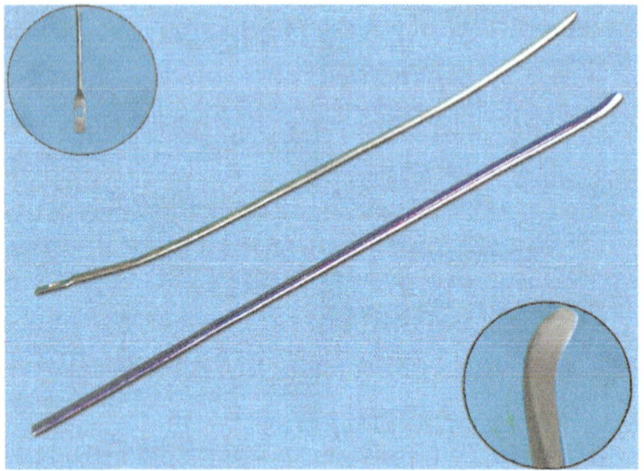

Fig. 17.11: Ender's nail and TENS nail.

- *These implants were primarily used for fracture fixation in trochanteric and sub trochanteric area of femur.*
- *Disadvantages*:
  - Do not provide rotational stability.
  - No locking mechanism.
  - Titanium made elastic nails are commonly used nowadays, called TENS.

Kuntscher's Cloverleaf Nail (Gerhard Kuntscher from Germany) (Figs. 17.12A and B)

- *Anatomy of nail*:
  - *Two blunt ends with eye*: Blunt end reduces chance of cortex penetration.
  - *A hollow shaft*: Allows bone marrow continuity and guidewire passage if needed.
  - *Cloverleaf cross section*: Provide some rotational stability.
  - *Eye*: For nail extraction,
- *Principle*:
  - *Three point fixation*
  - *Longitudinal slot*: Lies anterolaterally and allows bend along tensile surface of bone.
  - *Longitudinal metal bar opposite to slot*: Accommodate body weight along compressible surface of bone (Fig. 17.12B).
- *Determination of length*:
  - Tip of greater trochanter to knee joint line—2 cm.

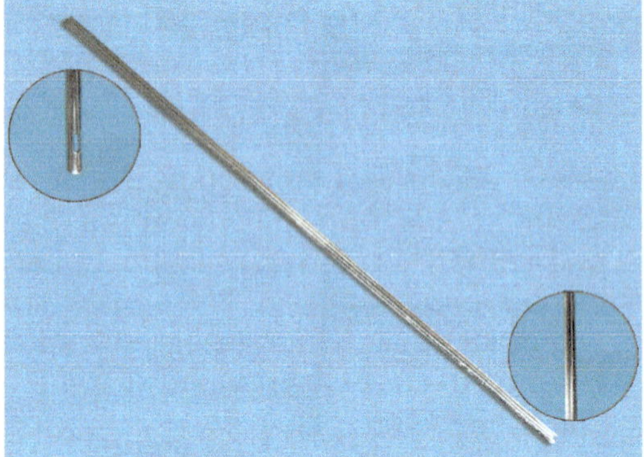

Fig. 17.12A: Kuntscher's cloverleaf nail.

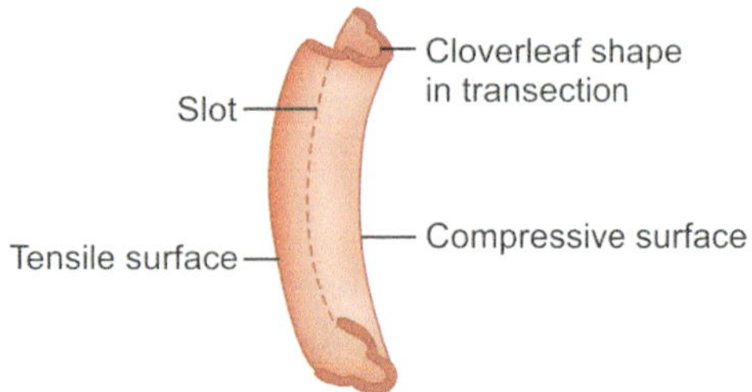

Fig. 17.12B: Effect of loading on cloverleaf nail.

  - Tip of greater trochanter to upper pole of patella.
  - Greater trochanter to metaphyseal scar (seen in X-ray)
- *Method of nail insertion*:
  - Retrograde entry (from fracture site).
  - Anterograde entry (piriformis fossa).
- *Disadvantages*:
  - Do not provide rotational stability.
  - No locking mechanism.
- *Complication with K-nailing*:
  - Splintering of cortex
  - Proximal and distal migration of nail
  - Stucking of nail
  - Nail bending and breakage
  - Knee joint stiffness.
- Commonly available in 6–15 mm diameter (variation 1 mm) of various length.

CANNULATED CANCELLOUS HIP SCREW (FIG. 17.13)

- *Screw description*:
  - Partially threaded, cannulated, and cancellous screw.

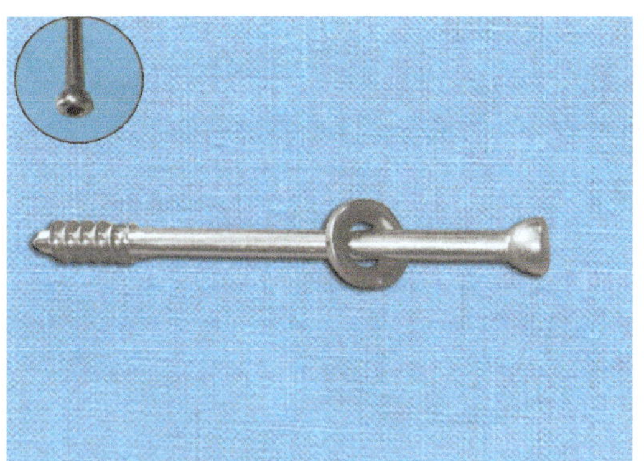

Fig. 17.13: Cannulated cancellous screw with washer.

- *Diameter*: 6.5 mm and 7.0 mm.
- *Diameter of guidewire used*: 2.0 mm.

- *Use*: Fracture neck of femur where physis are fused.
- *Screw configuration*:
  - Reverse triangle—why most common? Due to maximum bone density area.
  - *Diamond configuration*: For comminuted fracture.

DYNAMIC HIP SCREW (DHS) PLATE (FIG. 17.14)

- *Barrel*:
  - Short barrel—25 mm.
  - Standard barrel—38 mm.
- *Plate*:
  - 4.5 mm screw.
  - Hole arrangement—staggered. Why?
    - Even distribution of stress over plate and bone when limb is loaded.
    - Hence, prevent implant breakage and weakening of bone.
- *Angle between barrel and plate*: 130° and 135° (commonly available).
- *Sliding screw*:
  - Screw length—50-130 mm at interval of 5 mm.
  - Core diameter—8 mm.
  - Thread length—22 mm.
  - Thread diameter—12.5 mm.
- *Mode of action*: Sequential collapse at the fracture site when joint is loaded.

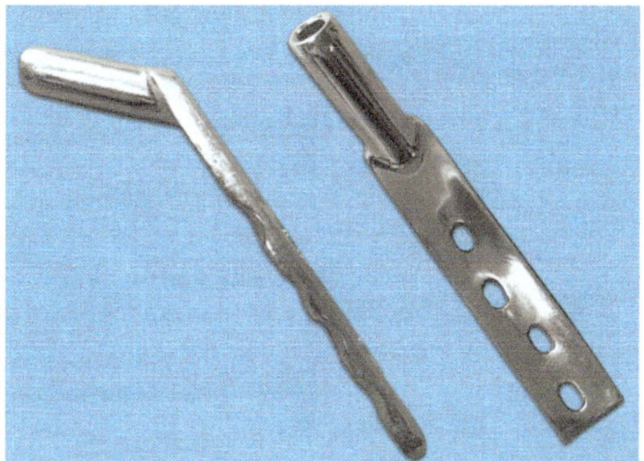

Fig. 17.14: Dynamic hip screw (DHS) plate.

- *Uses*:
  - Intertrochanteric fracture.
  - Basal neck fracture.
  - Sometime in valgus osteotomy when wedge is less than 20°.

UNIPOLAR HIP PROSTHESIS: AUSTIN-MOORE AND THOMPSON PROSTHESIS (FIG. 17.15)

Comparison between Austin-Moore and Thompson prosthesis has been shown in Table 17.4.

- *Advantages of smooth, quadrangular, and tapered end design*:
  - Easy insertion.
  - Snugly fits in medullary cavity and check rotation.

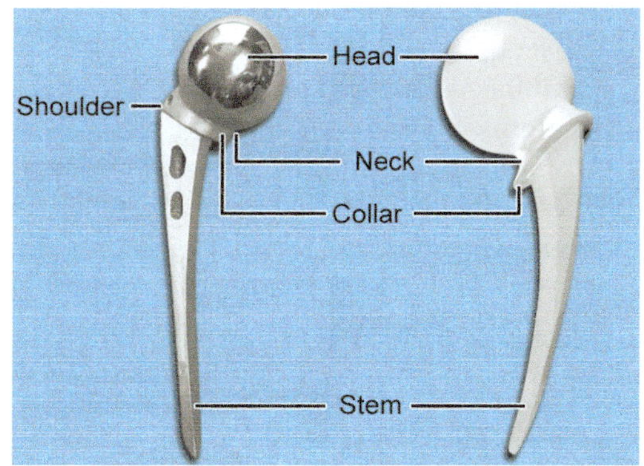

Fig. 17.15: Austin-Moore and Thompson prosthesis.

Table 17.4: Comparison between Austin-Moore and Thompson prosthesis.

	Austin-Moore prosthesis	Thompson prosthesis
Parts of implant	Head, neck, collar, and stem	Head, neck, collar, and stem
Role of collar	Collar sits over calcar	No such provision
Holes in implant	• Collar hole for anteversion maintenance and implant removal • Two stem hole for bone ingrowth • Holes also make the implant lighter	No hole
Shoulder	Shoulder fits at medial aspect of greater trochanter in medullary cavity and prevents rotation	No provision of shoulder
Mechanism of fixation with bone	Fixation due to bone ingrowth	Fixation with cement
Indication	Where calcar is left of at least 1.5 cm	Where calcar is deficient or less than 1 cm

- Prevent peroperative fracture of lateral cortex of femur.

Note: The stem hole of Austin-Moore prosthesis is filled with bone graft taken from extracted femoral head that induces the process of bone ingrowth.

TALWALKAR'S BIPOLAR PROSTHESIS (FIG. 17.16)

- **Bateman** was pioneer in development of bipolar prosthesis.
- *Parts of prosthesis*:
  - Head within head—big outer metallic head lined by polyethylene liner and a smaller metallic head inside it. Inner head moves in interprosthetic joint but outer head rotates in acetabulum, i.e. why it is called bipolar prosthesis.
  - Neck—fixed length.
  - Collar—sits over calcar.
  - Stem—smooth and tapered.
- *Mechanism of fixation*: Cemented; but very frequently used as uncemented prosthesis in good bone-stock.

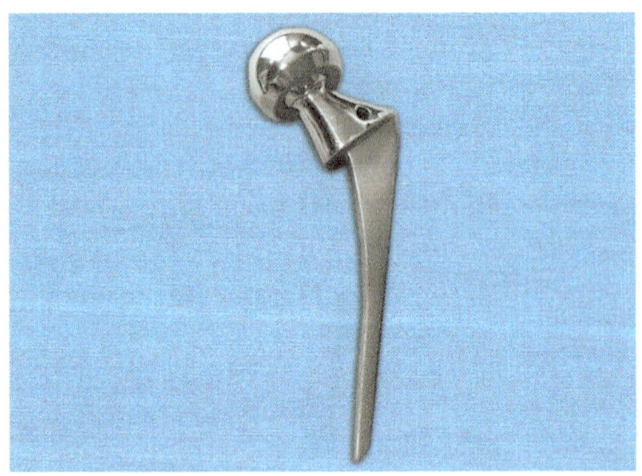

Fig. 17.16: Talwalkar bipolar prosthesis.

- Used for hemiarthroplasty hip
- *Advantages of bipolar prosthesis*:
  - Increased range of motion
  - Less acetabular wearing.

Note: Is it truly a bipolar prosthesis? It is proved in various studied that articulation between outer and inner head is lost in few months (3 months) after surgery and bipolar prosthesis becomes unipolar. To overcome this issue bicentric bipolar prosthesis has been designed.

4

Section

Some Common Orthopedic Radiographs

- Radiographs from Trauma
- Radiographs of Common Bone Tumors
- Radiographs of Common Infective, Rheumatic and Metabolic Disorders

Chapter

18

Radiographs From Trauma

X-RAY: FRACTURE PATTERNS AND MECHANISM OF INJURY (FIGS. 18.1A TO F)

- *Various patterns of fracture*:
  - Transverse fracture
  - Oblique fracture
  - Spiral fracture
  - Comminuted fracture
  - Butterfly fragment
  - Segmental fracture.

Comparisons of various fracture patterns and mechanism of injury are shown in Table 18.1.

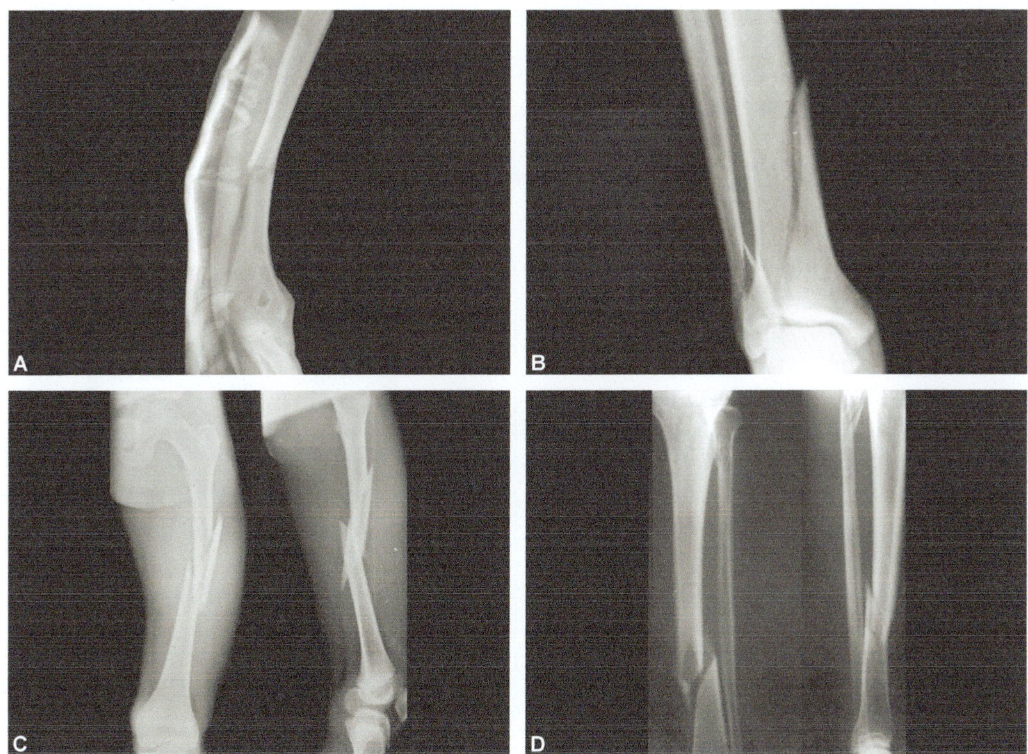

Figs. 18.1A to D

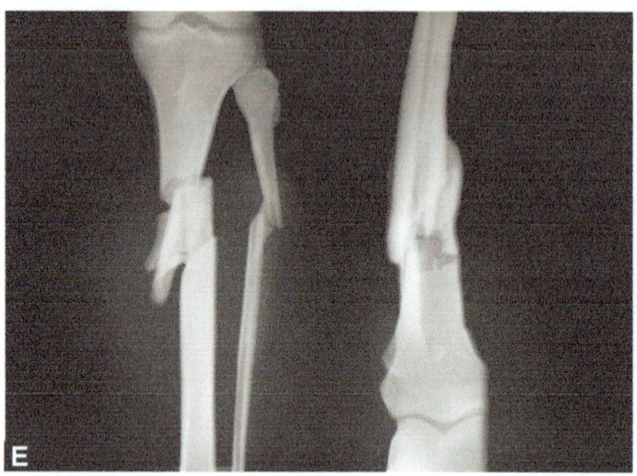

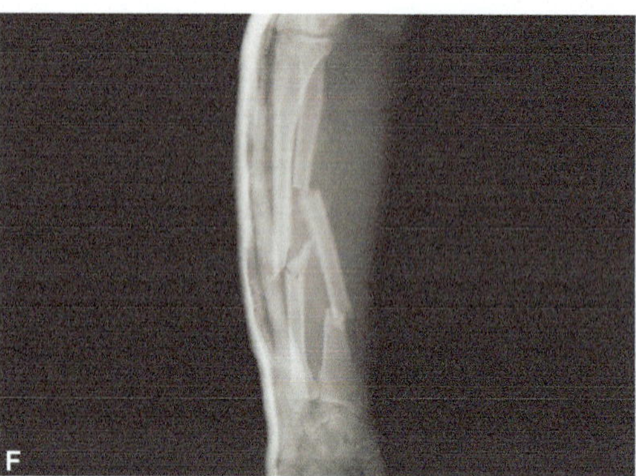

Figs. 18.1A to F: X-ray: Various fracture patterns: A. Oblique fracture; B. Transverse fracture; C. Butterfly fragment; D. Spiral fracture; E. Comminuted fracture; F. Segmental fracture.

(*Courtesy*: Dr Tarun Solanki)

Table 18.1: Comparisons of various fracture patterns and mechanism of injury.

Fracture patterns	Fractures line	Loading forces	Energy of trauma
Transverse fracture	Makes an angle less than 30° with a line perpendicular to long axis of bone	Bending force	Low energy
Oblique fracture	Makes an angle more than 30° with a line perpendicular to long axis of bone	Bending and compression forces	Moderate energy
Butterfly	A broad triangular fracture fragment present in diaphyseal comminuted fracture	Bending and compression forces	Moderate energy
Spiral fracture	Three-dimensional	Torsional forces	Low energy
Comminuted fracture	Multiple small fragments at fracture site	Variable torsion	High energy
Segmental fracture	More than two fracture fragments	Impact at more than one site	High energy

X-RAY: STRESS FRACTURE (FIG. 18.2)

- Repetitive stress in professional like dancers, athlete, and military persons
- Zone of callus formation visible
- Faint hairline undisplaced fracture
- Transverse fracture pattern
- Bone scan is diagnostic
- Common sites are metatarsals (shaft of 2nd most common), tibia, and fibula
- Retreatment options are restriction of activities, immobilization of the part, analgesics, and calcium with vitamin D supplements.

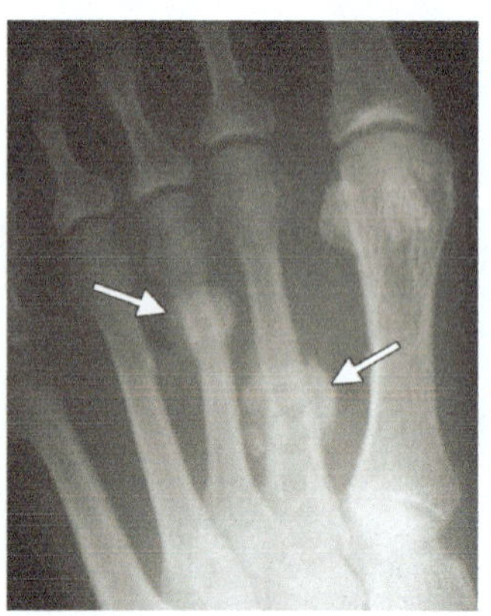

Fig. 18.2: X-ray: Stress fracture.

X-RAY: PATHOLOGICAL FRACTURES (FIGS. 18.3A AND B)

- *Etiological classification of pathological fracture*:
  - *Infective disorder*:
    - Chronic pyogenic osteomyelitis
    - Chronic tubercular osteomyelitis.
  - *Tumorous disorder*:
    - Cystic lesion like simple bone cyst and ABC
    - Malignant tumor, e.g. osteosarcoma, chondrosarcoma, and multiple myeloma.
  - *Metabolic disorder*: Osteoporosis and hyperparathyroidism
  - *Genetic and dysplastic disorder*:
    - Fibrous dysplasia
    - Osteogenesis imperfecta and osteopetrosis.
  - **Mirel criteria** (site, pain, lesion nature, and size) are used for prediction of pathological fracture and prophylactic fixation.
- *Treatment options*:
  - Treatment of underlying pathology
  - Improvement of bone stock
  - Prophylactic or definitive fixation of pathological bone.

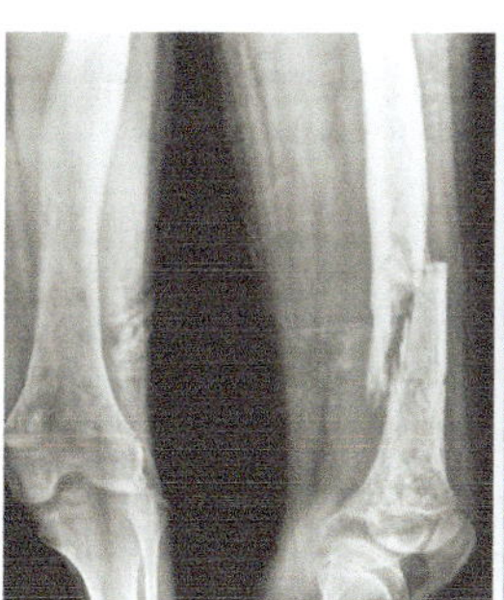

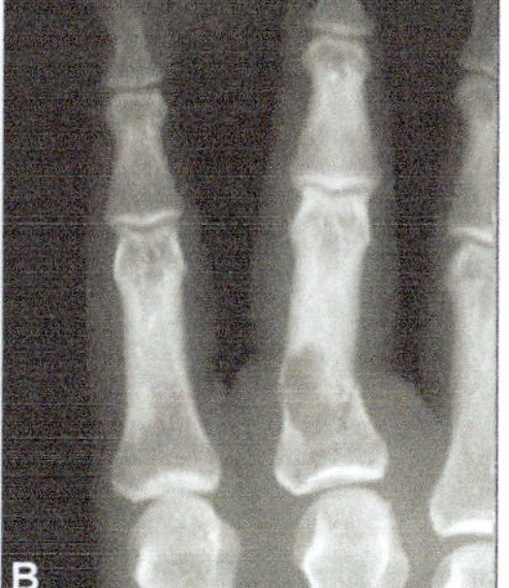

Figs. 18.3A and B: X-ray: Pathological fractures: A. Chronic osteomyelitis; B. Tumor.

(*Courtesy*: Dr DK Taneja)

X-RAY: PEDIATRIC FRACTURE (FIGS. 18.4A TO D)

- *Characteristics of pediatric fracture*:
  - Due to great elasticity and thick periosteum, incomplete fractures are common

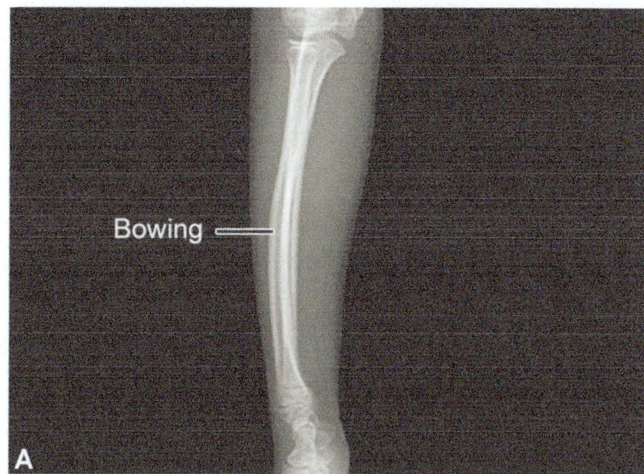

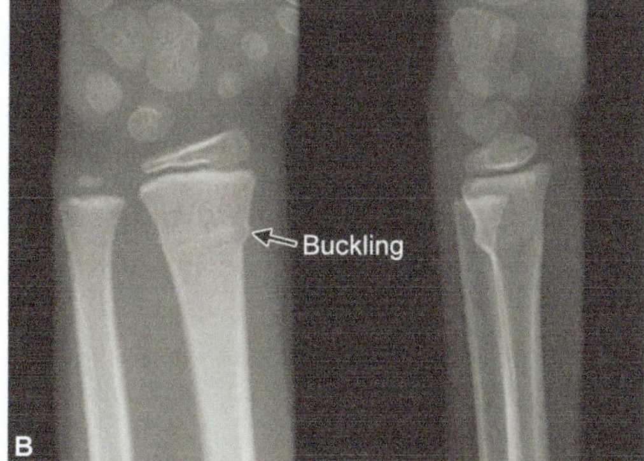

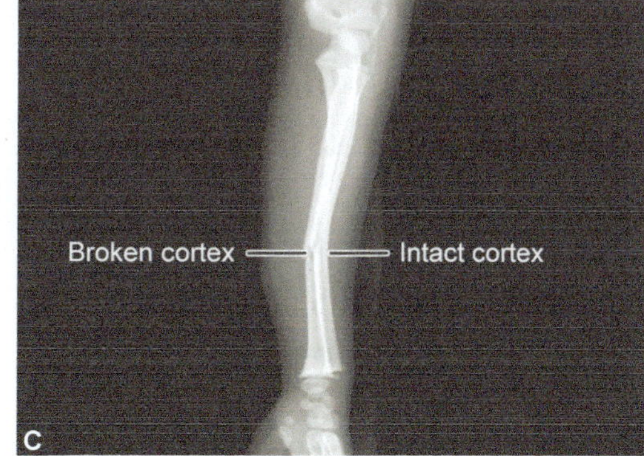

Figs. 18.4A to C: X-ray: Pediatric fracture: A. Plastic deformation; B. Torus fracture; C. Green stick fracture.

(*Courtesy*: Dr Govind Ballav Joshi)

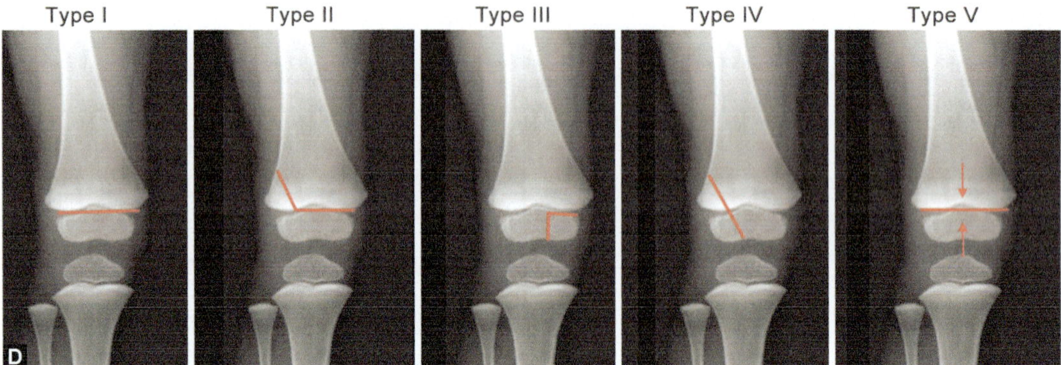

Fig. 18.4D: Salter-Harris classifications.

- Due to weak physeal zone, avulsions are more common
- Due to high growth potency, fracture healing is faster
- Maximum remodeling capacity around fracture
- Minimal periarticular stiffness.

- *Pediatric fracture classification (Figs. 18.4A to C)*:
  - *Bowing*: Here only plastic deformation of bone
  - *Torus*: Only buckling of cortex
  - *Green stick fracture*: Here only one cortex is broken other is intact
  - *Epiphyseal fracture (Fig. 18.4D).*
- *Treatment options*:
  - Closed reduction and immobilization.
  - Closed reduction and percutaneous fixation (K-wire or screw).
  - Open reduction and fixation.

Salter-Harris classification of pediatric fracture.

Type I: Transverse fracture running through the physis.
Type II: The most common pattern of epiphyseal injury where fracture line run through the physis and the metaphysis, producing a beak like corner. **Thurston Holland** sign or shiny corner sign.
Type III: Fracture line running through physis and epiphysis.
Type IV: Here fracture line passes through the physis, metaphysis, and epiphysis.
Type V: It is a compression fracture of the physis.
Type VI: It is an injury of peripheral portion of the physis **(Mercer Rang-1969)**.

REVIEW OF COMMON FRACTURES AND DISLOCATIONS

X-RAY: FRACTURE CLAVICLE (FIG. 18.5)

- Most common fracture at birth.
- Mechanism of injury: Fall on shoulder or fall on outstretched hand.
- *Features*:
  - Middle 1/3rd is the most common site for fracture and lateral 1/3rd fracture are prone to be unstable.
  - Medial fragment displaces upward (under effect of sternocleidomastoid) and lateral fragment displaces downward (under effect of gravity and pectoralis major pull) leading to tenting of overlying skin.
  - Complications: Malunion, neurovascular injury, and less commonly non-union.
- *Management*:
  - Conservative method: Mainstay of treatment. Simple cuff and collar sling for 3–4 weeks is sufficient. Other methods are clavicular bracing, *figure 8 bandage* having hardly any importance.
  - Surgical method: Indications are—(1) compound fracture, (2) fracture with neurovascular compromise, (3) fracture having 2 cm overriding or gross displacement in active adult, (4)

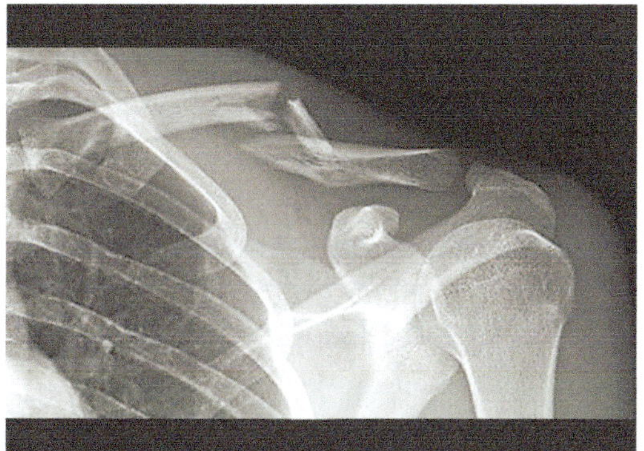

Fig. 18.5: X-ray: Fracture clavicle.

nonunion, (5) *floating shoulder*, i.e. fracture clavicle with fracture scapular neck, and (6) unstable lateral 1/3rd fracture. Modalities used for fixation are clavicular plate and sometime elastic nail.

X-RAY: ANTERIOR SHOULDER DISLOCATION (FIG. 18.6)

- Anterior shoulder dislocation is the most common one. Others are posterior and inferior.
- Mechanism of injury: Sudden anterior jerk in already abducted and externally rotated shoulder as person standing anywhere by holding an overhead support or direct anterior impact on shoulder from posterior side.
- Features:
  - On the basis of location of head it might be: (1) subcoracoid, (2) subglenoid, and (3) subclavicular.
  - Patient remains in attitude of helplessness as holding his affected limb with normal hand and leaning towards affected side.
  - Deltoid bulge flattened and head is palpable anteriorly.
  - Few clinical observations are: (1) **Duga's test**—patient is unable to touch opposite shoulder. (2) **Hamilton ruler test**—a ruler can touch the acromion process and lateral condyle of humerus simultaneously when it is placed by the side of arm in affected side. It is normally impossible due to deltoid bulge. (3) **Callaways test**—the circumference of axilla is increased in affected side. (4) **Bryant test**—the anterior axillary fold is broader and lower in affected side. (5) Military badge sign.

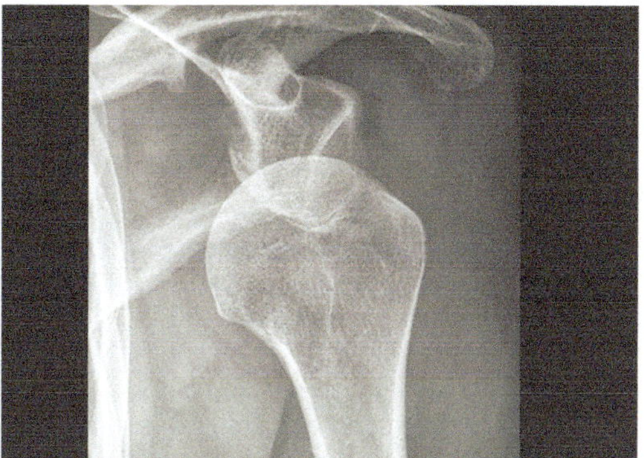

Fig. 18.6: X-ray: Shoulder dislocation.

- Complications: (1) Recurrent dislocation—most common, (2) Axillary nerve neuropraxia—early complication.
- Treatment:
  - Conservative method: Close reduction under general anesthesia is mainstay of treatment. Some methods are: (1) **Hippocrates method**—an abduction traction force is applied by surgeon by keeping his foot against affected axilla. It is the oldest and a crude method but helpful when no assistant is there. (2) **Kocher maneuver**—maneuver is done as follow with a simultaneous countertraction by an assistant: Traction → external rotation → adduction → internal rotation (TEAI). (3) **Stimson gravity method**—here patient is asked to lie prone and hanging his hand by the side of table. Approximately a 2.5 kg weight is fastened in his hand and reduction occurs in 30 minutes. (4) **A.K. Saha method**—here patient's affected limb is abducted to 145° and then flexed

to 65° (zero position), reduction is achieved. Postreduction: After reduction shoulder is maintained in adducted and internal rotation posture with help of universal shoulder immobilizer or arm chest bandage for 4 weeks.
- Surgical method: Open reduction is reserved for close reduction failure cases and old/unreduced dislocation with or without any fracture.

X-RAY: FRACTURE PROXIMAL HUMERUS (FIG. 18.7)

- Proximal humerus is divided into four distinct part as articular humeral head, greater tuberosity, lesser tuberosity, and surgical neck.
- Mechanism of injury: Fall on shoulder or fall on outstretched hand.
- Features:
  - Fracture is classified **(Neer's)** as: (1) Undisplaced; (2) displaced—2 parts, 3 parts, and 4 parts; and (3) fracture dislocation.
  - Fracture is said to be displaced when there is 1 cm displacement and 45° angulation.
  - Complications: Axillary nerve involvement, stiffness, and avascular necrosis especially in 4 parts fracture.
- Management: X-ray AP and lateral view
  - Conservative method: (1) Undisplaced fracture is managed with a cuff and collar sling or arm chest bandage only. (2) If displaced fracture is possible to approximate, it can be immobilized in U-slab. 3–4 weeks is sufficient period for immobilization.
  - Surgical method: Indications are unreducible fractures, reduction might be closed or open and modalities for fracture fixation are K-wires and proximal humerus plate.

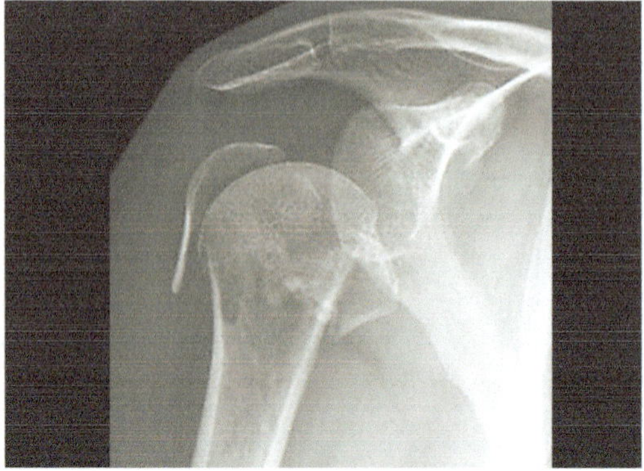

Fig. 18.7: X-ray: Fracture humeral head.

X-RAY: FRACTURE SHAFT HUMERUS (FIG. 18.8)

- As humerus has good muscle bulk, hence it can hide the deformity of humerus to some extent. Side by side radial nerve is in close proximity with humerus, hence much vulnerable to be injured.
- Mechanism of injury: Fall on outstretched hand and direct trauma.
- Features:
  - Displacement: If fracture occurs above deltoid attachment, proximal fragment is adducted under effect of pectoralis major. And if fracture occurs below, the proximal fragment is abducted under effect of deltoid.
  - **Holstein-Lewis fracture:** Fracture at junction of middle 1/3rd and lower 1/3rd humerus, spiral or long oblique, and entrapping radial nerve, especially during reduction.

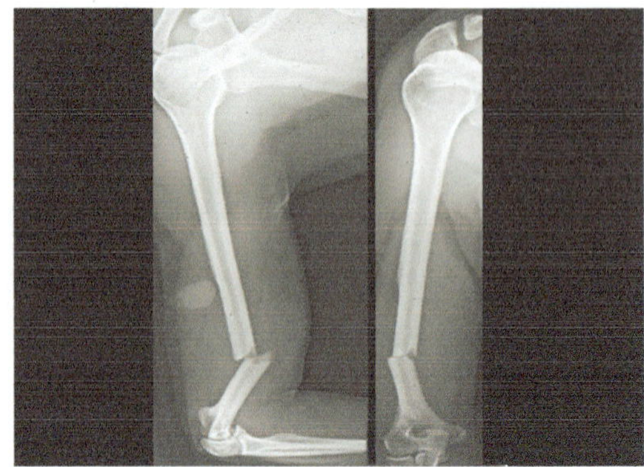

Fig. 18.8: X-ray: Fracture shaft humerus.

- Complications: Radial nerve injury, nonunion, and malunion.
- Management: X-ray AP and lateral view
  - Conservative method: Undisplaced fracture or displaced fractures having possibilities of acceptable approximation can be maintained in U-slab or cast. 3–4 weeks is sufficient period for immobilization.
  - Surgical method: Indications are unreducible fractures and modalities are dynamic compression plating (DCP), interlocking nailing, and rush nailing.

X-RAY: FRACTURE SUPRACONDYLAR AND INTERCONDYLAR HUMERUS (FIGS. 18.9A AND B)

Differences between supracondylar fracture and intercondylar fracture has been shown in Table 18.2.

X-RAY: POSTERIOR DISLOCATION OF ELBOW (FIG. 18.10)

- Posterior shoulder dislocation is most common among all types. Others are lateral, anterior, and medial.

Table 18.2: Differences between supracondylar fracture and intercondylar fracture.

Supracondylar fracture	Intercondylar fracture
• Common in children (5–8 years). • Mechanism of injury: Fall on outstretched hand. • Features: ➢ Fracture may be extension type (97%) or flexion type (3%). **Gartland classification** for extension type fracture: – Undisplaced – Partially displaced with posterior cortex intact – Fully displaced. ➢ Displacement: – Proximal shift – Medial tilt or shift and sometime lateral shift – Posterior tilt or shift – Internal rotation. ➢ Three point bony relationship (Chapter 6) is maintained ➢ Complications: Malunion (cubitus varus deformity or *gunstock deformity*), nerve injury: Anterior-interosseous most commonly involved, radial nerve in post-medial rotation, median nerve in post-lateral rotation, ulnar nerve in flexion type, elbow stiffness. • Management: X-ray AP and lateral view ➢ Conservative method: – Undisplaced fracture: Above elbow slab application in flexed and supine elbow. – Displaced fracture: Close reduction and above elbow slab in flexed and pronated elbow to lock the reduction. Maintain slab for 3–4 weeks. ➢ Surgical method: Indications are unreducible fractures. Reduction might be closed or open and modality for fracture fixation is K-wire.	• Common in adult. • Mechanism of injury: Due to fall on elbow point. • Features: ➢ Fracture classification: **Muller et al.** – Extra-articular – Partial articular (unicondylar) – intra-articular. ➢ Common fracture pattern: – T-pattern – Y-pattern ➢ Three bony point relationship altered ➢ Complications: Malunion and elbow stiffness. • Management: X-ray AP and lateral view ➢ Conservative-method: Limited role, only for undisplaced fracture: Above elbow slab application in flexed and supine elbow. Maintain slab for 3 weeks and start mobilization. ➢ Surgical method: Mainstay of treatment, modalities for fracture fixation are K-wire, tubular plates, reconstruction plates or locking plates.

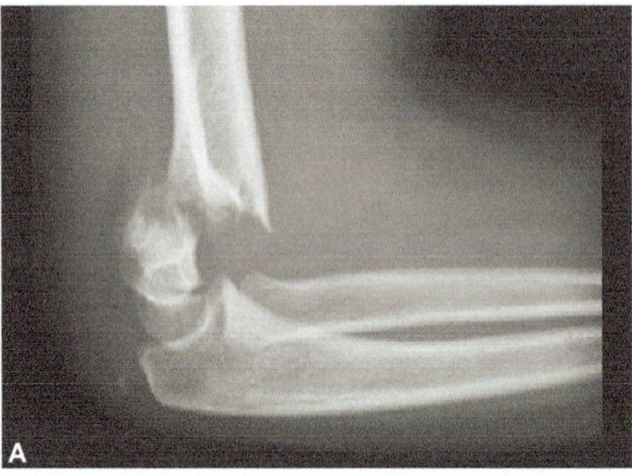

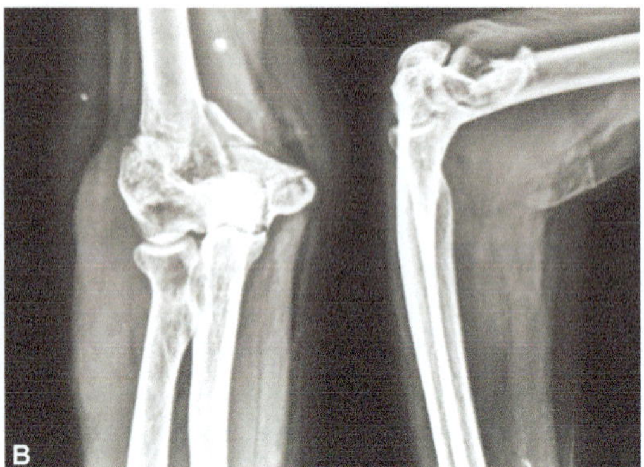

Figs. 18.9A and B: A. Fracture supracondylar humerus; B. Fracture intercondylar humerus.

- Mechanism of injury: Fall in outstretched hand in slightly flexed elbow.
- Features:
  - Posterior dislocation may be associated with soft tissue injury like collateral ligaments and capsular tear side by side fracture coronoid process and radial head are also seen sometimes.
  - Elbow remains in attitude of slight flexion and supination.
  - Olecranon process is prominent and a dimple is visible adjacent to it.
  - Three bony point relationship is reversed.
  - **Terrible triad of Hotchkiss:** Posterior dislocation of elbow along with fracture radial head and fracture coronoid process.

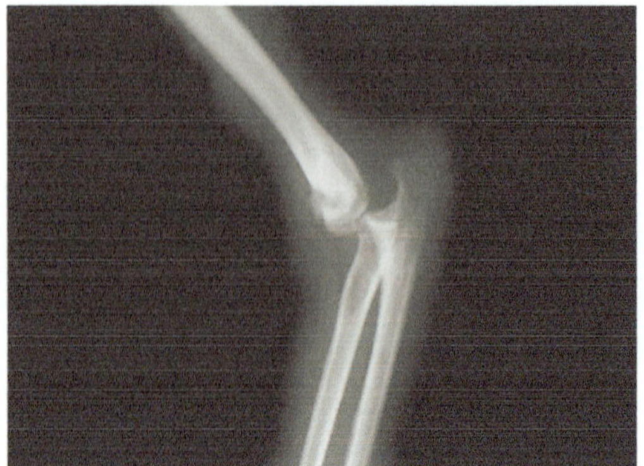

Fig. 18.10: X-ray: Posterior dislocation of elbow.

  - Complications: (1) Nerve injury, i.e. ulnar nerve > median nerve and (2) elbow stiffness.
- Treatment:
  - Conservative method: Close reduction is the mainstay of treatment. Maintain reduction in above elbow slab with elbow flexed and supinated position for 3–4 weeks.
  - Surgical method: Surgery is reserved for failed close reduction, neglected, and unstable elbow.

X-RAY: FRACTURE RADIAL HEAD (FIGS. 18.11A AND B)

- Radial head fracture is common in adult and radial neck fracture is common in children.
- Mechanism of injury: Fall on outstretched hand.
- Features:
  - Classification: **(Masson)** Type I—undisplaced, Type II—marginal fracture with displacement, Type III—comminuted, and Type IV—associated with elbow dislocation
  - **Essex-Lopresti fracture**: Fracture radial head, disruption of interosseous membrane and DRU joint
  - Complications: (1) Elbow stiffness and (2) arthritis.

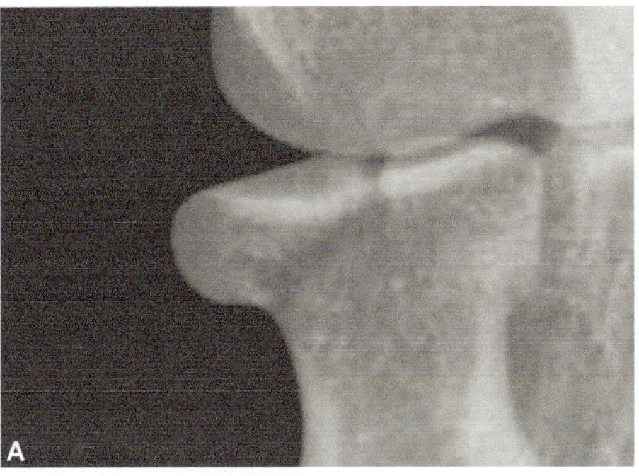

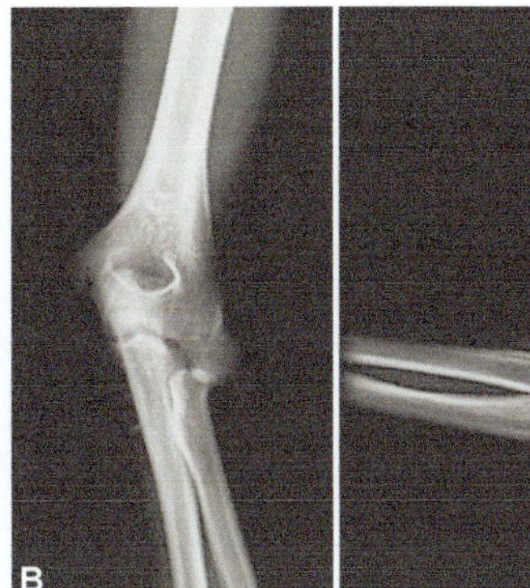

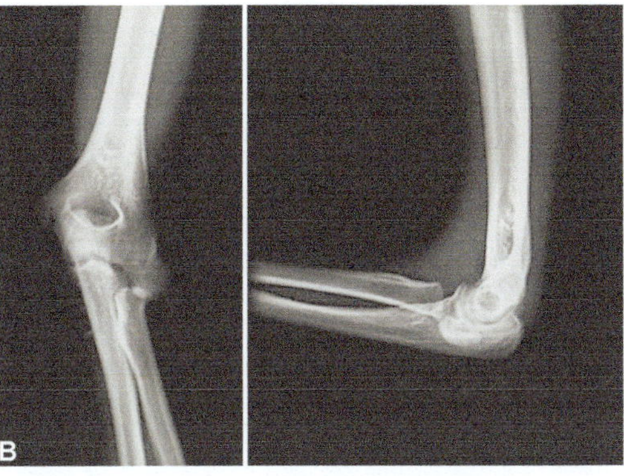

Figs. 18.11A and B: X-ray: Fracture radial head and neck.

- Management: X-ray AP and lateral view
  - Conservative method: Indications are: (1) Undisplaced radial head fracture, (2) displaced fracture where approximation of fragment is possible by manipulation, and (3) tilted neck fractures (<40°) are treated by above cuff and collar sling or elbow slab for 3–4 weeks.
  - Surgical method: (1) Unreducible radial head fracture should be treated with open reduction and screw or T-plate fixation. (2) Comminuted radial head fracture with stable elbow should be addressed with radial head excision. (3) If elbow is unstable then radial head excision must be followed by radial head prosthesis.

X-RAY: FRACTURE OLECRANON PROCESS (FIG. 18.12)

- Although it is subcutaneous, hence always remains on risk of injury.
- Mechanism of injury: Fall on elbow point directly or fall in partially flexed elbow position.
- Features:
  - Olecranon base is the most common site of fracture and pattern may be transverse, oblique or comminuted.
  - Triceps pull is reason for displacement.
  - **Hume's fracture:** Fracture olecranon along with radial head dislocation.

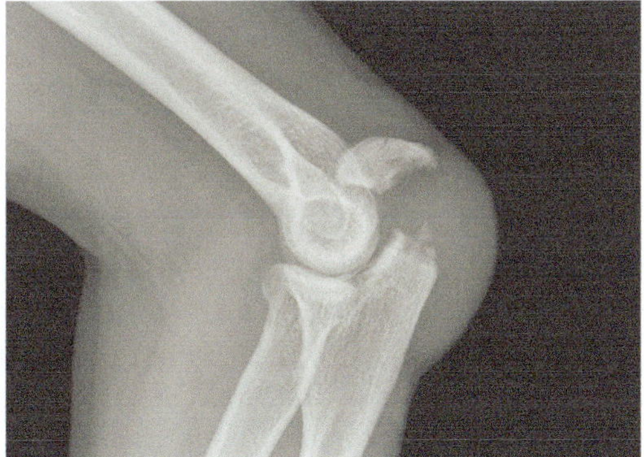

Fig. 18.12: X-ray: Fracture olecranon process.

  - Complications: Nonunion and elbow stiffness.
- Management: X-ray AP and lateral view
  - Conservative method: Undisplaced fractures are treated with above elbow slab in 20–30° of elbow flexion for 3–4 weeks.
  - Surgical method: All displaced fractures are treated with tension band wiring.

X-RAY: FRACTURE RADIUS AND ULNA (FIGS. 18.13A TO C)

- Mechanism of injury: Fall on outstretched hand.
- Features:
  - Displacement:
    - Fracture above insertion of pronator teres: Proximal fragment is flexed

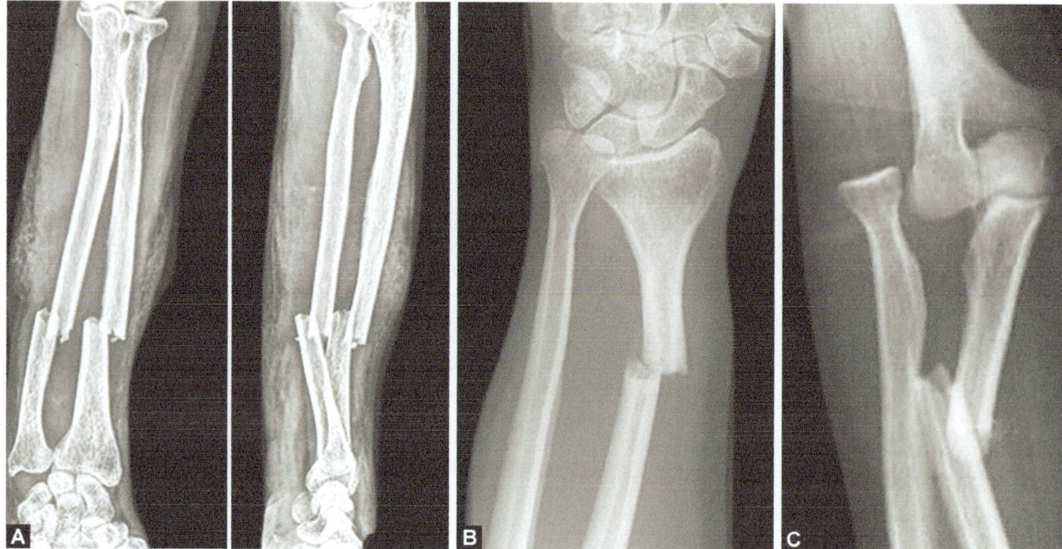

Figs. 18.13A to C: A. Fracture radius and ulna; B. Galeazzi fracture dislocation; C. Monteggia fracture dislocation.

and supinated under action of biceps brachii and supinator, respectively.

- Fracture below insertion of pronator teres: Distal fragment is pronated under effect of pronator quadratus.
- **Monteggia fracture dislocation:** Fracture upper 1/3rd ulna along with subluxation or dislocation of superior radioulnar joint.
- **Galeazi fracture dislocation:** Fracture lower 1/3rd radius along with subluxation of inferior radioulnar joint.
- *Night stick fracture*: Isolated undisplaced fracture of ulna is called night stick fracture.
- Complications: (1) Nonunion, (2) malunion, and (3) crossunion.

- Management: X-ray AP and lateral view
  - Conservative method: Undisplaced or closely reducible and maintainable fractures are treated with above elbow cast for 4–6 weeks followed by physiotherapy. Fracture level and position of forearm:
    - If fracture is in upper 1/3rd portion: Position of forearm is fully supinated
    - If fracture is in middle 1/3rd portion: Position of forearm is midprone.
    - If fracture is in lower 1/3rd portion: Position of forearm is fully pronated.
    - Surgical method: If conservative method fails then reduce the fracture by close method and stabilize with elastic nails or reduce the fracture by open method and fix with dynamic compression plates.
    - For Monteggia and Galeazzi fracture dislocation: Conservative method should be tried only in pediatric cases otherwise open reduction and dynamic compression plate fixation is treatment of choice.

X-RAY: FRACTURE DISTAL RADIUS (COLLES FRACTURE) (FIG. 18.14)

- This is common in elderly female and at corticocancellous junction of bone approximately 2 cm from wrist joint.
- Mechanism of injury: Fall on outstretched hand.
- Features:

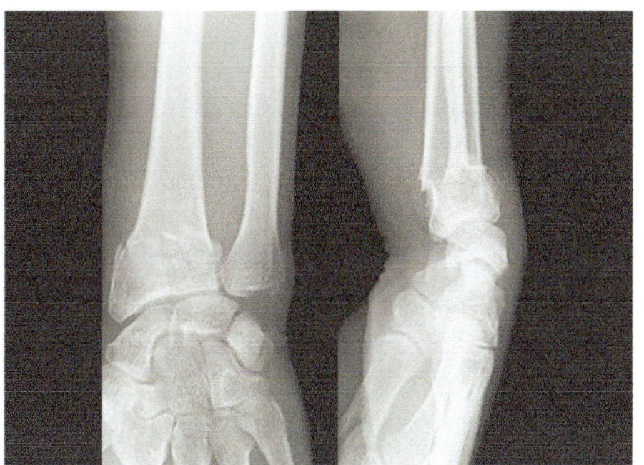

Fig. 18.14: X-ray: Colles fracture.

- Displacement of distal fragment: (1) Proximal impaction, (2) dorsal tilt, (3) dorsal shift, (4) radial shift, (5) radial shift, and (6) supination. These peculiar displacements produce atypical dinner fork deformity at wrist.
- The tip of both styloid processes is at same level, although normally tip of radial styloid process lies 1 cm distal to ulnar styloid process.
- **Barton fracture:** Coronal intra-articular split fracture. It might be volar or dorsal.
- *Chauffeur's fracture:* Isolated radial styloid fracture, e.g. Generator man wrist injury.
- Complications: (1) Stiffness, (2) malunion, (3) reflex sympathetic dystrophy, (4) rupture of extensor pollicis longus, and (5) carpal tunnel syndrome.

• Management: X-ray AP and lateral view
  - Conservative method: Close reduction and Colles cast application for 4–6 weeks followed by physiotherapy is mainstay of treatment. Radiography at 1 week after cast application is mandatory to check the status of reduction or collapse at fracture site.
  - Surgical method: Surgery is reserved for cases having fear of collapse at fracture site and modalities of fixation are K-wire or distal radius volar plates.

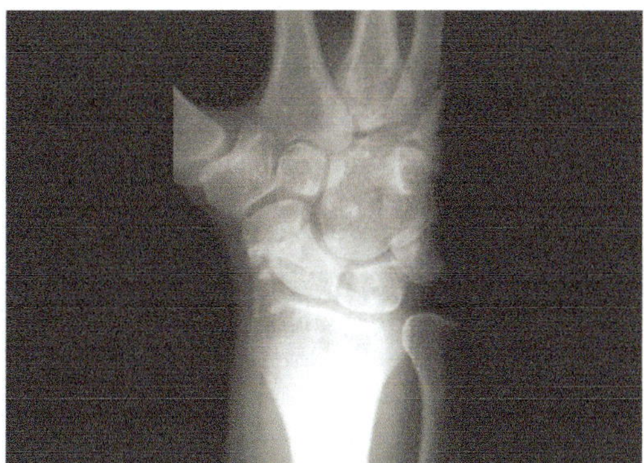

Fig. 18.15: X-ray: Scaphoid fracture.

X-RAY: FRACTURE SCAPHOID (FIG. 18.15)

- This is the most common carpal bone to be fractured and waist is the site having maximum occurrence. Its blood supply is precarious.
- Mechanism of injury: Fall on outstretched hand in radially deviated wrist.
- Features:
  - Displacement of distal fragment: (1) Proximal impaction, (2) dorsal tilt, (3) dorsal shift, (4) radial shift, (5) radial shift, and (6) supination. These peculiar displacements produce atypical dinner fork deformity at wrist.
  - Tenderness in anatomical snuffbox is classical finding.
  - Pressure tenderness can be elicited at scaphoid tubercle on volar aspect of wrist.
  - Complications: (1) Nonunion, (2) avascular necrosis, and (3) wrist arthritis.
- Management: X-ray scaphoid view—wrist is dorsally and ulnar ward deviated. Impacted fractures are not visible in plain radiographs immediately after injury hence CT scan is needed in such suspicious cases to confirm the diagnosis. After 2 weeks the fracture line could be visible in plain radiographs due to osteolysis at fracture

site. MRI can comment on vascularity of bone.

- Conservative method: Scaphoid cast in glass holding position for 2 months followed by physiotherapy is the mainstay of treatment.
- Surgical method: Surgical fixation (Herbert screw) is reserved for displaced and unstable fractures.

X-RAY: FRACTURE BASE OF 1ST METACARPAL (FIG. 18.16)

- Bennett's and Rolando's are the two common intra-articular fracture pattern found at base of 1st metacarpal.
- Mechanism of injury: Direct injury at site in closed fist position, e.g. Boxer.
- Features:
  - **Bennett's fracture:** It is actually a chip fracture with significant displacement under effect of abductor pollicis longus.
  - **Rolando's fracture:** It is relatively undisplaced fracture having T or Y fracture pattern.
  - Complication: (1) Malunion and (2) 1st CMC joint arthritis.
- Management: X-ray AP and lateral view
  - Conservative method: Only thumb spica as definitive treatment has limited role in such fractures.
  - Surgical method: Reduction either closed or open followed by K-wire fixation is the mainstay of treatment.

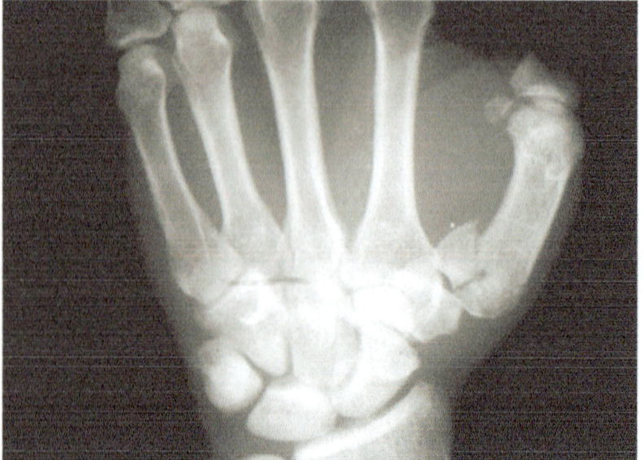

Fig. 18.16: X-ray: Fracture base of 1st metacarpal.

X-RAY: DISLOCATION OF HIP (FIG. 18.17)

- Posterior hip dislocation is the most common among all; others are anterior and central fracture dislocation.
- Mechanism of injury: A violent posterior force against flexed and adducted hip position, e.g. dashboard injury in RTA.
- Features:
  - Posterior dislocation of hip may be associated acetabular rim/wall fracture.
  - Affected limb remain in attitude of flexion, adduction, and internal rotation.
  - Femoral head is palpable in gluteal region as a smooth bulge.
  - Complications: (1) Sciatic nerve injury—foot drop, (2) avascular necrosis of femur head, (3) myositis ossificans, and (4) osteoarthritis hip.
- Management: X-ray AP and lateral view
  - Conservative method: Close reduction under general anesthesia is mainstay of treatment. Some methods are:
    - **Allis's method:** Here patient is asked to lies over floor in supine position. Maintain approximately 70° flexion at hip joint and apply longitudinal

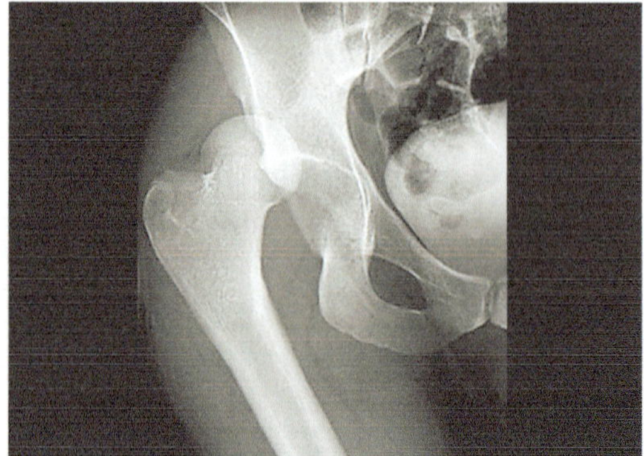

Fig. 18.17: X-ray: Dislocation of hip.

traction. Side by side a gentle internal and external rotation is done to achieve reduction.

- **Bigelow method:** Adducted limb is flexed to 90° and dislocated head is reduced by applying forces in opposite direction as abduction, external rotation, and extension.
- Stimson gravity method: Here patient lies on a couch in prone position and affected limb hangs over the side of couch in such a way that hip and knee maintain 90° flexion. Now, a downward fore is applied on calf in line of femur to reduce the dislocation. Reduction is maintained in skin and sometime skeletal traction for 4 weeks.
- Surgical method: Open reduction is reserved for close reduction failure cases and old/unreduced dislocation with or without acetabular wall fracture.

X-RAY: FRACTURE NECK FEMUR (FIG. 18.18)

- Fracture neck femur is common in elderly after 50 years.
- Mechanism of injury: (1) Trivial fall in elderly and (2) direct or rotational violence at hip in younger.

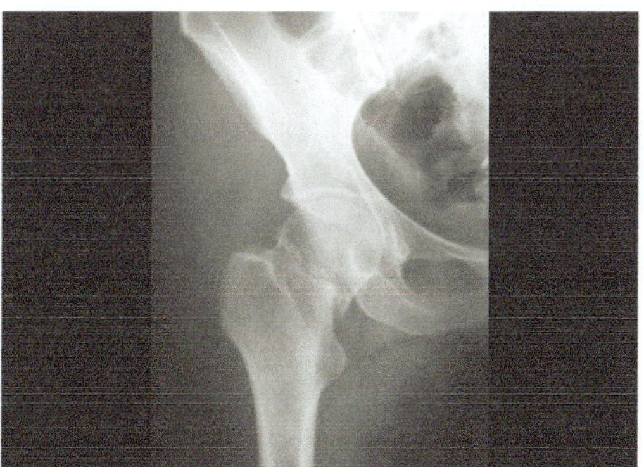

Fig. 18.18: X-ray: Fracture neck femur.

- Features:
  - Anatomically fracture may be subcapital, transcervical, and basal. **Garden's** classification: (1) Incomplete fracture, (2) complete but undisplaced fracture, (3) complete fracture with partial displacement, and (4) complete fracture with total displacement.
  - Tenderness in Scarpa's triangle (Chapter 12), external rotation attitude (<45°), and shortening (<1 inch) are some key clinical findings.
  - Complications: Avascular necrosis of head of femur, nonunion, and hip arthritis.
- Management: X-ray AP pelvis showing both hip joint in 15° internal rotation (for complete neck visibility) and lateral view of affected hip. **Pauwel's angle:** This is an angle formed by fracture line with horizontal plane in AP view. It keeps the fracture in three groups as; Type I—Pauwel angle < 30°, Type II—Pauwel angle 30–50°, and Type III—Pauwel angle > 50°.
  - Conservative method: In children, undisplaced fractures are treated under hip spica for 4 weeks. Adults having impacted fracture neck femur are candidate for conservative treatment by restricting mobilization and weight bearing, e.g. by application of derotation bar.
  - Surgical method: Surgery is the mainstay of treatment. In children—closed or open reduction followed by fixation with Moore's pin or 4 mm partially threaded cancellous screw in children. In adult:
    - Patient below 60 years: Closed or open reduction followed by fixation with 6.5 mm partially threaded cancellous screw or sometime valgus osteotomy
    - Patient above 60 years: Hemiarthroplasty and sometime total hip arthroplasty.

X-RAY: FRACTURE TROCHANTER FEMUR (FIG. 18.19)

- Fracture trochanter femur is common in elderly after 60 years.
- Mechanism of injury: Significant trauma either directly or indirectly.
- Features:
  - Classification **(Boyd and Griffith)**. Type I: Intertrochanteric simple fracture, Type II: Intertrochanteric fracture with communication in coronal plane, Type III: Reverse oblique fracture, and Type IV: Intertrochanteric fracture with subtrochanteric extension. Fractures may be stable or unstable.
  - Broadening and tenderness in greater trochanteric area, external rotation attitude (>45°) and shortening (>1 inch) are some key clinical findings.
  - Complications: Malunion is the most common complication.
- Management: X-ray AP view of pelvis of affected hip
  - Conservative method: This method is used for medically unfit patient. Here a continuous upper tibial skeletal traction is given on Bohler-Braun splint with appropriate countertraction (by raising leg end of couch) for 6 weeks in 45° abducted hip position. After that first partial then full weight-bearing is given.
  - Surgical method: Closed or open reduction followed by fixation with dynamic hip screw (DHS) or proximal femoral nailing (PFN).

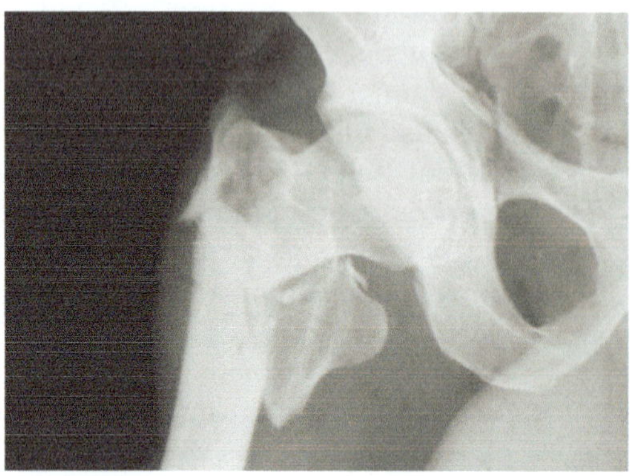

Fig. 18.19: X-ray: Fracture trochanter.

X-RAY: FRACTURE SHAFT FEMUR (FIG. 18.20)

- Femur is the main load-bearing bone having good muscle bulk. Its fracture might produce shock due to loss of 1–2 liters of blood.
- Mechanism of injury: (1) Fall from height and (2) high velocity direct impact as in road traffic accidents.
- Features:
  - Displacement: (1) Upper 1/3rd fracture—proximal fragment is flexed and abducted under effect of iliopsoas and gluteus medius and minimus, respectively. (2) Lower 1/3rd fracture—distal fragment sags posteriorly due to pulling effect of gastrocnemius and may endanger the popliteal vessels.
  - Association: Femoral or popliteal vasculature injury in distal 1/3rd fracture.
  - Complications: (1) Fat embolism, (2) nonunion, and (3) malunion.
- Management: X-ray AP and lateral view
  - Conservative method: It is reserved for pediatric fractures. Here fracture is maintained with help of skin traction

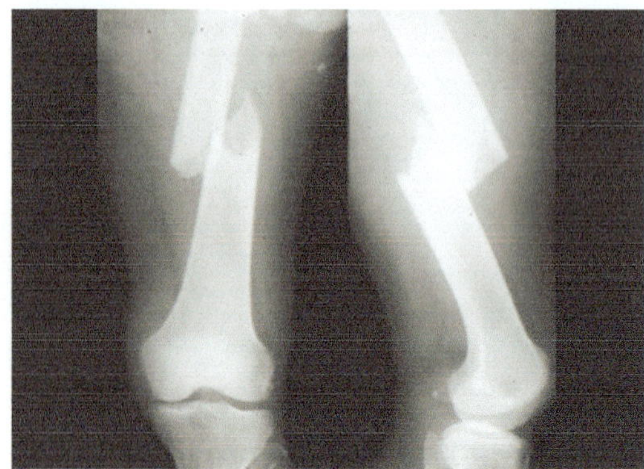

Fig. 18.20: X-ray: Fracture shaft femur.

over Thomas splint and Buck pulley (Chapter 14). When fracture becomes sticky (3 weeks) hip spica is applied for 4–6 weeks. After that knee mobilization exercises and weight-bearing started.
- Surgical method: Main stay of treatment, nowadays. Open or close reduction followed by intramedullary nailing (Ender nail, K-nail, and interlocking nails) and sometimes screws and plates.

X-RAY: FRACTURE SUPRACONDYLAR AND INTERCONDYLAR FEMUR (FIGS. 18.21A AND B)

- Periarticular distal femur fractures are common in young population.
- Mechanism of injury: (1) Direct trauma and (2) axial loading with valgus or varus forces acting at knee.
- Features:
  - Classification **(Muller et al.)**: (1) Type A—extra-articular supracondylar. (2) Type B—partial articular, i.e. unicondylar. (3) Type C—complete articular, i.e. bicondylar.
  - Associated injury: Injury of femoral or popliteal artery may be associated with this fracture.
  - Complications: (1) Malunion, (2) malalignment, i.e. varus or valgus at knee, (3) knee stiffness, and (4) knee arthritis.
- Management: X-ray AP and lateral view
  - Conservative method: Only stable and undisplaced fracture can be treated with above knee cast for 6 weeks followed by knee mobilization exercises.
  - Surgical method: Displaced and unstable fractures are treated by open reduction and internal fixation (ORIF) and implant commonly used are cancellous screw, metaphyseal plates or supracondylar nail.

X-RAY: FRACTURE PATELLA (FIG. 18.22)

- Patella is largest sesamoid bone developed under quadriceps tendon. Being subcutaneous it is very much exposed for injury.
- Mechanism of injury: (1) Direct trauma and (2) indirect—sudden forcible contraction

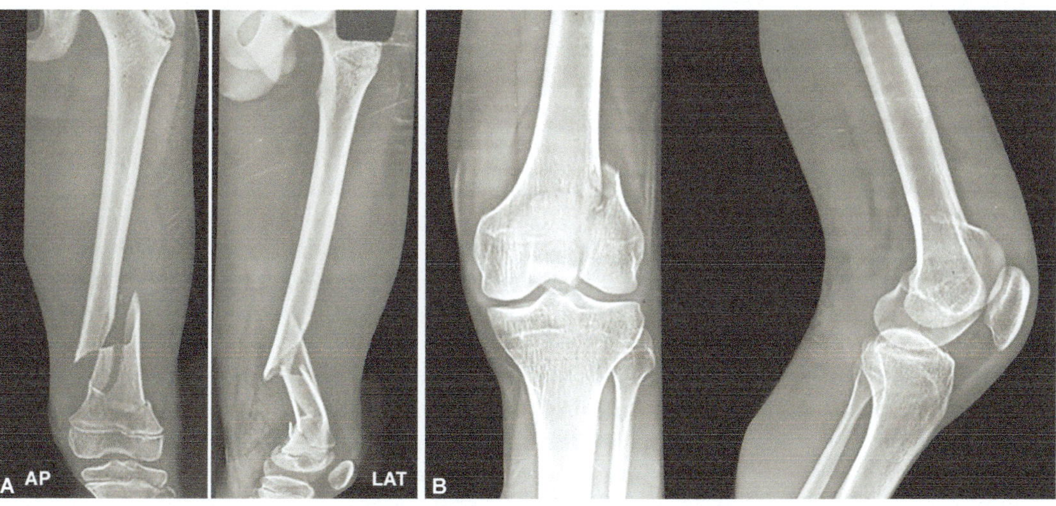

Figs. 18.21A and B: A. Fracture supracondylar femur; B. Fracture intercondylar femur.

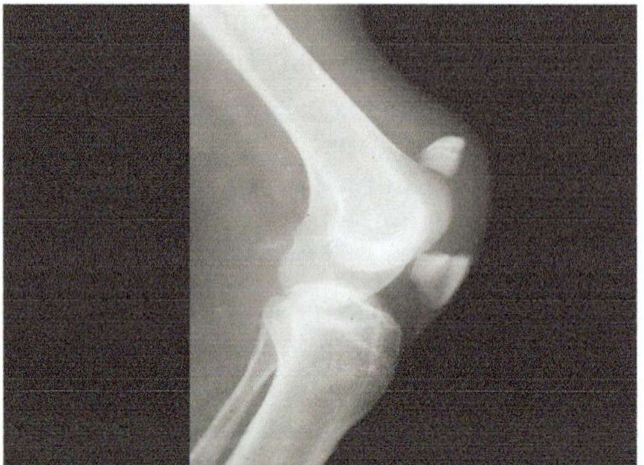

Fig. 18.22: X-ray: Fracture patella.

of quadriceps in semiflexed knee position (falling position).

- Features:
  - Displacement: Under effect of quadriceps pull.
  - Fracture pattern: (1) Transverse, (2) vertical, (3) polar, (4) stellate, and (5) osteochondral.
  - Association: Medial and lateral retinaculum rupture is commonly associated with fracture patella.
  - Palpable gap is often found at fracture site.
  - Complications: (1) Knee stiffness and (2) knee arthritis.
- Management: X-ray AP and lateral view
  - Conservative method: Undisplaced fracture is treated by a cylindrical cast of 6 weeks followed by knee mobilization exercises.
  - Surgical method: All displaced fractures are treated surgically. (1) Transverse fractures are fixed with tension band wiring. (2) For comminuted fracture cerclage wiring is preferred. (3) Partial or complete patellectomy when patella could not be saved. Any intra-articular step at under surface of patella must be checked before fixation.

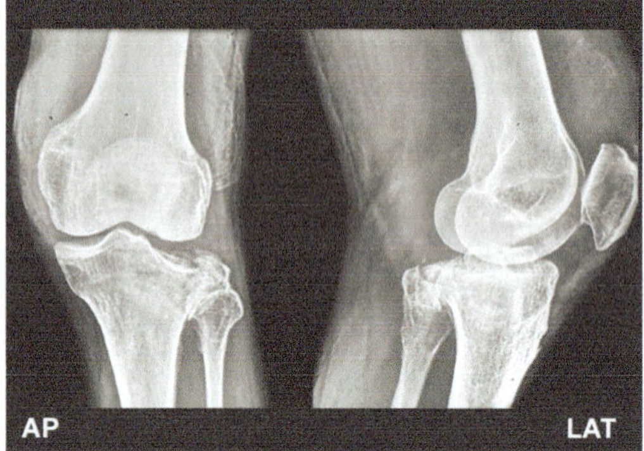

Fig. 18.23: X-ray: Fracture proximal tibia (plateau fracture).

X-RAY: FRACTURE PROXIMAL TIBIA (FIG. 18.23)

- Proximal tibia fracture is also called Bumper's fracture.
- Mechanism of injury: Direct trauma, e.g. road traffic accident.
- Features:
  - Classification **(Schatzker)**:
    - Type I—lateral split
    - Type II—lateral split depression
    - Type III—lateral pure depression
    - Type IV—medial plateau fracture
    - Type V—bicondylar fracture
    - Type VI—metaphyseal-diaphyseal fracture dissociation.
  - Association: Tibial plateau may be associated with injury of cruciate ligaments, menisci or collateral ligaments that produces instability of joint.
  - Complications: (1) Knee stiffness and (2) malunion—varus or valgus deformity.
- Management: X-ray AP and lateral or oblique view
  - Conservative method: Undisplaced and stable fracture having less than 5 mm intra-articular step are treated by above knee cast for 6 weeks followed by partial weight-bearing and knee mobilization exercises.

- Surgical method: All displaced, unstable or fracture having more than 5 mm intra-articular step must be treated surgically and modality of fixation is proximal tibial plates (buttress plates) or cancellous screw or combination.

X-RAY: FRACTURE SHAFT TIBIA AND FIBULA (FIG. 18.24)

- Most common long bone to be fractured. As it is less supported by soft tissue in anterior aspect of leg hence fracture both bone legs are very prone for compounding (open fracture).
- Mechanism of injury: (1) Direct impact in road traffic accident and (2) fall from height.
- Features:
  - Displacement: In proximal 1/3rd tibial fracture there is chances of anterior displacement of proximal fragment due to action of ligamentum patellae.
  - Associated injury: Most of the cases of tibial fractures are associated with fibula fracture too.
  - Complications: (1) Nonunion, (2) malunion, and (3) adjacent joint stiffness.
- Management: X-ray AP and lateral view
  - Conservative method: Undisplaced and closely reducible and maintainable fractures are treated with above knee cast for 4–6 weeks followed by patellar tendon-bearing (PTB—Chapter 13) brace.
  - Surgical method: Fractures those could not be treated conservatively are treated with intramedullary nailing (interlocking nailing or ender's nailing) and sometime plates and screw.

X-RAY: FRACTURE MALLEOLI (FIG. 18.25)

- Bimalleolar (medial malleoli and lateral malleoli) fractures are eponym as **Pott's fracture**.
- Mechanism of injury: Twisting injury around ankle.
- Features:
  - Fracture pattern of malleoli depends upon position of foot say supination or pronation and twisting force acting on ankle as adduction or abduction.
  - Associated injury: Ankle dislocation and tarsal bones fracture.
  - **Maisonneuve fracture:** Proximal fibular fracture associated with malleoli fracture and syndesmotic injury.
  - Complications: (1) Nonunion, (2) malunion, (3) joint stiffness, and (4) osteoarthritis.
- Management: X-ray—AP, lateral, and mortise view (mortise view: X-ray in 30° internal rotation).

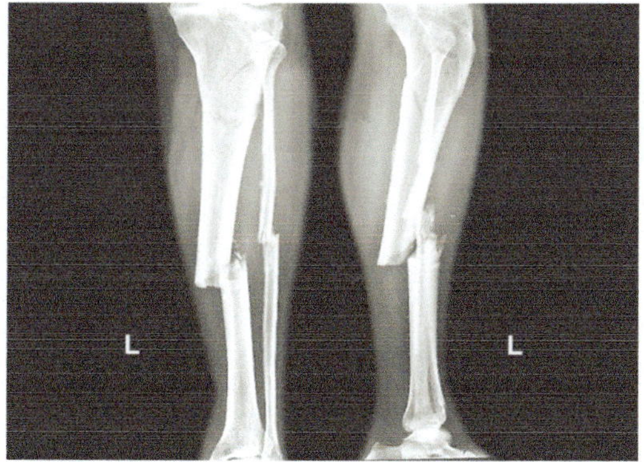

Fig. 18.24: X-ray: Fracture shaft of tibia and fibula.

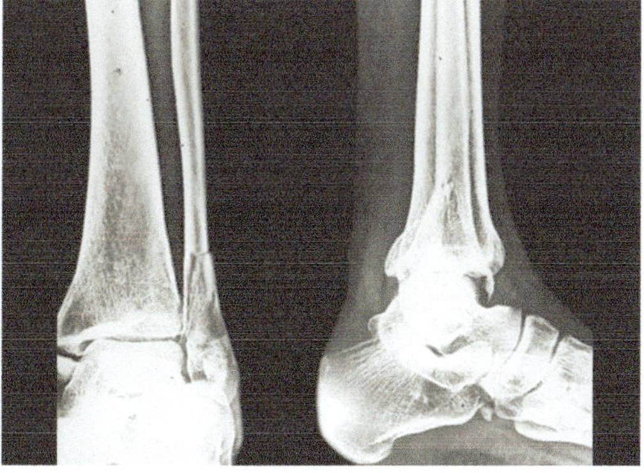

Fig. 18.25: X-ray: Fracture malleoli of ankle.

- Conservative method: Only for impacted fracture in the form of below knee cast.
- Surgical method: (1) Fibular fracture are addressed with rush nail or tubular plates and sometime partially threaded 4 mm cancellous screw. (2) Medial malleolar fracture is treated with 4 mm cancellous screw or tension band wiring if fracture piece is small. In case of syndesmotic injury represented by ankle subluxation or dislocation a separate screw is applied running from fibula to tibia called syndesmotic screw.

X-RAY: FRACTURE CALCANEUS (LOVER'S FRACTURE) (FIGS. 18.26A AND B)

- Most common fracture among tarsals bone.
- Mechanism of injury: (1) Fall from height and (2) direct impact.
- Features:
  - Classification: (1) Extra-articular fracture and (2) intra-articular fracture.
  - Associated fracture: Spine, hip, and other lower limb bone.
  - Widening of heel is characteristic feature.
  - Complications: Malunion is the most common complication.
- Management: X-ray axial view and lateral view (**Bohler angle:** 20–40°, **Gissane angle:** 100–1,140°); Bohler angle decreases and Gissane angle increase in calcaneal fracture.
  - Conservative method: Undisplaced and closely reducible fractures are treated by below knee cast for 8–10 weeks followed by ankle mobilization.
  - Surgical method: All depressed intra-articular fractures need closed or open reduction and fixation (calcaneal plates/ screws) with or without bone-grafting.

X-RAY: FRACTURE BASE OF 5TH METATARSAL (JONES FRACTURE) (FIG. 18.27)

- Most common fracture among metatarsals bone.
- Mechanism of injury: Sudden inversion of foot.
- Features:
  - Fracture pattern: (1) Avulsion fracture/pseudo-Jones fracture and

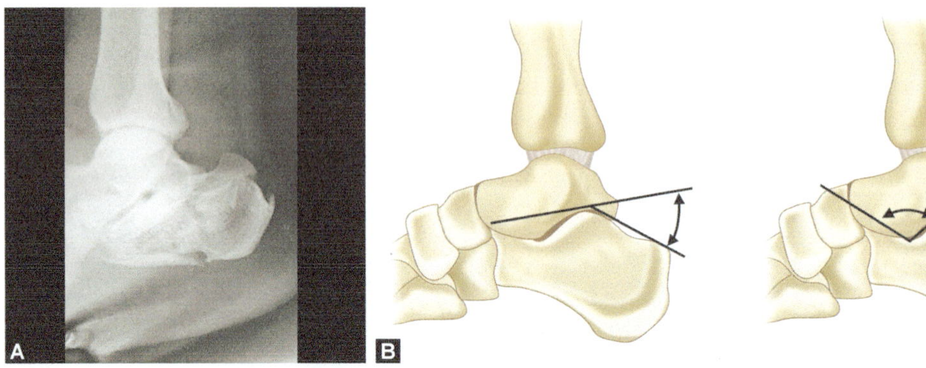

Figs. 18.26A and B: A. X-ray: Fracture calcaneus; B. Bohler angle and Gissane angle.

(2) metaphyseal-diaphyseal junction fracture—true Jones fracture.
- *Dancer's fracture*: Fracture having oblique or spiral pattern commonly occurring in dancers performing over ball of toes.
- Complications: Nonunion sometimes.

- Management: X-ray AP and lateral view
  - Conservative method: Boot cast for 6–8 weeks is mainstay of treatment.
  - Surgical method: Screw fixation is only reserved for significantly displaced fracture.

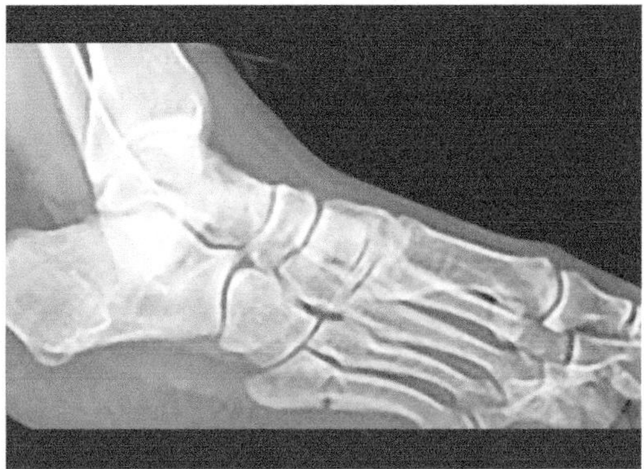

Fig. 18.27: X-ray: Fracture base of 5th metatarsal (Jones fracture).

Chapter

19

Radiographs of Common Bone Tumors

DESCRIPTION OF A TUMOR RADIOGRAPH (FIGS. 19.1A TO D)

- *Tumor location*:
  - Epiphyseal
  - Diaphyseal
  - Metaphyseal.
- *Destruction pattern*:
  - *Geographical*—well-demarcated lesion, easily differentiated from normal bone, wide zone of transition, and homogeneous matrix if any
  - *Moth-eaten*—multiple scattered holes in apparently normal bone, wide zone of transition, and matrix homogenous or heterogeneous
  - *Permeative*—poorly demarcated lesion, not distinguishable from adjacent normal bone, zone of transition lost, and matrix mostly heterogeneous.
- *Periosteal reaction*: It is a reactive new bone formation which takes 1–3 weeks to appear radiologically.

Various types of periosteal reaction are given in Table 19.1.

- *Soft tissue extension*:
  - Absent (cortex intact)
  - Present (cortex breached).

Table 19.1: Various types of periosteal reaction.

Broad categories	Subtypes	Examples
Solid shell periosteal reaction: When slow growing lesion erode endosteal bone which is replenished by subperiosteal bone deposition	Smooth shells	Benign neoplasm
	Septated ridge shells	Aneurysmal bone cyst
Continuous periosteal reaction: Here cortex is intact	Solid	Osteoid osteoma
	Lamellar	Ewing sarcoma
Interrupted periosteal reaction: Here cortex is breach	Buttress	Benign neoplasm
	Codman triangle	Any aggressive bony reaction
Spiculated periosteal reaction: Bone formation with radial neovascularization	Divergent spiculated appearance	Sunburst pattern of osteosarcoma
	Parallel spiculated appearance	Hair on end appearance of Ewing sarcoma

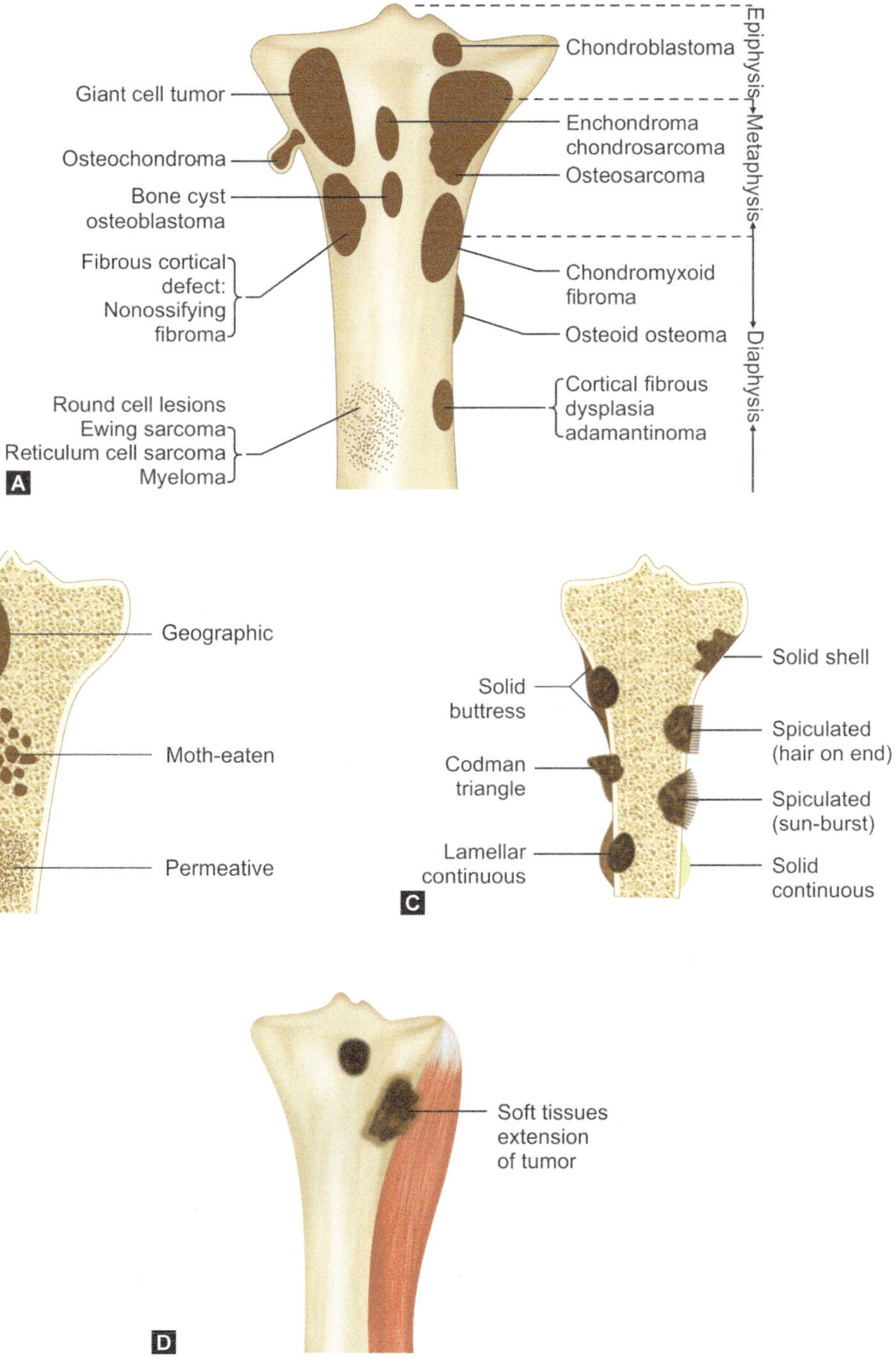

Giant cell tumor
Osteochondroma
Bone cyst
osteoblastoma
Fibrous cortical
defect:
Nonossifying
fibroma
Round cell lesions
Ewing sarcoma
Reticulum cell sarcoma
Myeloma
Chondroblastoma
Enchondroma
chondrosarcoma
Osteosarcoma
Chondromyxoid
fibroma
Osteoid osteoma
Cortical fibrous
dysplasia
adamantinoma
Epiphysis
Metaphysis
Diaphysis
A
Geographic
Moth-eaten
Permeative
B
Solid
buttress
Codman
triangle
Lamellar
continuous
Solid shell
Spiculated
(hair on end)
Spiculated
(sun-burst)
Solid
continuous
C
Soft tissues
extension
of tumor
D

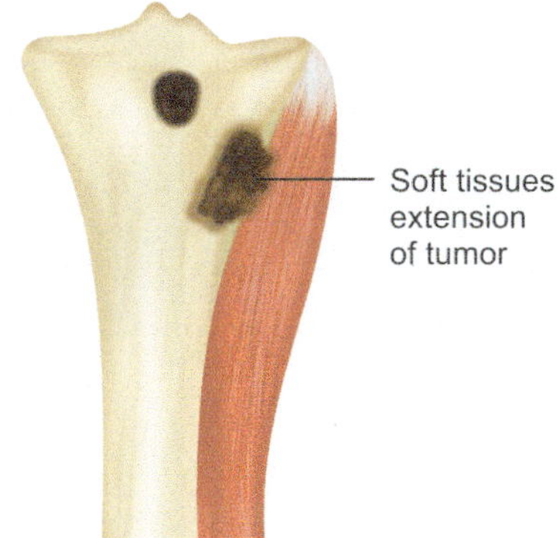

Figs. 19.1A to D: Description of a tumor radiographs: A. Tumor location; B. Destruction pattern; C. Periosteal reaction; D. Soft tissue extension.

X-RAY: OSTEOCHONDROMA/ EXOSTOSIS (FIG. 19.2)

- *Osteochondroma:* Not a true tumor, a hamartoma, also called exostosis, arises from peripheral part of growth plate adjacent to metaphysis.
  - *Age:* 2nd decade
  - *Site:* Distal femur > proximal tibia > proximal humerus
  - Risk percentage for malignant transformation in exostosis—chondrosarcoma
    - Solitary exostosis—1%
    - Multiple exostosis—5–6%
  - Epiphyseal site osteochondroma is called **Trevor's disease.**
- *Description of a tumor radiographs*:
  - *Tumor location*: Metaphyseal outgrowth directed away from the joint
  - *Growth pattern*: Well defined, pedunculated or sessile, *cortical part of tumor* is continuous with cortex of parent bone and *medullary part of growth* is also continuous with medullary cavity of parent bone
  - *Periosteal reaction:* Absent
  - *Soft tissue extension:* Absent.

Note: Radiological sign of malignant transformation in exostosis—chondrosarcoma

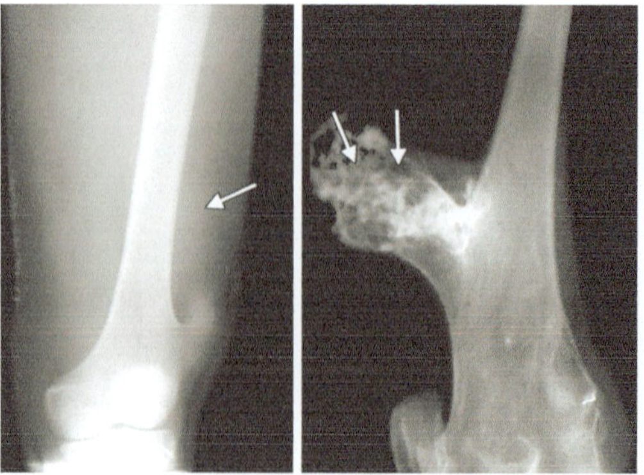

Fig. 19.2: X-ray: Osteochondroma (distal femur). (*Courtesy*: Dr DK Taneja)

- Stippled calcification in cartilage cap
- Margin of tumor becomes ill defined
- Soft tissue extension
- Cartilaginous cap size more than 2 cm in CT or MRI (normally thickness of cartilage cap is more in children, i.e. up to 2 cm than adult, i.e. in few millimeters.

- *Treatment options*: Extraperiosteal resection of tumor, i.e. excision of exostosis along with periosteum lying over it.

X-RAY: SIMPLE BONE CYST AND ANEURYSMAL BONE CYST (FIGS. 19.3A AND B)

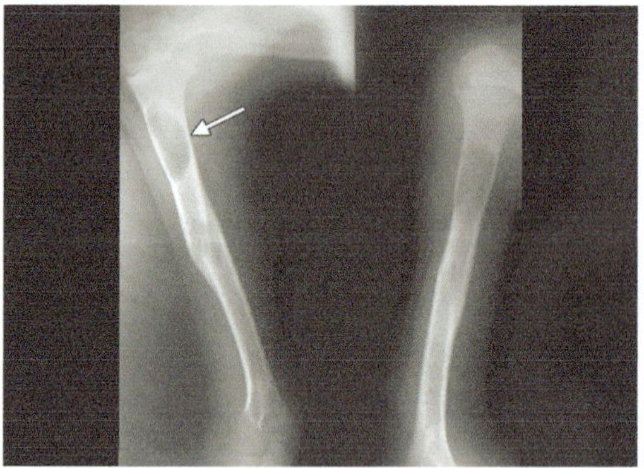

Fig. 19.3A: X-ray: Simple bone cyst (proximal humerus). (*Courtesy*: Dr John Mukhopadhyay)

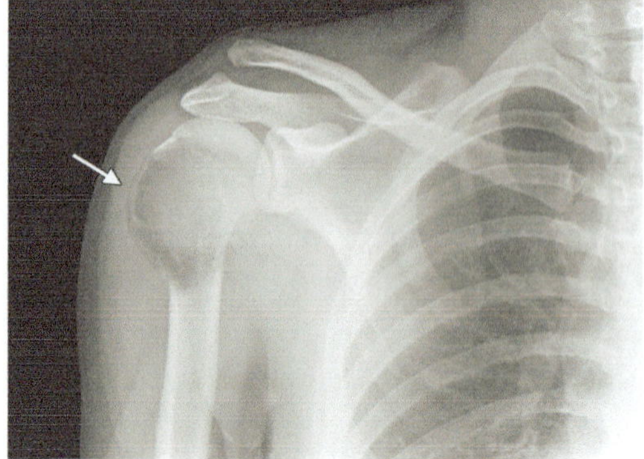

Fig. 19.3B: X-ray: Aneurysmal bone cyst (proximal humerus).

	Simple bone cyst	Aneurysmal bone cyst
About tumor	• Also called unicameral bone cyst; cyst formation occur due to transient failure of physeal ossification. • *Age:* 1st to 2nd decade. • *Site:* Proximal humerus > proximal femur > proximal tibia. • When tumor lies nearer to physis, it is called active tumor and it migrates towards diaphysis it becomes inactive tumor.	• A vasocystic tumor formed following arteriovenous malformation in metaphysis (most accepted theory). • *Age*: 1st to 2nd decade. • *Site*: Proximal humerus > proximal femur >proximal tibia > spinous process. • ABC of spinous process closely resembles osteoblastoma.
Tumor radiograph description	• *Tumor-location*: Metaphyseal/diaphyseal, centrally placed. • *Destruction pattern*: *Well defined,* lytic thinned cortex. • *Periosteal reaction*: Absent (present only with pathological fracture). • *Soft tissue extension*: Absent. *Note*: *Fallen fragment sign* in X-ray is pathognomonic feature for simple bone cyst with fracture.	• *Tumor location:* Metaphyseal/diaphyseal, eccentric. • *Destruction pattern:* Well defined, lytic, expansile, cortex thinned out and egg shell. • *Periosteal reaction:* Present (solid-soap bubble septation). • *Soft tissue extension:* Absent.
Treatment options	• *If pathological fracture*: Spontaneous resolution following conservative treatment. • Aspiration of cyst and intralesional injection of steroids. • Curettage and bone grafting.	• *If pathological fracture*: Spontaneous resolution following conservative treatment. • Curettage and bone grafting. • *Inaccessible tumor and for shrinkage of larger tumors*: Repeated arterial embolization.

X-RAY: FIBROUS DYSPLASIA (FIG. 19.4)

- *Fibrous dysplasia*: Failure of normal lamellar bone formation and abundance of fibrous tissue with flecks of immature bone. May be mono or polyostotic.
  - *Age*: 1st to 3rd decade
  - *Site*: Proximal femur > proximal tibia
  - *Common association*:
    - **McCune Albright syndrome**—polyostotic fibrous dysplasia with precocious puberty
    - **Mazabraud's syndrome**—fibrous dysplasia with myxoma
    - **Cherubism (leontiasis ossea)**—fibrous dysplasia of jaw.
- *Description of a tumor radiographs*:
  - *Tumor location*: Epiphysis/metaphyseal/diaphyseal

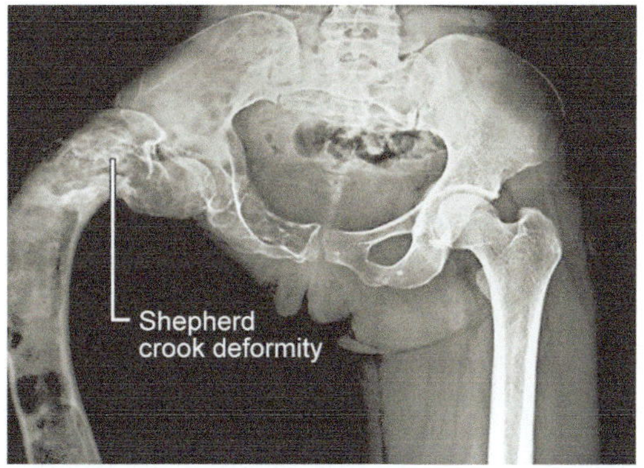

Fig. 19.4: X-ray: Fibrous dysplasia. Proximal femur.

(*Courtesy*: Dr John Mukhopadhyay)

  - *Destruction pattern: Well defined,* lytic, cortex is thinned but may sclerosed at some places, and ground-glass matrix
  - *Periosteal reaction*: Present (continuous-solid periosteal reaction)
  - *Soft tissue extension*: Absent.

Note: A peculiar deformity in fibrous dysplasia involving proximal femur is called **Shepherd crook** deformity.

- *Treatment options*:
  - *Cystic lesion*: Curettage and bone grafting
  - *If pathological fracture*: ORIF and bone grafting
  - *Bone deformity*: Osteotomy and fixation with bone grafting
  - *Polyostotic disease*: Intravenous bisphosphonate like pamidronate.

X-RAY: GIANT CELL TUMOR (FIGS. 19.5A AND B)

- *Giant cell tumor*: A tumor due to overproliferation of osteoclast cell, hence its other name is osteoclastoma.
  - *Age*: 20–40 years (a tumor of mature skeleton)
  - *Site*: Distal femur > proximal tibia > distal radius
  - The aneurysmal bone cyst is one of the tumors of giant cell group that may exist with osteoclastoma.
- *Description of a tumor radiographs*:
  - *Tumor location*: Epiphyseal, metaphyseal in skeletally immature (less common)
  - *Destruction pattern*: Well defined, lytic, eccentric and abutting to joint cartilage, cortex thinned but may breached in locally malignant tumor (*soap bubble appearance*)
  - *Periosteal reaction*: Minimal or absent
  - *Soft tissue extension*: Absent/present.
- *Treatment options*:
  - Extended curettage—when curettage is followed by cauterization by following ways:
    - Phenol
    - Liquid nitrogen
    - Burr
    - Electrical
    - Argon laser
  - Dead space management with bone graft (auto and allo), bone substitute, and bone cement
  - En block excision and reconstruction by turn-o-plasty or bone grafting
  - *Inaccessible lesion*: Radiotherapy.

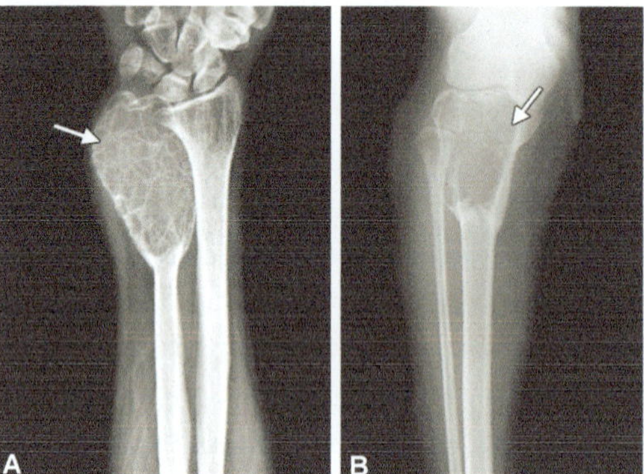

Figs. 19.5A and B: X-ray: Giant cell tumor: A. Distal ulna; B. Proximal tibia.

(*Courtesy*: Dr Chandan Sekhar)

X-RAY: OSTEOSARCOMA (FIGS. 19.6A AND B)

- *Osteosarcoma*: A malignant osteoid producing tumor.
  - *Age*: Primary 2nd decade, secondary 5th decade

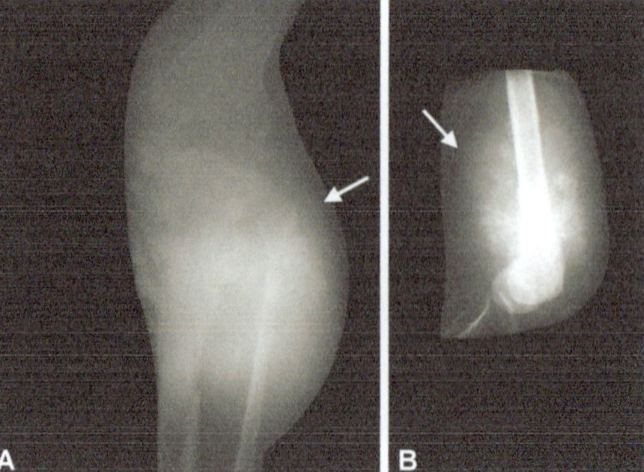

Figs. 19.6A and B: X-ray: Osteosarcoma: A. Proximal tibia; B. Distal femur.

(*Courtesy*: Dr John Mukhopadhyay)

- *Site*: Distal femur > proximal tibia > proximal humerus
- Parosteal osteosarcoma closely resembles myositis ossificans. Characteristic of parosteal osteosarcoma:
  - Common in female
  - Common site—posterior aspect of distal femur
  - Slow growing and painless
- *Description of a tumor radiographs*:
  - *Tumor location*: Metaphyseal
  - Destruction pattern: Ill defined, permeative, breached cortex with heterogeneous matrix with wide zone of transition
  - *Periosteal reaction*: Interrupted type **(Codman triangle)** and divergent spiculated type (*sun burst appearance*)
  - *Soft tissue extension*: Present.
- *Treatment options*:
  - Neoadjuvant chemotherapy followed by wide resection of tumor and postoperative chemotherapy
    - T-10 a/b regimen are commonly followed as T-10 a (methotrexate, Adriamycin, ifosfamide, and dexamethasone)
    - T-10 b (above drugs + cisplatin)
  - Reconstruction with bone graft (autograft and allograft) and endoprosthesis
  - Resection arthrodesis and rotationplasty
  - Amputation of limb.

X-RAY: EWING SARCOMA (FIGS. 19.7A AND B)

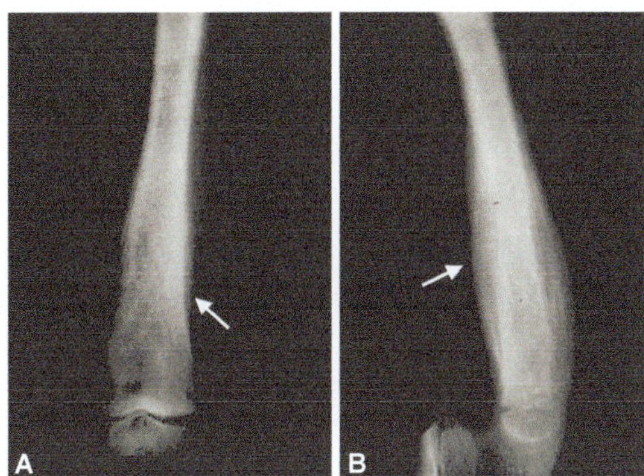

Figs. 19.7A and B: X-ray: Ewing sarcoma (femur).

(*Courtesy*: Dr John Mukhopadhyay)

- *Ewing sarcoma*: A tumor of neuroectodermal origin
  - *Age*: 1st to 3rd decade (10–20 years)
  - *Site*: Flat bones > long bones
  - These tumors can be mistaken for acute osteomyelitis.
- *Description of a tumor radiographs*:
  - *Tumor location*: Metaphyseal/diaphyseal
  - *Destruction pattern*: Ill defined, permeative, breached cortex, wide zone of transition, heterogeneous matrix
  - *Periosteal reaction*: Present (continuous—lamellated periosteal reaction or *onion peel appearance*, Parallel spiculated type—*hair on end appearance.*)
  - *Soft tissue extension*: Present (massive).
- *Treatment options*:
  - Radiotherapy for local control
  - Chemotherapy for micrometastasis control
  - Wide resection of tumor and limb salvage procedure
  - Amputation of limb.

Chapter 20

Radiographs of Common Infective, Rheumatic and Metabolic Disorders

X-RAY: CHRONIC OSTEOMYELITIS (FIGS. 20.1A AND B)

- *Chronic osteomyelitis*: To ascertain a bone suffering from chronic osteomyelitis; there should be a dead bone surrounded by thick periosteum and fibrosed muscle and subcutaneous tissue.
- *X-ray description*:
  - Cortical thickening
  - Cortical irregularity
  - Cortical sclerosis
  - Obliteration of medullary cavity
  - Sequestrum
  - Involucrum.
- *Treatment principles*:
  - Debridement of necrotic part (sequestrectomy and saucerization)
  - Dealing with dead space by bone graft or bone cement
  - Soft tissue coverage by skin grafting or flap
  - Stabilization of bone by some external fixator if required
  - Antibiotics
  - *Other methodologies are*:
    - Debridement and closed suction irrigation
    - Ilizarov method
    - Excision of bone, e.g. fibula
    - Amputation.

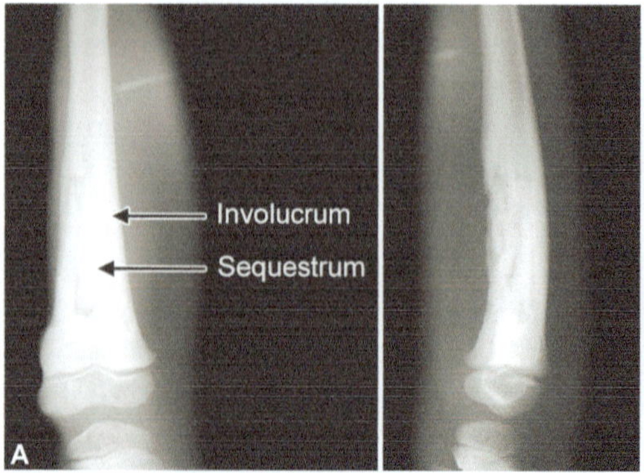

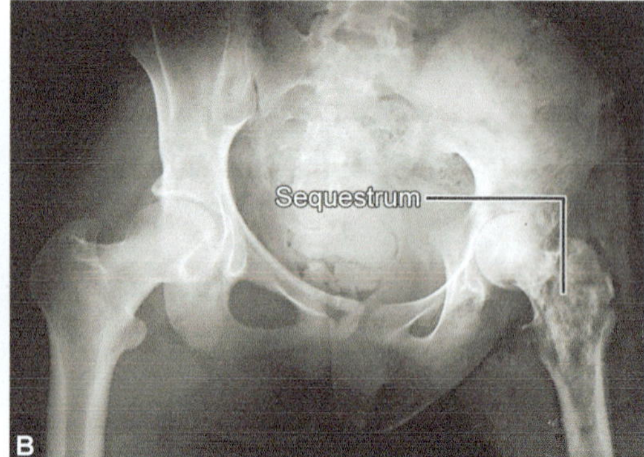

Figs. 20.1A and B: X-ray: Chronic osteomyelitis: A. Distal femur; B. Proximal femur.

(*Courtesy*: Dr John Mukhopadhyay)

X-RAY: OSTEOARTICULAR TUBERCULOSIS (FIGS. 20.2A TO C)

- *Tuberculosis of joints*: Tubercular arthritis is always secondary with primary foci either in lung or lymph node.
- *X-ray description*:
  - **Phemister's triad**
    - Gradual diminution of joint space
    - Juxta-articular osteoporosis
    - Osseous erosion
  - Sequential changes in radiographs as TB advances from synovitis—to arthritis—to erosive stage
    - Increased joint space due to effusion
    - Periarticular osteoporosis
    - Gradual narrowing of joint space
    - Subchondral erosion
    - Joint subluxation and dislocation
    - Fibrous ankylosis in peripheral joint
    - Bony ankylosis in spine
  - Tubercular dactylitis—spina ventosa (air filled small bones)
    - Diaphyseal location
    - Expansile lesion
    - Periosteal reaction rare
    - Cortical sclerosis present in healing phase
- *Treatment principle*:
  - Antitubercular treatment
  - Traction and splintage
  - Incision and drainage
  - Debridement
  - Stabilization of bone.

X-RAY: DEGENERATIVE ARTHRITIS (FIGS. 20.3A TO C)

- *Degenerative arthritis*: A disease of joint cartilage destruction and new bone formation.
- *X-ray description*:
  - *Characteristic radiological feature of degenerative joint*:
    - Narrowing of joint space
    - Subchondral sclerosis
    - Subchondral cyst formation
    - Osteophyte formation (horizontal osteophyte)
    - Loose bodies
    - Collapse of weight-bearing bone
    - Joint subluxation
    - Deformity at joint.
- *Treatment options*:
  - Analgesics (NSAIDs and opioids)
  - Cartilage forming drugs
  - Physiotherapy and habit changes
  - Joint debridement
  - Intra-articular injections (viscosupplement and steroids)
  - Osteotomy, arthrodesis, and arthroplasty.

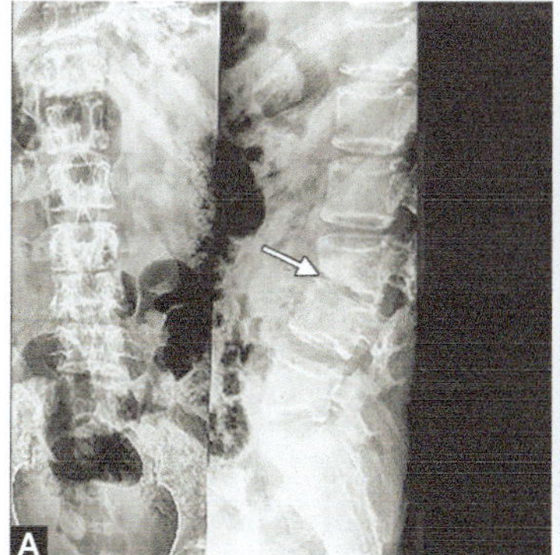

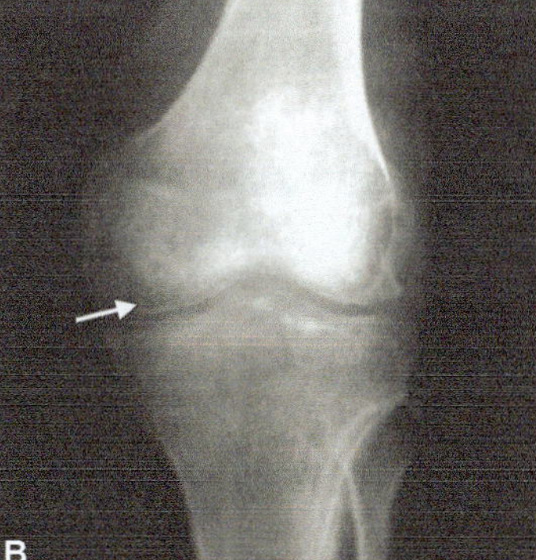

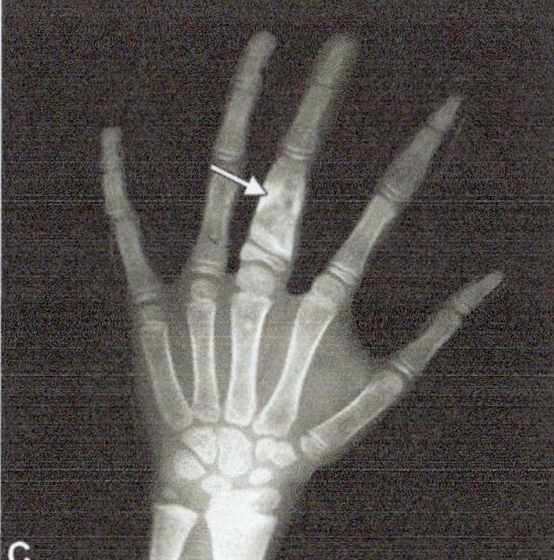

Figs. 20.2A to C: X-ray: Osteoarticular tuberculosis: A. Pott's spine; B. TB knee; C. Spina ventosa.

(*Courtesy*: Dr Shailendra Gupta)

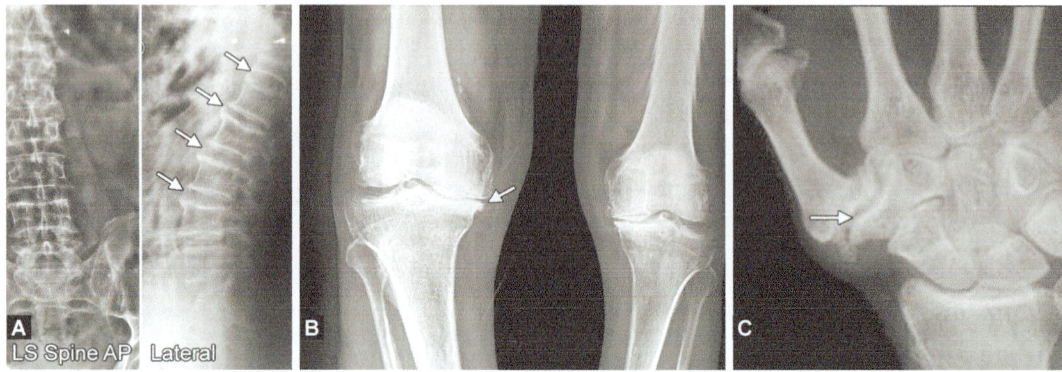

Figs. 20.3A to C: X-ray: Degenerative arthritis: A. Lumbar spondylosis; B. Osteoarthritis knee; C. First carpometacarpal arthritis.

(*Courtesy*: Dr Ajay Rajput)

X-RAY: RHEUMATOID ARTHRITIS (FIGS. 20.4A TO C)

- *Rheumatoid arthritis*: A polyarthralgia of autoimmune etiology primarily involving synovium (pannus formation) and leading to joint destruction. Pannus formation is the inflammatory hyperplasia of synovium under effect of inflammatory mediators.
- *X-ray description*:
  - *Characteristic radiological feature of rheumatoid joint*:
    - Soft tissue swelling—earliest changes
    - Juxta-articular osteoporosis
    - Symmetrical diminution of joint space
    - Marginal erosion—due to pannus formation
    - Subchondral cyst may present
    - Joint subluxation and dislocation
    - Joint deformity
  - *Radiology of rheumatoid hand*:
    - **Swan neck** deformity (flexion at dip joint and hyperextension at pip joint of fingers)
    - **Boutonniere** deformity(extension at dip joint and hyperflexion at pip joint of fingers)

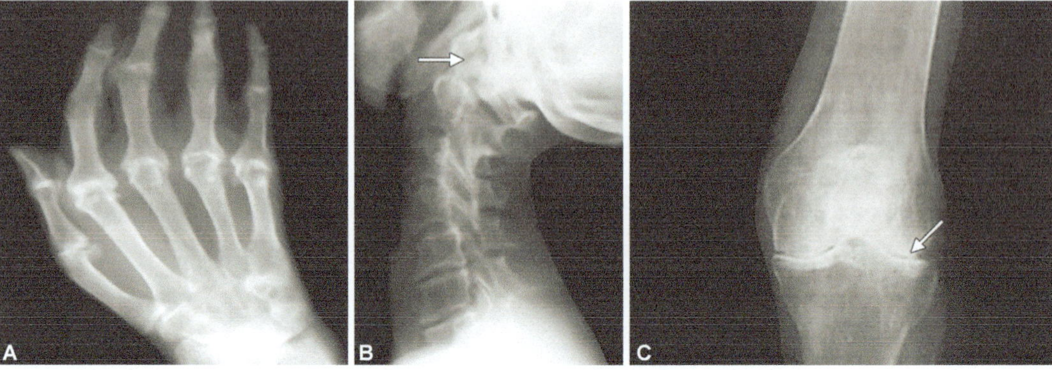

Figs. 20.4A to C: X-ray: Rheumatoid arthritis: A. Rheumatoid hand; B. Rheumatoid upper cervical spine; C. Rheumatoid knee.

(*Courtesy*: Dr Khuswant Rathore)

  - Ulnar deviation of fingers at metacarpophalangeal joint
  - Z-deformity of fingers
  - Hitchhiker's thumb (hyperextension at interphalangeal joint)
  - Ankylosis of small joints
  - Instability of wrist
- In Juvenile rheumatoid arthritis unlike adult, growth retardation along with epiphyseal over growth (prominent condyles) is a main feature.

• *Treatment options*:
  - Analgesics (NSAIDs and opioids)
  - Disease modifying drugs
  - Biologics
  - Physiotherapy and habit change
  - Osteotomy, arthrodesis, and arthroplasty.

X-RAY: ANKYLOSING SPONDYLITIS (FIGS. 20.5A AND B)

• *Ankylosing spondylitis*: A seronegative spondyloarthropathy involving both sacroiliac joints, spine hip, etc. also called **Bechterew's** disease or **Marie-Strumpell** syndrome. Enthesitis, i.e. inflamation of tendon or ligament at bone interface is chief pathology of this disease.
• *X-ray description*:
  - *Characteristic radiological feature of sacroiliac joint*:
    - Blurring of joint margins
    - Erosion
    - Sclerosis
    - Ankylosis.
  - *Characteristic radiological feature in hip and pelvic bone*:
    - Concentric reduction of joint space
    - Osteopenia with changes like erosion, sclerosis, and ankylosis
    - Whiskering—it is radiological appearance for lace like new bone formation at the site of enthesopathies.
  - *Characteristic radiological feature of spine*:
    - Squaring of dorsolumbar vertebrae body (earliest change)
    - *Syndesmophyte formation: Vertical new bone formation)*
    - *Bamboo spine appearance: Due to ossification of anterior and posterior longitudinal ligament, facet joint*
    - *Diffuse osteoporosis*
    - *Pathological fracture with pseudo-arthrosis*
• *Treatment options*:
  - Analgesics (NSAIDs and Opioids)
  - Disease modifying drugs (sulfasalazine) and biologics
  - Physiotherapy and habit change
  - Osteotomy, arthrodesis, and arthroplasty.

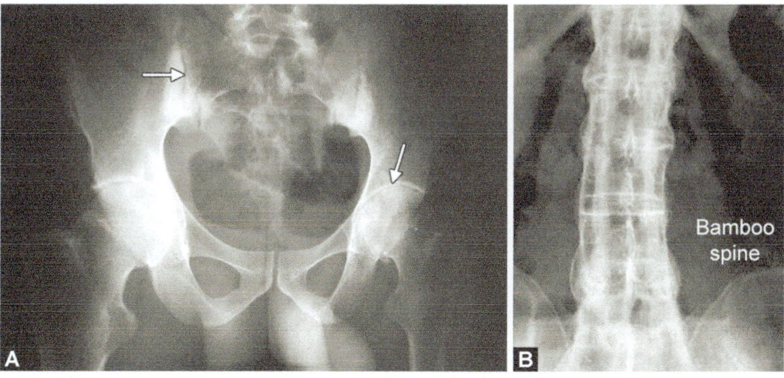

Figs. 20.5A and B: X-ray: Ankylosing spondylitis: A. Hip and sacroiliac joint; B. Bamboo spine.

(*Courtesy*: Dr John Mukhopadhya)

X-RAY: NUTRITIONAL RICKETS (FIGS. 20.6A AND B)

- *Rickets*: Failure of mineralization of osteoid matrix in immature skeleton.
- *X-ray description*:
  - *Common feature*: Generalized rarefaction (*ground glass appearance*).
  - *Skull*:
    - Frontal bossing
    - Craniotabes.
  - *Rib cage*:
    - Pectus carinatum (*pigeon chest*)
    - Rachitic rosary.
  - *Spine:*
    - Kyphoscoliosis
    - Increased lumbar lordosis (*Pott's belly*).
  - *Long bone*:
    - Bowing of bone
    - Changes in end of long bone as cupping, fraying and splaying
    - Deformities like genu valgus, varus, or wind swift deformity (valus at one knee and varus at another).
- *Treatment options*:
  - Drugs (calcium and vitamin D supplement)
  - Sunbath
  - Splintage
  - Epiphysiodesis
  - Osteotomy.

X-RAY: OSTEOMALACIA (FIG. 20.7)

- *Osteomalacia*: Failure of mineralization of osteoid matrix in mature skeleton
- *X-ray description*:
  - *Common feature:* Generalized rarefaction (*ground glass appearance*)
  - *Long bone:* Bowing of shaft
  - *Spine*:
    - Kyphoscoliosis
    - Biconcave vertebrae (*cod fish/fish mouth appearance*)

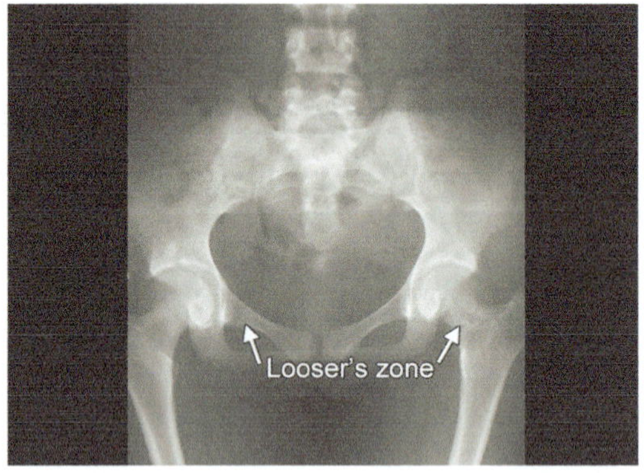

Fig. 20.7: X-ray: Osteomalacia (pelvis).
(*Courtesy*: Dr Nitesh Rustagi)

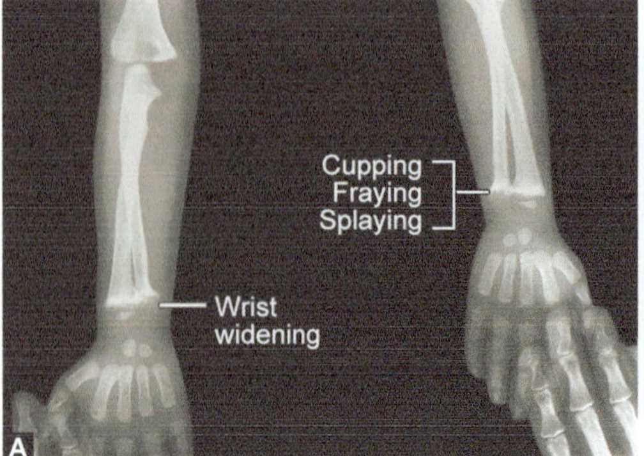

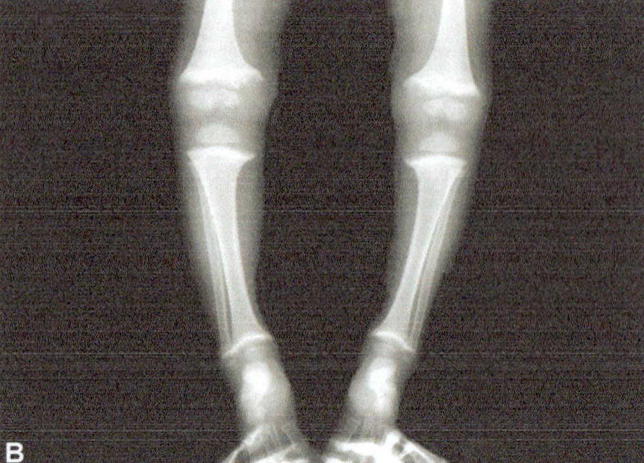

Figs. 20.6A and B: X-ray: Nutritional rickets: A. Wrist; B. Knee and ankle.
(*Courtesy*: Dr Naresh Chandra)

- *Pelvis*:
  - Protrusio acetabuli
  - Trefoil pelvis (*champagne glass pelvis*)
- *Looser's zone*:
  - Pseudofracture or *Milkman's fracture*
  - *Common sites are*: Ribs, scapula, pubic rami, ischium, and neck of femur
  - *Characteristic of Looser's zone are*:
    - Incomplete and transverse fracture
    - Oftenly bilaterally symmetrical
    - Healing by inappropriate callus formation
- *Treatment options*:
  - Calcium and vitamin D supplementation
  - Dealing with complication.

X-RAY: OSTEOPOROSIS (FIG. 20.8)

- *Osteoporosis*: Deficient bone matrix with normal mineralization.
- *X-ray description*:
  - *Common feature*: Generalized rarefaction (*ground glass appearance*)
  - *Long bone*:
    - Pencil thin cortex
    - Pathological fracture
  - *Spine*:
    - Kyphoscoliosis
    - Vertical compression of vertebrae
    - Anterior wedge compression of vertebrae
    - Biconcave vertebrae (*Typical cod fish/fish mouth appearance*).
- *Treatment options*:
  - Calcium and vitamin D supplementation
  - Bisphosphonates
  - Calcitonin
  - Hormone replacement therapy
  - Bracing
  - Dealing with complication
  - Physiotherapy and habit change.

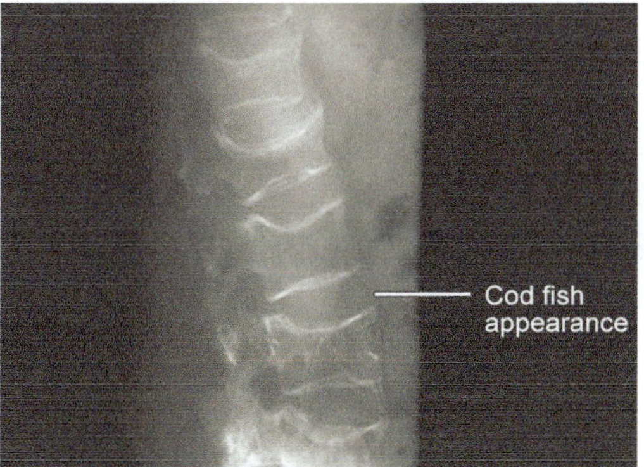

Fig. 20.8: X-ray: Osteoporosis (spine).

X-RAY: SCURVY (FIG. 20.9)

- *Scurvy*: Occur due to dietary deficiency of vitamin C, also called Barlow's disease. The combined deficiency of vitamin C and D is called **Barton's** disease.
- *X-ray description*:
  - *Common feature*: Generalized rarefaction (common in adult)
  - *Long bones*:
    - Pencil thin cortex (common in adult)
    - Periosteal reaction following subperiosteal hemorrhage.

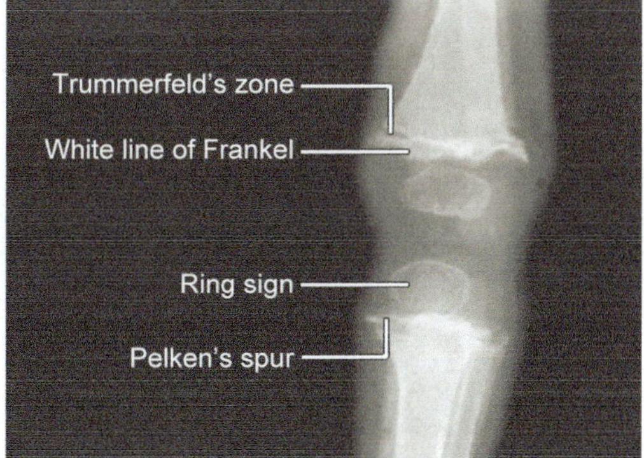

Fig. 20.9: X-ray: Scurvy (knee).

(*Courtesy*: Dr Nitesh Rustagi)

- *Chest X-ray*: Scorbutic rosary
- *Periarticular changes*:
  - *Ring sign of* ***Wimberger***: A radiodense area around epiphyseal ossification center
  - *White line of* ***Frankel***: A dense and wide zone of provisional calcification
  - *Zone of* ***Trummerfeld***: A radiolucent area adjacent to Frankel line
  - ***Pelken spur***: Metaphyseal corner formed due to splaying.
- *Treatment options*:
  - Analgesics (NSAIDs and opioids)
  - Vitamin C supplementation
  - Vitamin C rich diet.

X-RAY: LOOSE BODIES OF KNEE (FIG. 20.10)

- *Loose bodies of knee*: Loose bodies are small fragments of varying size (mm to cm) freely moving in the joint space. They can restrict the motion of joint and produces a special feeling of crepitations. These moving bodies are harmful for joint cartilage and arthritis may ensue.
- *X-ray description*:
  - Multiple radio-opaque flakes scattered around knee joint
  - Radiological feature underlying disease as osteoarthritis knee, osteochondritis dissecans, etc.

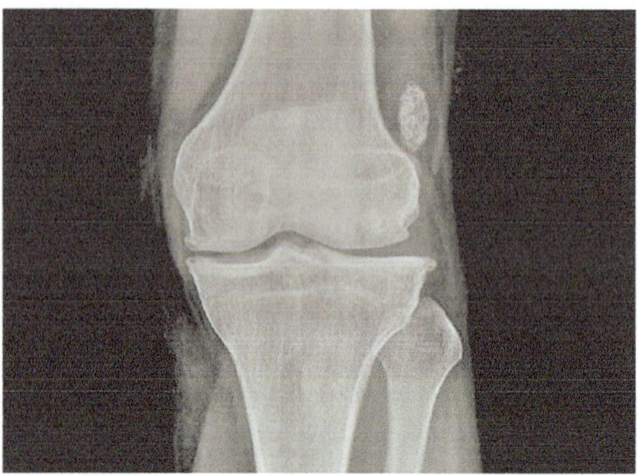

Fig. 20.10: X-ray: Loose body in knee joint.
(*Courtesy*: Dr Deepak Kumar, Patna)

Etiological classification for loose bodies.
Traumatic: Cartilaginous fragment, osteochondral fragment
Infective: Tuberculous (fibrinous)
Degenerative: OA knee (osteochondral)
Inflammatory disease: RA (osteochondral)
Ischemic: Osteochondritis dissecans of knee (osteochondral) most common
Metaplastic: Synovial chondromatosis (cartilaginous)
Neuropathic: Charcot joints (osteocartilaginous)

- *Treatment options*:
  - Analgesics and physiotherapy
  - Open arthrotomy and removal of loose bodies
  - Arthroscopic removal of loose bodies
  - Treatment of underlying cause.

5

Section

Bones Catalogue

Bones Catalogue

1. CLAVICLE

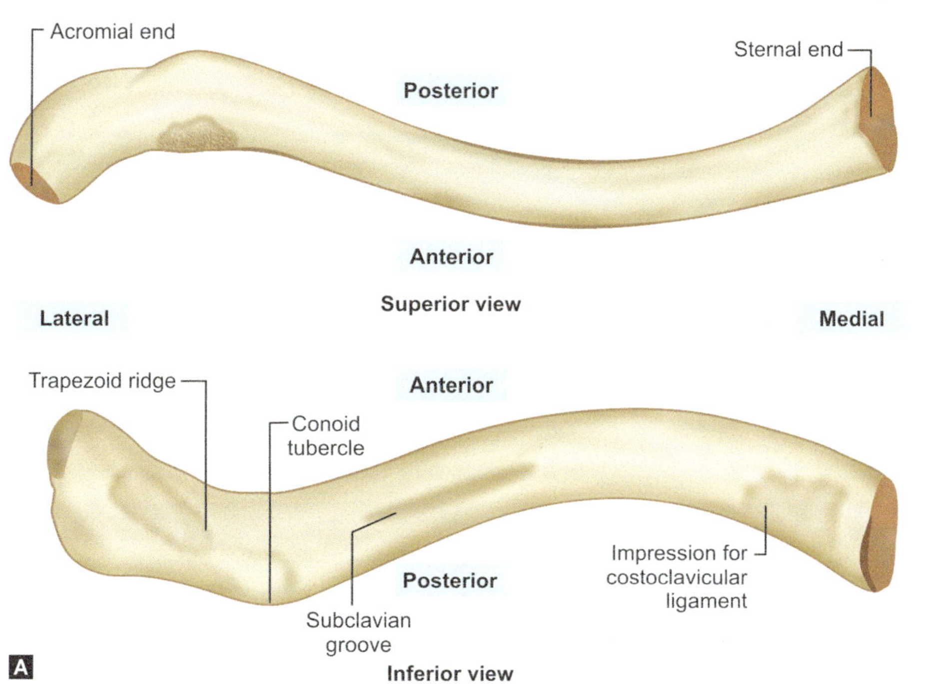

Fig. 1A: Morphology of clavicle.

(*Courtesy*: Inderbir Singh's Textbook of Human Anatomy)

Box 1: Points of orthopedic significance regarding clavicle

- Only long bone that lies horizontally.
- Subcutaneous throughout.
- First bone to start ossifying (but last to fuse).
- Only long bone with membranous ossification.
- Only long bone with two primary centers of ossification.
- Generally said to have no medullary cavity, not always true.
- Occasionally pierced by middle supraclavicular nerve.
- Only long bone connecting the axial to appendicular skeleton with skull n spine via sternocleidomastoid and trapezius and with rib cage via pectoralis major and subclavius.

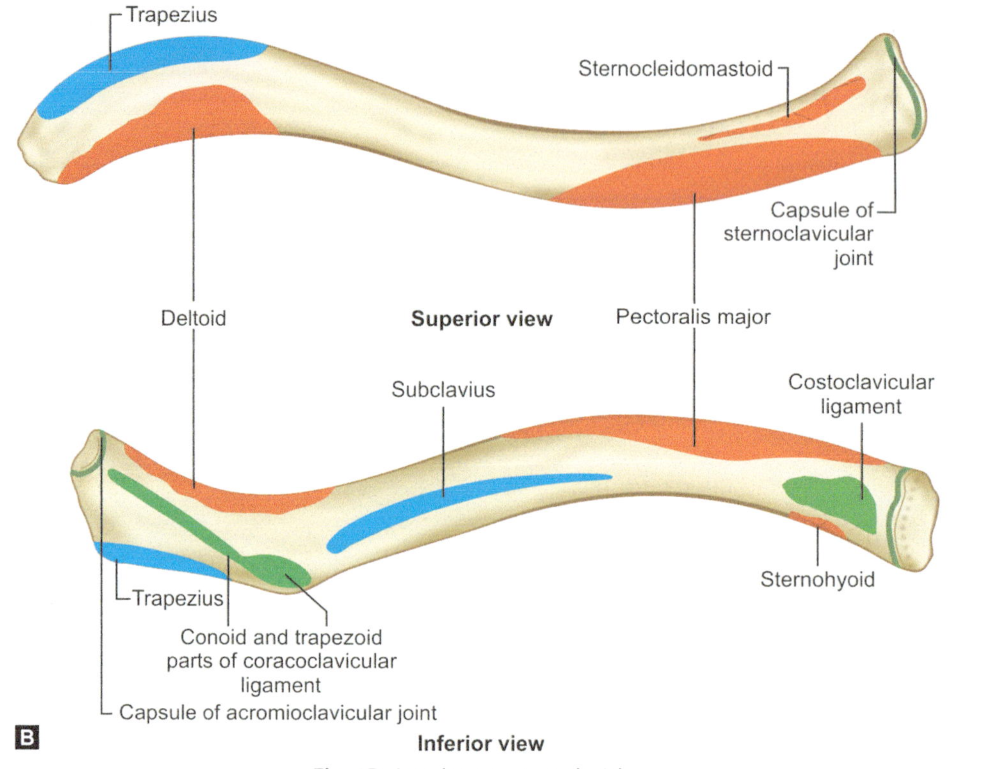

Fig. 1B: Attachments over clavicle.

(*Courtesy*: Inderbir Singh's Textbook of Human Anatomy)

2. SCAPULA

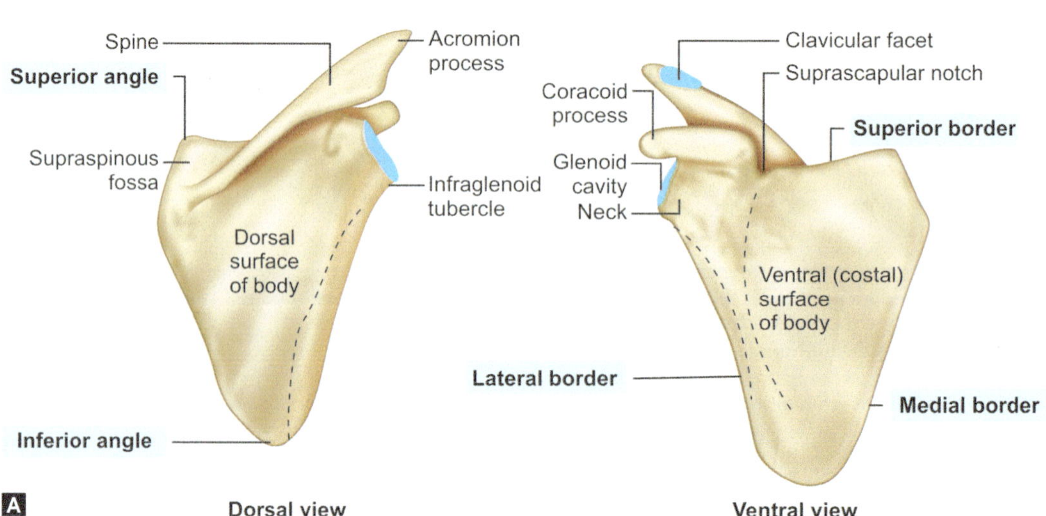

Fig. 2A: Morphology of scapula.

(*Courtesy:* Inderbir Singh's Textbook of Human Anatomy)

Box 2: Points of orthopedic significance regarding scapula

- *Suprascapular notch:*
  - Covered by transverse suprascapular ligament.
  - Suprascapular vessels run above this ligament.
  - Suprascapular nerve passes below this ligament.
- *Spinoglenoid notch:*
  - Covered by spinoglenoid ligament.
  - Suprascapular nerves and vessels pass through it.
  - Its compression leads to suprascapular impingement syndrome.
- With scapula is attached with spine by Levator scapulae, Rhomboidus, Latissimus dorsi and Trapezius.
- With scapula is attached with rib cage by Pectoralis minor

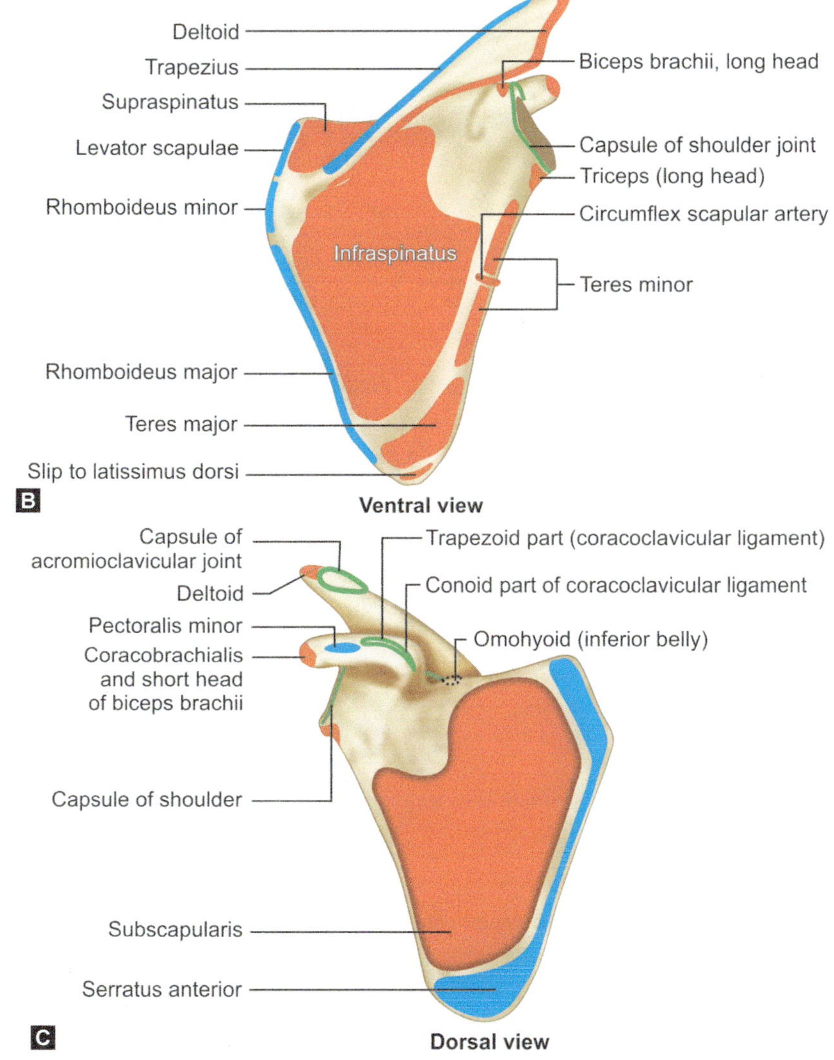

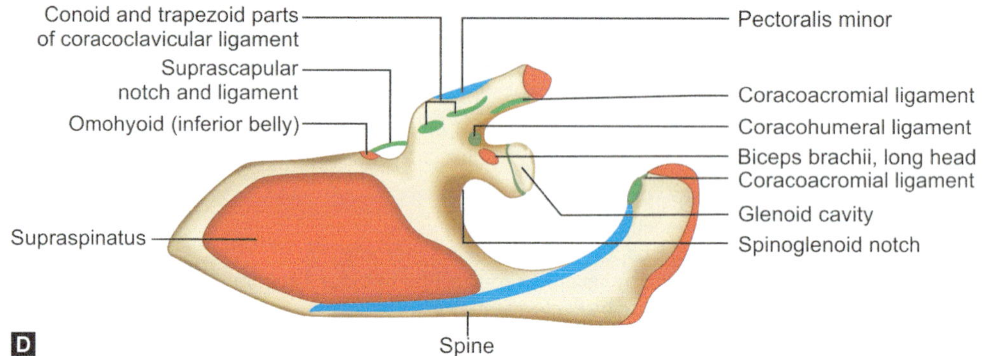

Figs. 2B to D: Attachments over scapula.

(*Courtesy*: Inderbir Singh's Textbook of Human Anatomy)

3. HUMERUS

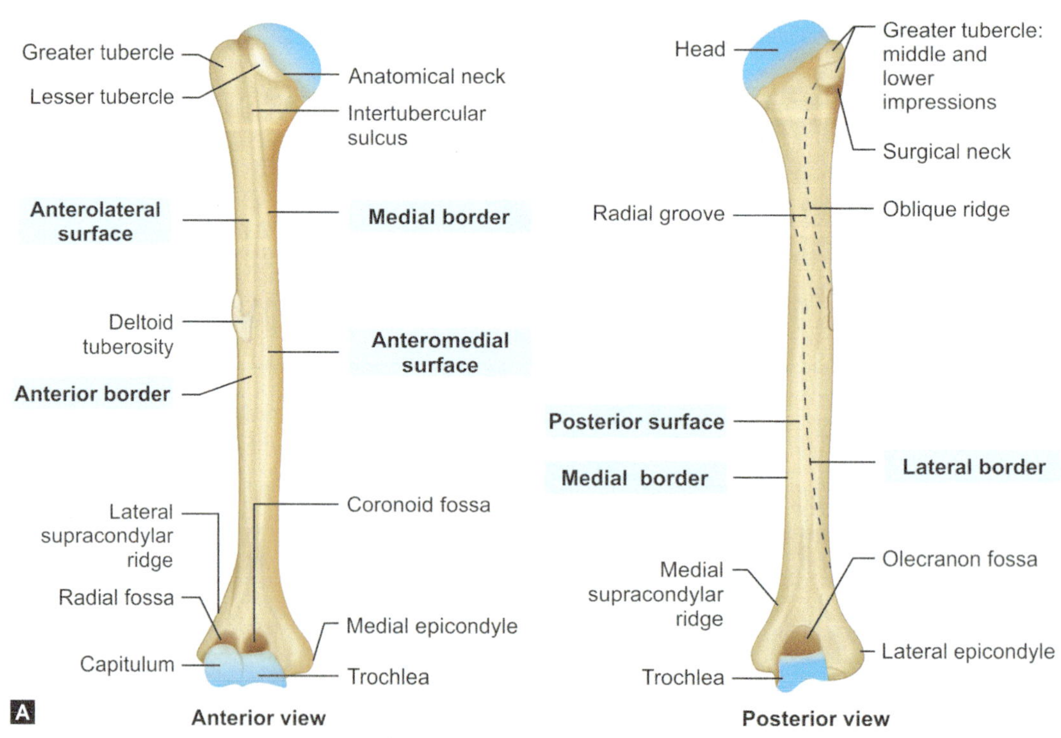

Fig. 3A: Morphology of humerus.

(*Courtesy*: Inderbir Singh's Textbook of Human Anatomy)

Box 3: Points of orthopedic significance regarding humerus

- *Angle of retroversion of head of humerus:* 20°–40° (average 30°).
- *Humeral head shaft angle:* 135°.
- *Surgical neck:* It connects diaphysis with proximal humerus, related to axillary nerve.
- *Anatomical neck:* It is boundary line between articular surface of head and rest of proximal humerus. It corresponds to synovial attachment.
- *Content of bicipital groove:* Long head of bicep brachii and ascending branch of anterior circumflex humeral artery.
- *Content of radial groove:* Radial nerve and profundabrachii vessels.
- *Content of ulnar groove:* Ulnar nerve.
- *Trochlear edges:* The medial edge of trochlea projects down 6 mm more than lateral edge.
- *Blood supply of head of humerus -by third part of axillary artery:-ant and post circumflex humeral artery.*

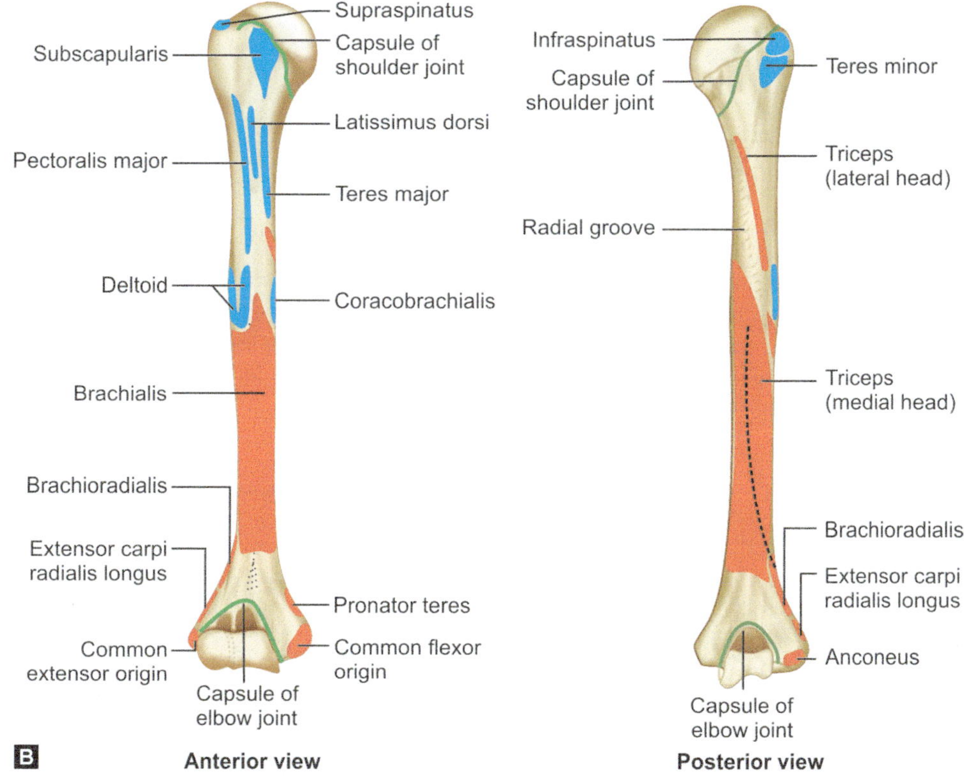

Fig. 3B: Attachments over humerus.

(*Courtesy*: Inderbir Singh's Textbook of Human Anatomy)

Box 4: Compartment of arm

- *Flexor compartment:*
  - Biceps-brachii
  - Brachialis
  - Coracobrachiolis—sometimes called medial compartment muscle.
- *Extensor compartment:*
  - Triceps—long head
  - Triceps—lateral head
  - Triceps—medial head..

4. RADIUS AND ULNA

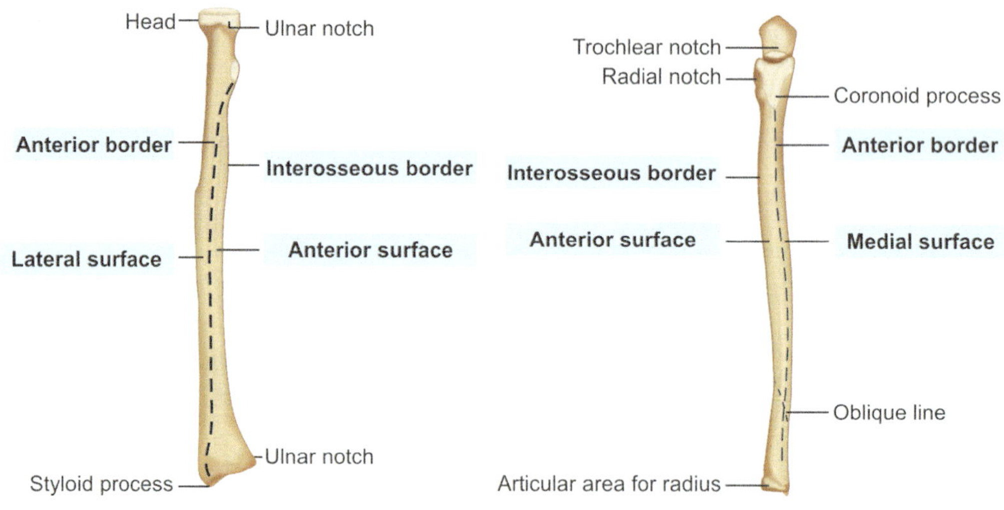

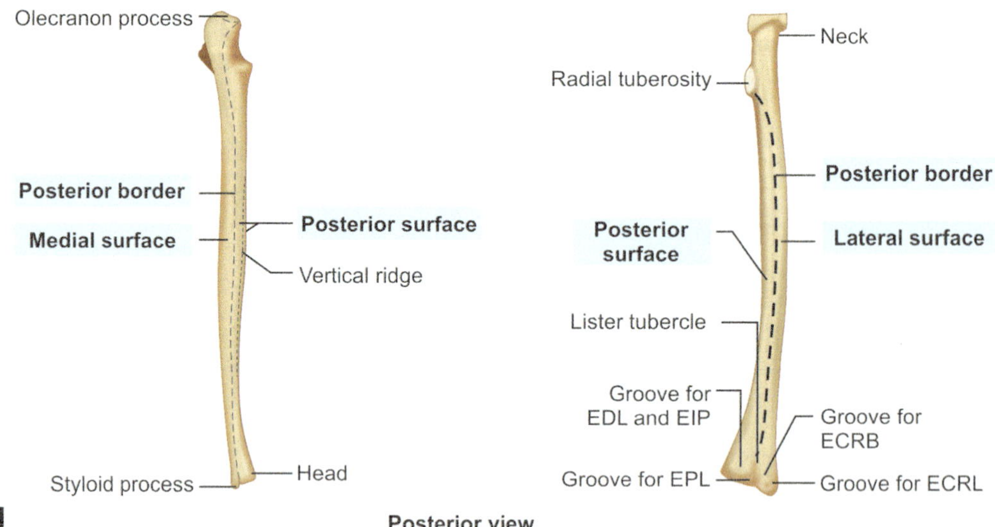

Fig. 4A: Morphology of radius and ulna.

(*Courtesy*: Inderbir Singh's Textbook of Human Anatomy)

Abbreviations: ECRB, extensor carpi radialis brevis; ECRL, extensor carpi radialis longus; EDL, extensor digitorum longus; EIP, extensor indicis proprius; EPL, extensor pollicis longus

Box 5: Points of orthopedic significance regarding radius and ulna

- *Radial neck correlation:* Posterior interosseous nerve run around neck of radius.
- *Lister tubercle:* EPL (extensor policislongus) tendon lies medial to lister tubercle.
- *Content of dorsal compartment of wrist* (6 compartment): (I) Abductor pollicislongus and extensor pollicisbrevis, (II) Extensor carpi radialislongus and extensor carpi radialis brevis. (III) Extensor pollicis longus. (IV) Extensor digitorum communis, extensor indici sproprius, posterior interosseous nerve and anterior interosseous artery. (V) Extensor digiti minimi. (VI) Extensor carpi ulnaris.

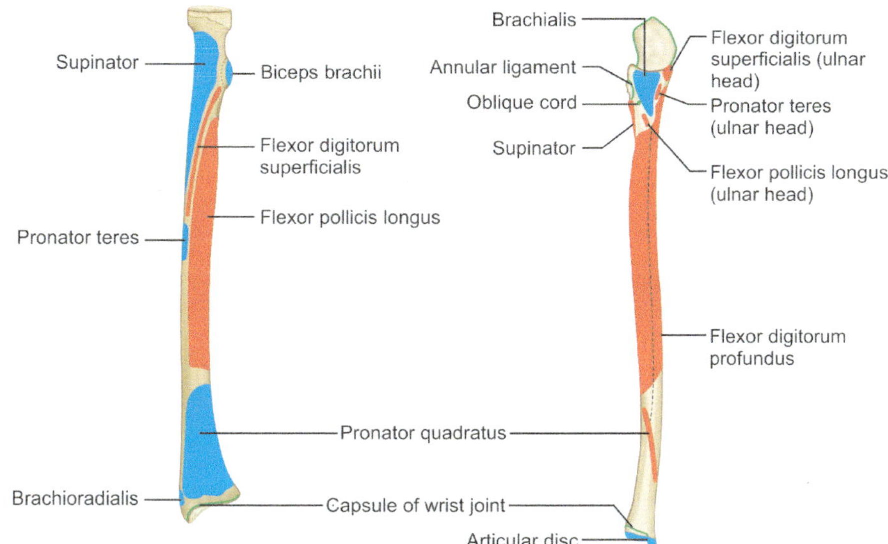

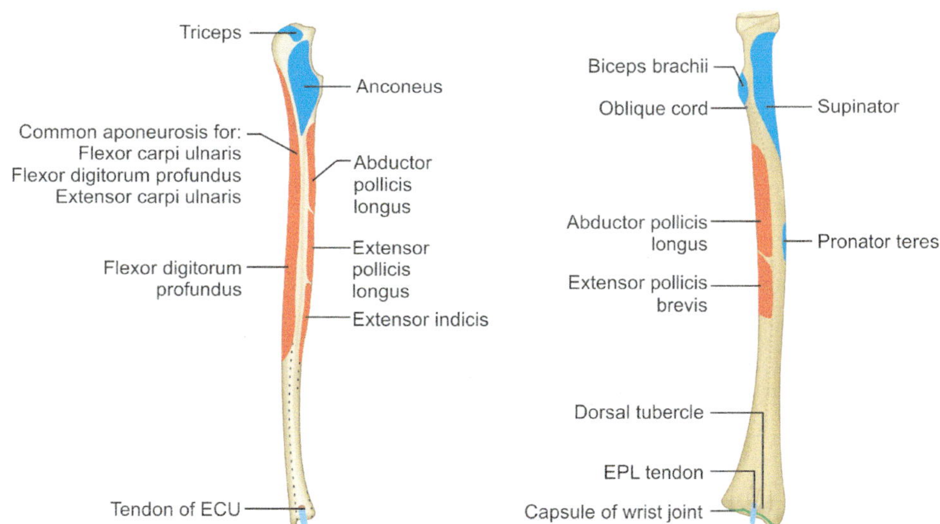

Fig. 4B: Attachments over radius and ulna.

(*Courtesy*: Inderbir Singh's Textbook of Human Anatomy)

Abbreviations: ECU, extensor carpi ulnaris; EPL, extensor pollicis longus

Box 6: Compartment of forearm

• *Flexor compartment:* Five superficial muscles	• *Flexor compartment:* Three deep muscles	• *Extensor compartment:* Seven superficial muscles	• *Extensor compartment:* Five deep muscles
1. Pronator teres 2. Flexor carpi radialis 3. Palmaris longus 4. Flexor carpi ulnaris 5. Flexor digitorum-superficialis	1. Flexor digitorum profundus 2. Flexor pollicis longus 3. Pronator quadratus	1. Anconeus 2. Brachioradialis 3. Extensor carpi radialis longus 4. Extensor carpi radialisbrevis 5. Extensor digitorum (communis) 6. Extensor digiti minimi 7. Extensor carpi ulnaris.	1. Supinator 2. Abductor pollicislongus 3. Extensor pollicisbrevis 4. Extensor pollicislongus 5. Extensor indicis (proprius)

5. PELVIC BONE

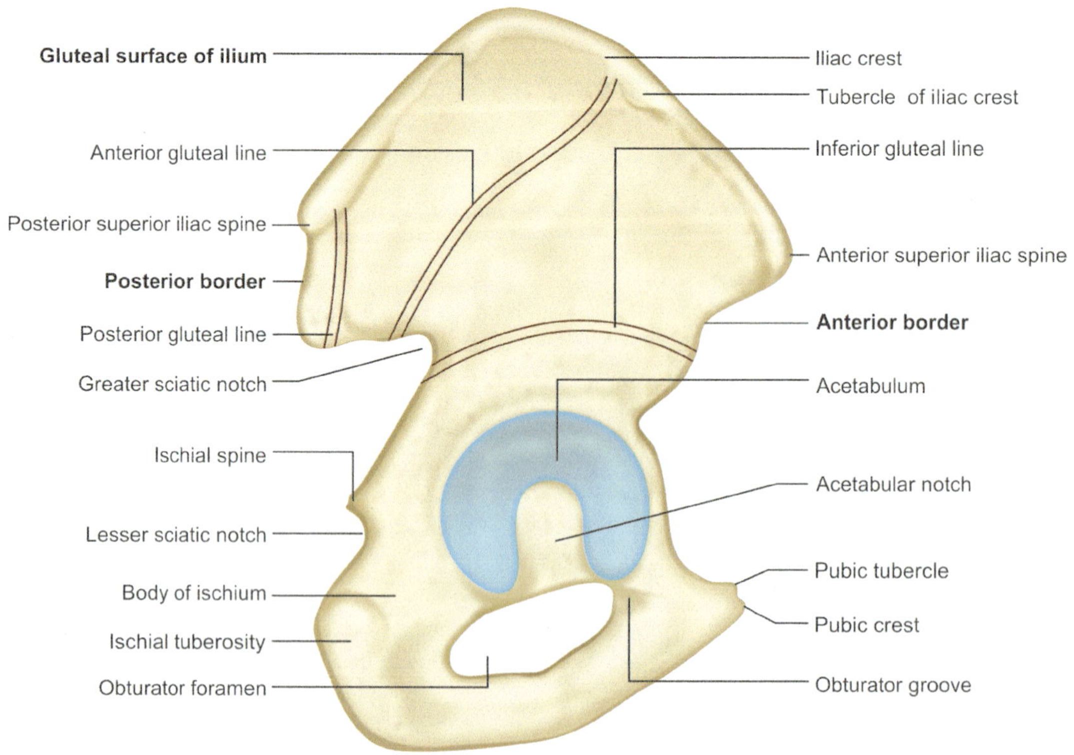

Fig. 5A: Morphology of pelvic bone.

(*Courtesy*: Inderbir Singh's Textbook of Human Anatomy)

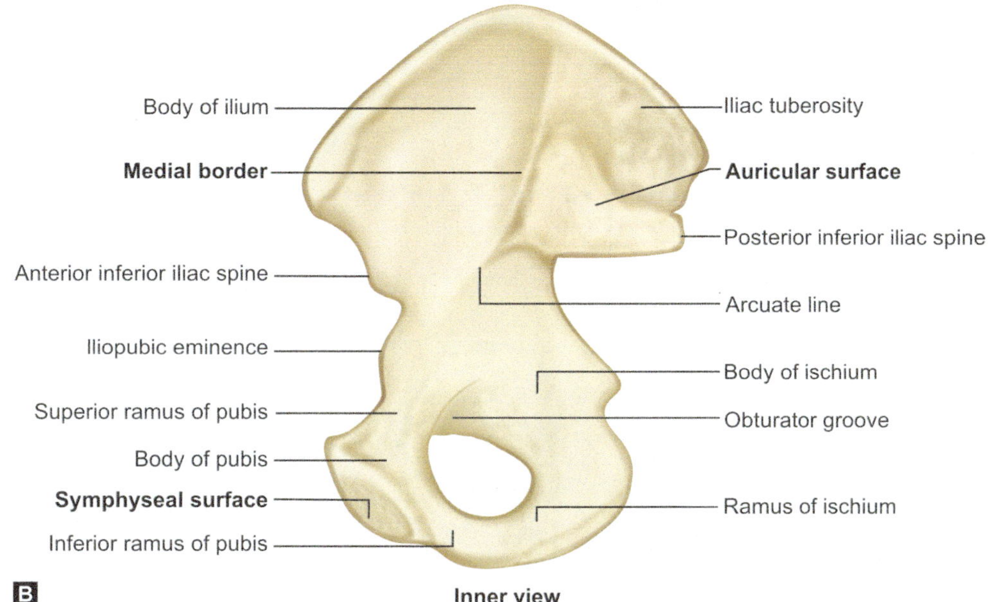

Fig. 5B: Morphology of pelvic bone.

(*Courtesy*: Inderbir Singh's Textbook of Human Anatomy)

Box 7: Points of orthopedic significance regarding pelvic bone

- *It is a irregular bone which developed by fusion of 3 separate bone as ilium, ischium and pubis in acetabulum.*
- *Sacrosoinous ligament convert greater sciatic notch into greater sciatic foramen.*
- Piriformis muscle bisects greater sciatic foramen into two parts.
- *Sacrotuberus and sacrosoinous ligament convert lesser sciatic notch into lesser sciatic foramen.*
- *Larger gluteal muscles are:* Gluteus maximus, gluteus medius and gluteus minimus.
- *Smaller gluteal muscles:* Piriformis, quadratus femoris, gemelli superior, gemelli inferior, obturator internus, obturator externus

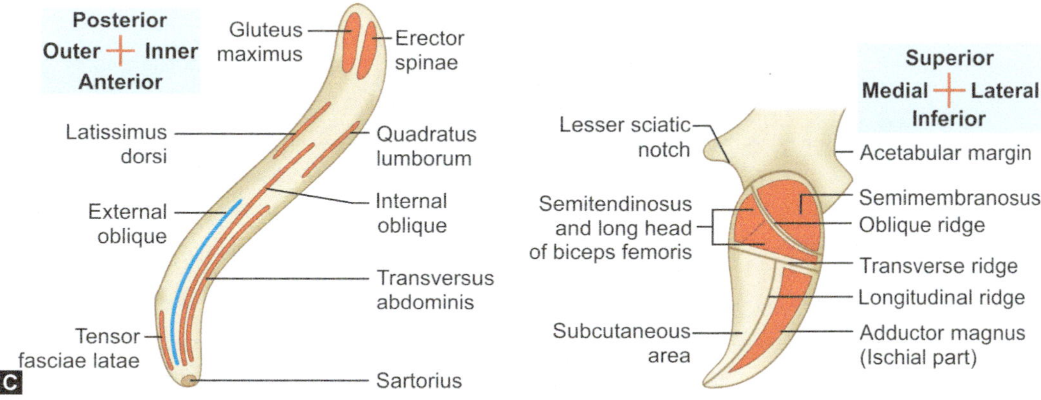

Fig. 5C: Attachments over pelvic bone (iliac crest and ischial tuberosity).

(*Courtesy*: Inderbir Singh's Textbook of Human Anatomy)

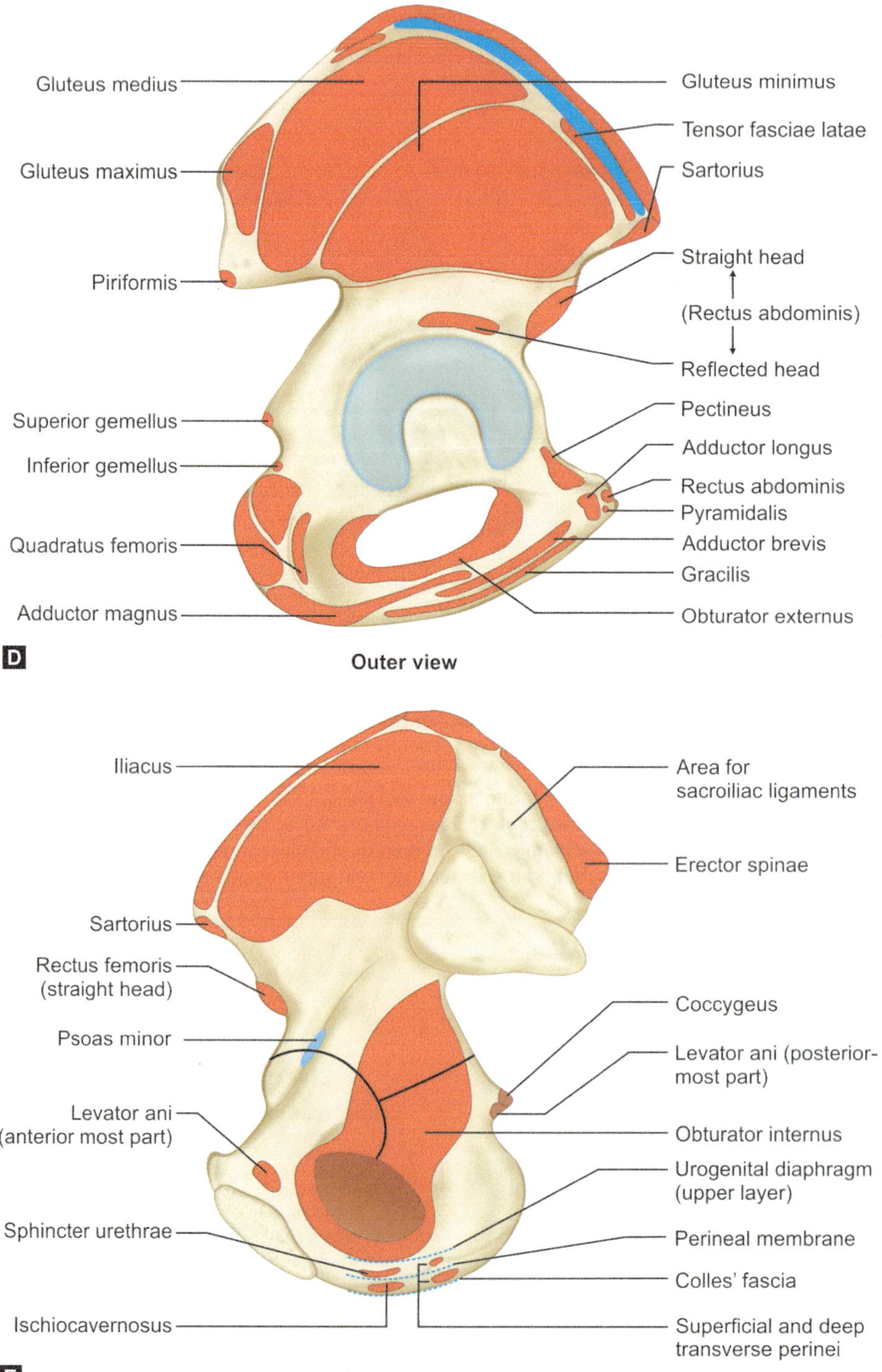

Figs. 5D and E: Attachments over pelvic bone.

(*Courtesy*: Inderbir Singh's Textbook of Human Anatomy)

6. FEMUR

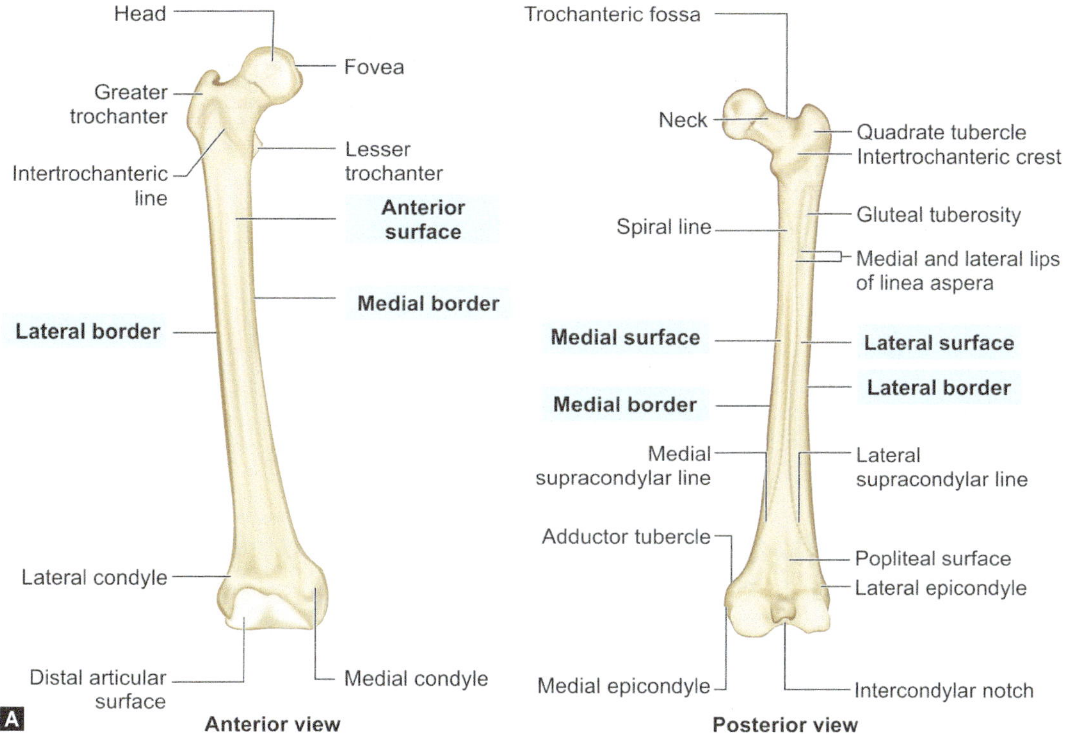

Fig. 6A: Morphology of femur.

(*Courtesy*: Inderbir Singh's Textbook of Human Anatomy)

Box 8: Points of orthopedic significance regarding femur

- *Angle of anteversion of femoral neck:*
  - At birth—40°
  - At age of 16 years settle at 15°.
- Femoral neck shaft angle—average 125°
- *Illiotibial band:*
  - Its two components are gluteus maximus and tensor fascia lata or femoris.
  - It is knee stabilizer in extension and partial flexion.
- *Blood supply of head of femur :*
  I. Retinacular vessels
  II. Artery to ligamentum teres.
  iii. Medullary supply

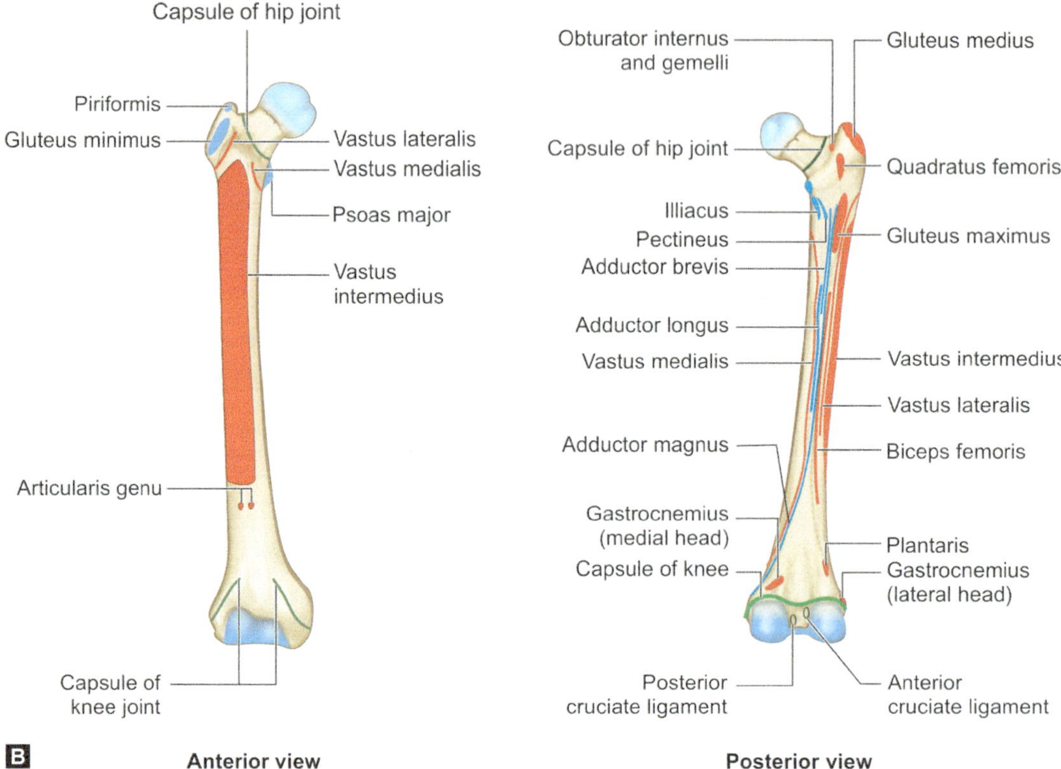

Fig. 6B: Attachments over femur.

(*Courtesy*: Inderbir Singh's Textbook of Human Anatomy)

Box 9: Compartment of thigh

- *Anterior compartment:*
  - Sartorius
  - Quadriceps femoris—rectus femoris, vastus lateralis, vastus medialis, vastus intermedius
- *Posterior compartment:*
  - Semitendinosus
  - Semimembranosus
  - Biceps femoris
  - Hamstring part of adductor magnus.
- *medial compartment:*
  - Adductor longus
  - Adductor brevis
  - Adductor magnus—only adductor part
  - Gracilis
  - Pectineus.

7. PATELLA

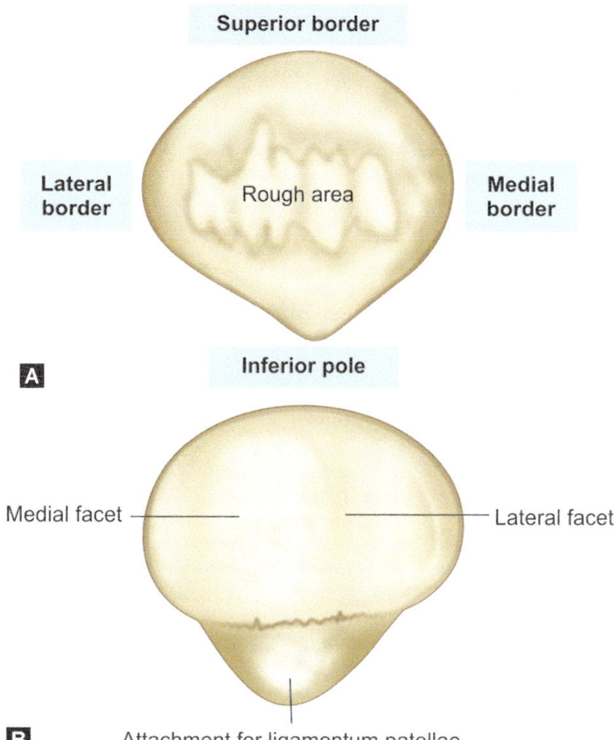

Fig. 7A and B: Anterior and posterior surface of patella.

(*Courtesy*: Inderbir Singh's Textbook of Human Anatomy)

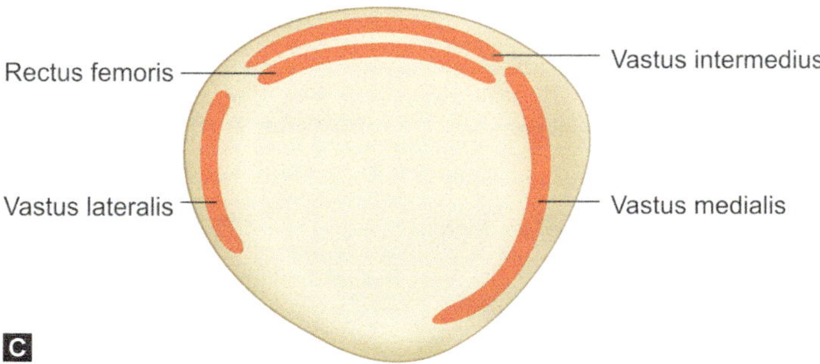

Fig. 7C: Muscle attachments on patella.

(*Courtesy*: Inderbir Singh's Textbook of Human Anatomy)

Box 10: Points of orthopedic significance regarding patella

- Largest sesamoid bone developed under tendon of quadriceps.
- Improves the lever action of quadriceps.
- *Extensor apparatus around patella is formed by:* i. Quadriceps femoris muscle ii. Ligamentum patellae iii. Medial retinaculum iv. Lateral retinaculum.

8. TIBIA AND FIBULA

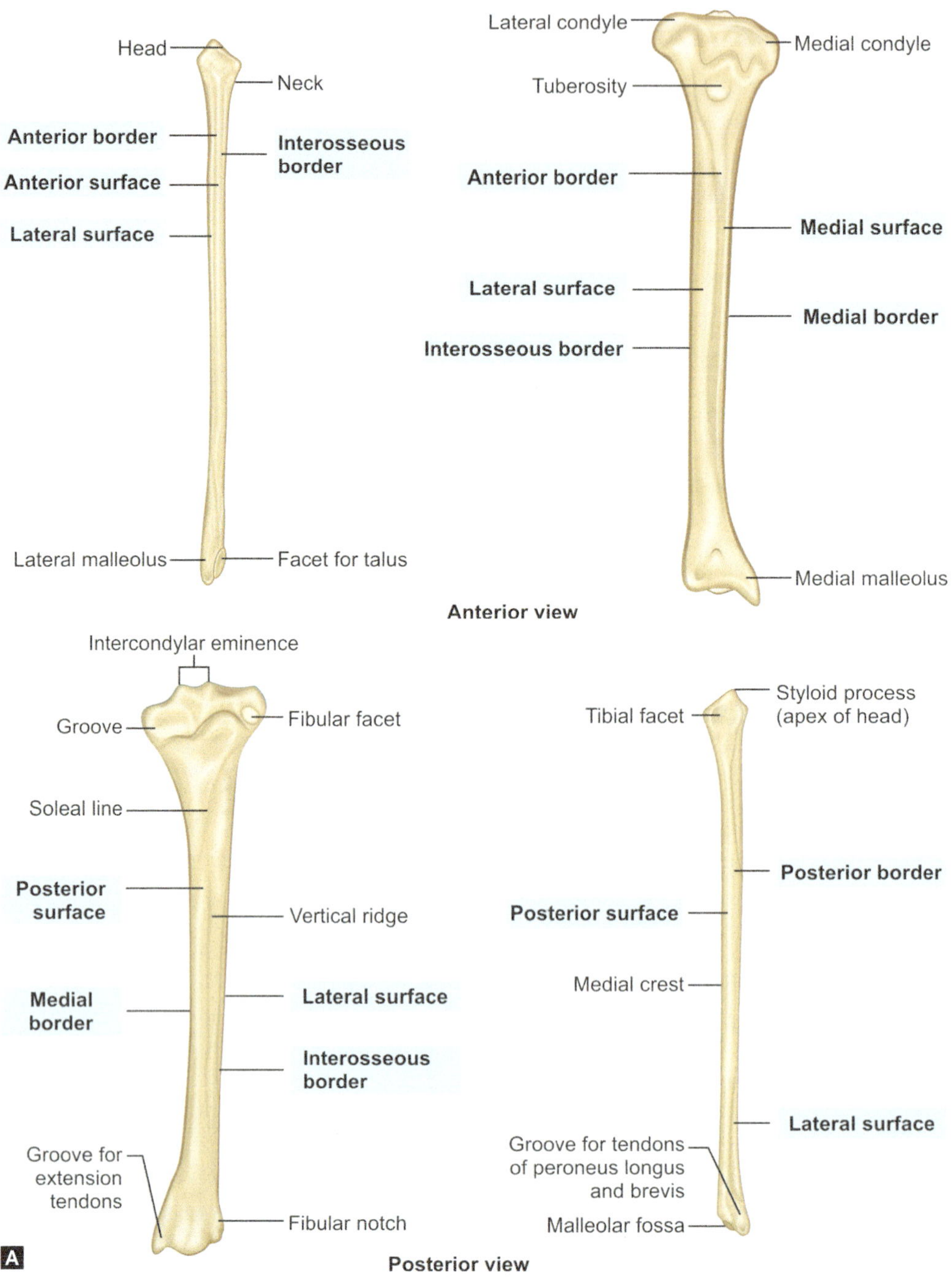

Fig. 8A: Morphology of tibia and fibula.

(*Courtesy*: Inderbir Singh's Textbook of Human Anatomy)

Box 11: Points of orthopedic significance regarding tibia and fibula

- *Guy ropes:*
  - It is formed by three muscle tendons originating from all three parts of pelvic bone (ilium, ischium, pubis) that holds the pelvis like rope of tent.
  - They represent the all three compartment of thigh.
  - They represent their separate nerve supply.
  - The muscles are as sartorius, gracillis, semitendinosus.
- *Anserine bursae:* There is a bursae around insertion of tendons of guy ropes called anserine bursae.

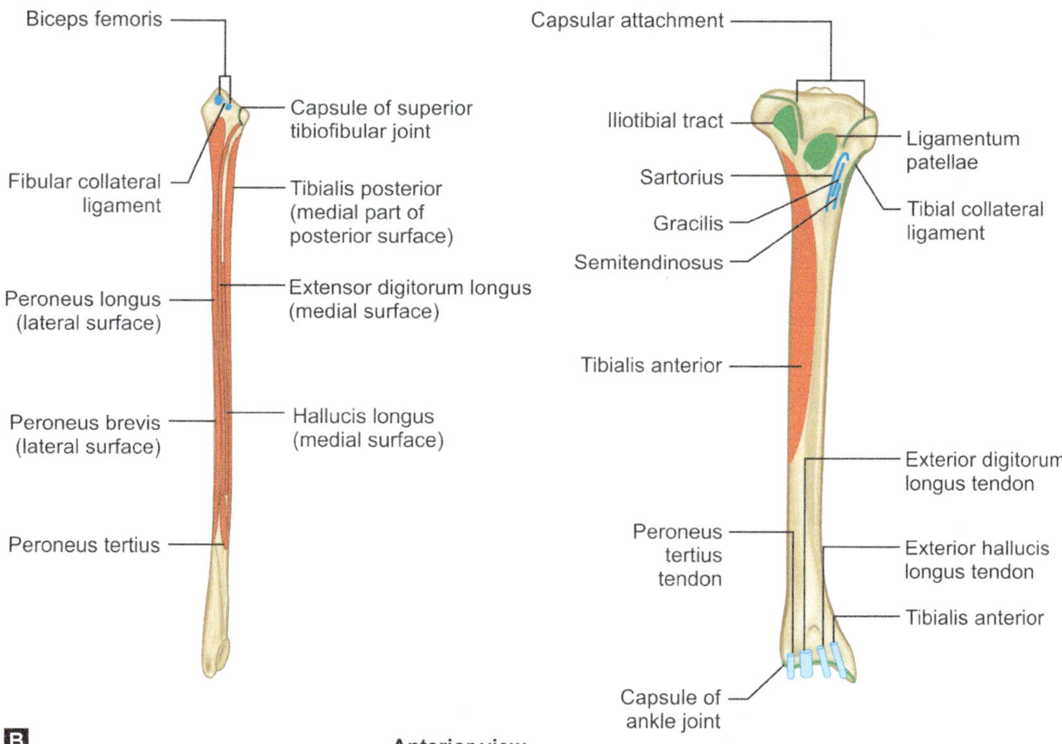

Fig. 8B: Attachments over tibia.

(*Courtesy*: Inderbir Singh's Textbook of Human Anatomy)

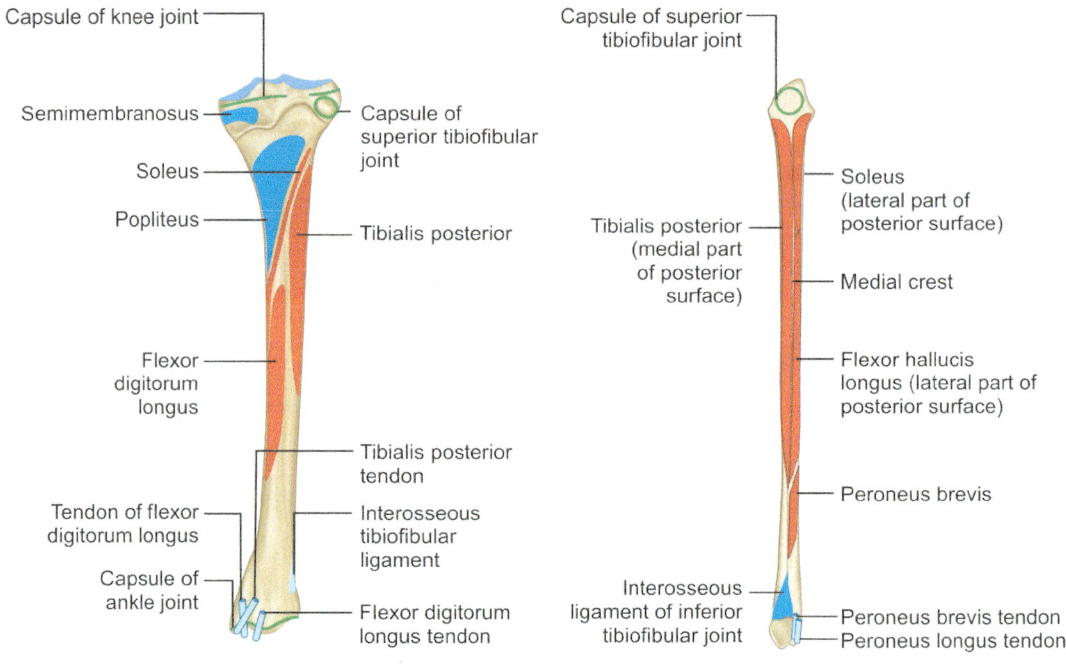

Fig. 8C: Attachments over fibula.

(*Courtesy*: Inderbir Singh's Textbook of Human Anatomy)

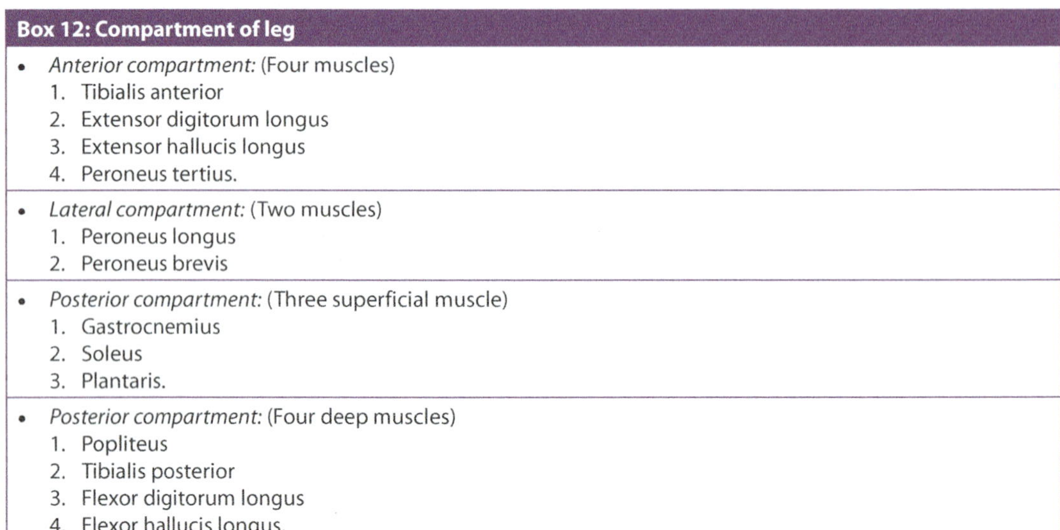

Box 12: Compartment of leg

- *Anterior compartment:* (Four muscles)
  1. Tibialis anterior
  2. Extensor digitorum longus
  3. Extensor hallucis longus
  4. Peroneus tertius.
- *Lateral compartment:* (Two muscles)
  1. Peroneus longus
  2. Peroneus brevis
- *Posterior compartment:* (Three superficial muscle)
  1. Gastrocnemius
  2. Soleus
  3. Plantaris.
- *Posterior compartment:* (Four deep muscles)
  1. Popliteus
  2. Tibialis posterior
  3. Flexor digitorum longus
  4. Flexor hallucis longus.

9. TYPICAL SPINE

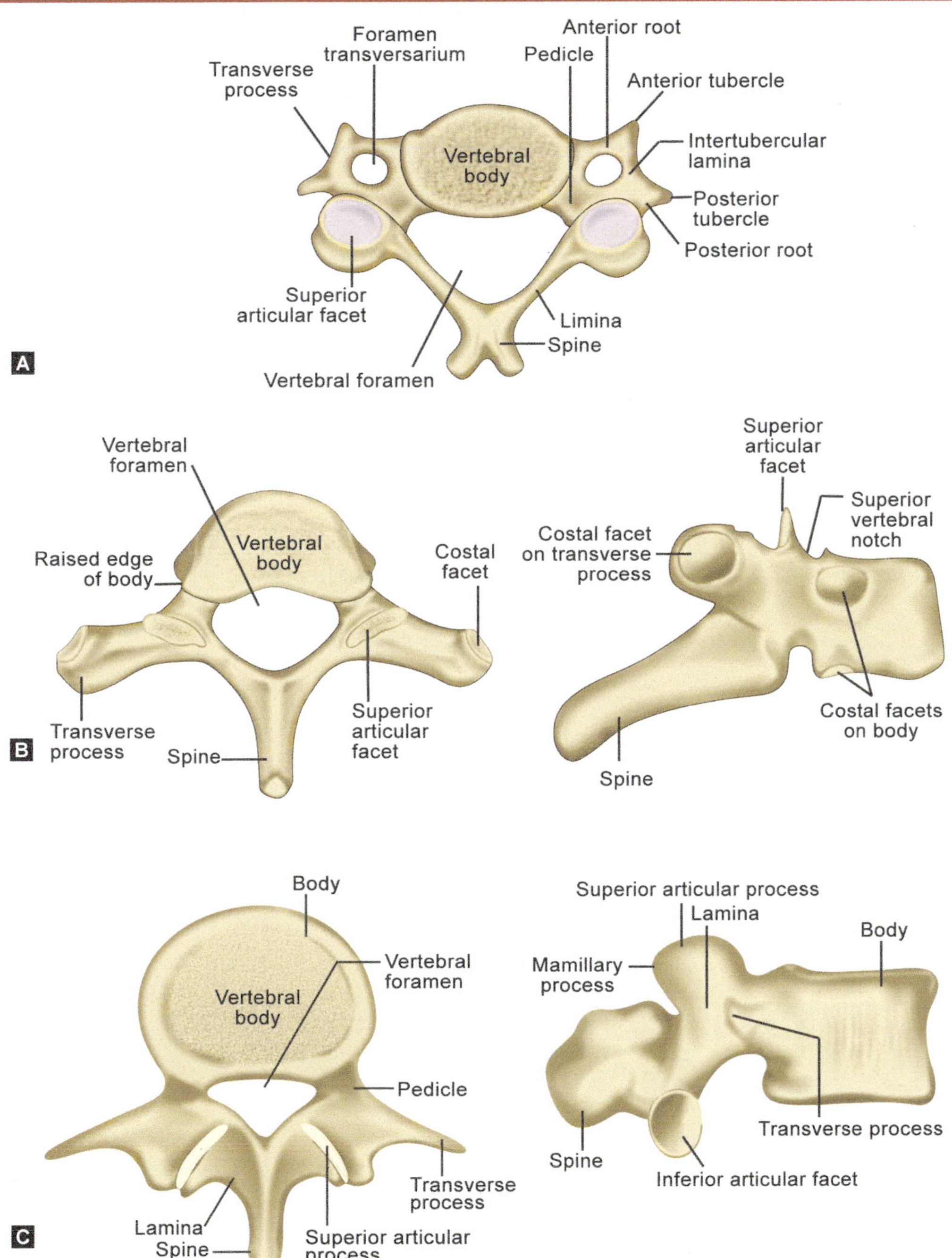

Figs. 9A to C: Typical spine: A. Typical cervical spine; B. Typical dorsal spine; C. Typical lumbar spine.

(*Courtesy*: Inderbir Singh's Textbook of Human Anatomy)

Box 13: Points of orthopedic significance regarding typical spine			
Comparison of cervical, thoracic and lumbar vertebrae			
Points	*Cervical*	*Thoracic*	*Lumbar*
Shape of body	Quadrangular	Heart shaped	Kidney shaped
Spinous-process	Bifid	Long and pointed	Short, blunt and broad
Articular facets	Almost horizontal	Coronal plane lie	Sagittal plane lie
Transverse process: • Costal element • Transverse element	 Anterior tubercle Posterior tubercle	 Ribs Transverse process proper	 Transverse process proper Accessory process
Others	Foramen transversarium for vertebral artery	Costal facets on vertebral body and transverse process	Mammillary body–a tubercle over posterior aspect of superior facet

Bibliography

1. AO/ASIF Instruments and Implants. Texhammar, Rigmor, Colton, Christopher.
2. Essentials of Prosthetics and Orthotics. AK Agarwal.
3. Inderbir Singh's Textbook of Anatomy. (Eds). Sudha Seshayyan.
4. Inderbir Singh's Textbook of Human Histology. (Eds). Neelam Vasudeva, Sabita Mishra.
5. Interpreting Orthopaedic Radiographs. Gemma Phillips.
6. Orthopedic Immobilization Techniques-Samuel A Brown, Frank Radja.
7. Orthopedic Radiography, Darryl Biery.
8. Orthoses, Prostheses and Assistive Devices for Physiotherapists. Akhoury Gourang Sinha, Subrat Kumar Tripathy, Raju Sharma.
9. Overview of Plaster Technique. Department of Orthopedic Surgery Stellenbosch University.
10. Principle of Traction Methods. Department of Orthopedic surgery-University Stellenbosch, South Afirca.
11. Splints and Cast: Indications and Methods, American Academy of Family Physician.
12. Synopsis of Medical Instruments and Procedures. Arora and Yadav.
13. Text Book of Rehabilitation. S Sunder.
14. The Closed Treatment of Common Fractures. John Charnley.
15. The Elements of Fracture Fixation. Anand J Thakur.
16. Traction and Orthopedic Appliances. John DM Stewart, Jeffrey P Hallet.
17. Treatment of Congenital Clubfoot using Ponsetti method. Cure International India.
18. Wound Dressing. Vanessa Jones, Joseph E Grey, Keith G Harding.

Index

Page numbers followed by *b* refer to box, *f* refer to figure, and *t* refer to table.

C

D

G

H

I

J

K

L

M

N

O

R

S

T

U

V

W

Z